Routledge Handbook of Clinical Supervision

The *Routledge Handbook of Clinical Supervision* provides a global 'state of the art' overview of clinical supervision, presenting and examining the most comprehensive, robust empirical evidence upon which to base practice.

This authoritative volume builds on a previous volume, *Fundamental Themes in Clinical Supervision*, whilst greatly expanding its coverage. It contains ten updated and 23 entirely new chapters, focusing on both areas of contemporary interest and hitherto under-examined issues. Divided into five parts, it discusses:

- education and training
- implementation and development
- experiences and practice
- research activity
- international perspectives

Containing chapters on Europe, the US, Canada and Australasia, the *Routledge Handbook of Clinical Supervision* has a multi-disciplinary approach to clinical supervision and includes chapters relevant to nurses, doctors, psychologists, psychiatrists and counsellors. It will be of interest to students, researchers and practitioners of clinical supervision in a range of health professions.

John R. Cutcliffe is Acadia Professor of Psychiatric and Mental Health Nursing at the University of Maine, US. He is also Adjunct Professor of Nursing at the University of Ulster, UK and the University of Malta, the Associate Editor (Americas) for the *International Journal of Mental Health* and an Assistant Editor for the *International Journal of Nursing Studies*.

Kristiina Hyrkäs is Director of the Center for Nursing Research and Quality Outcomes at Maine Medical Center and Adjunct Professor of Nursing at the University of Southern Maine, US. She is also the Editor of the *Journal of Nursing Management*.

John Fowler is Principal Lecturer in the School of Nursing and Midwifery at De Montfort University, UK. He has held recent joint appointment posts as an educational consultant and undertakes a number of consultancy posts with the NHS and the independent sector.

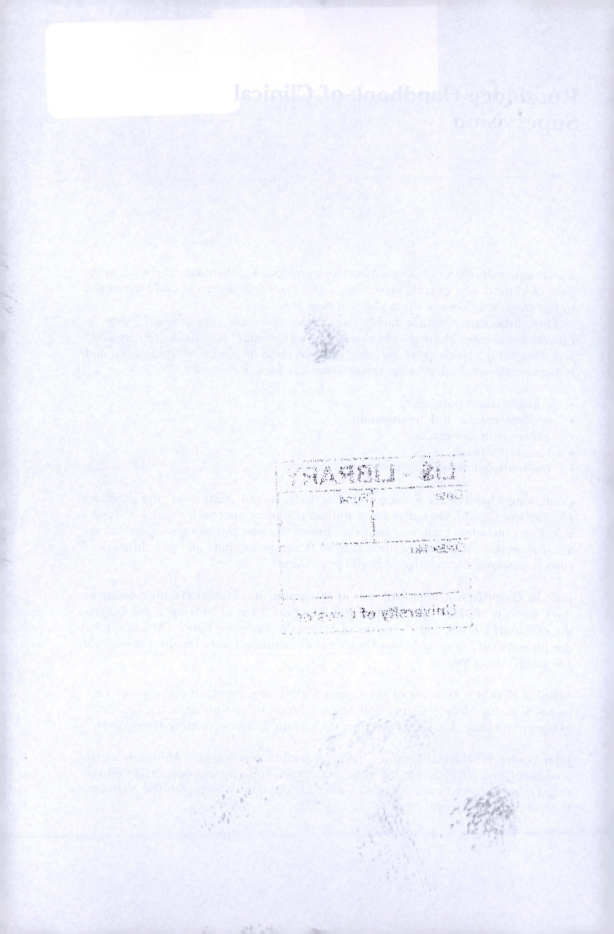

Routledge Handbook of Clinical Supervision

Fundamental international themes

**Edited by John R. Cutcliffe,
Kristiina Hyrkäs and John Fowler**

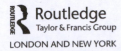

Routledge
Taylor & Francis Group

LONDON AND NEW YORK

First published in paperback 2016

First published in 2011
by Routledge
2 Park Square, Milton Park, Abingdon, Oxon OX14 4RN

and by Routledge
711 Third Avenue, New York, NY 10017

Routledge is an imprint of the Taylor & Francis Group, an informa business

British Library Cataloguing in Publication Data
A catalogue record for this book is available from the British Library

Library of Congress Cataloging in Publication Data
Routledge handbook of clinical supervision: fundamental international themes/edited by John Cutcliffe, Kristiina Hyrkäs, and John Fowler.
 p. cm.
 Other title: Handbook of clinical supervision
Includes bibliographical references.
 1. Nurses–Supervision of. I. Cutcliffe, John R., 1966– II. Hyrkäs, Kristiina. III. Fowler, John, RGN. IV. Title: Handbook of clinical supervision. [DNLM: 1. Administrative Personnel. 2. Organization and Administration. 3. Clinical Competence. 4. Evidence-Based Practice. 5. Internationality. 6. Leadership. W 88 R869 2011]
 RT86.45.R68 2011
 362.17′3068–dc22
    2010010178

ISBN: 978-0-415-77955-5 (hbk)
ISBN: 978-1-138-95490-8 (pbk)
ISBN: 978-0-203-84343-7 (ebk)

Typeset in Baskerville
by Wearset Ltd, Boldon, Tyne and Wear
Printed by Ashford Colour Press Ltd.

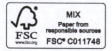

MIX
Paper from
responsible sources
FSC
www.fsc.org   FSC® C011748

This book is dedicated to all those whom we have encountered and work with on our individual clinical supervision journeys.

To Tony and David, we offer our thanks for your fine forewords and the work you have already done in clinical supervision.

And, from John Cutcliffe to my youngest daughter Charlotte Holly, this one is for you.

Contents

Illustrations

Boxes

Kristiina Hyrkäs PhD, LicNSc, MNSc, RN is currently the Director of the Center for Nursing Research and Quality Outcomes (CNRQO) at Maine Medical Center. Kristiina's clinical background has specialised in surgical and oncology nursing. She has worked at the University of Tampere, Finland, as a Planning Officer, a Senior Lecturer, Senior Assistant Professor in the Department of Nursing Science and a full time researcher. Kristiina has worked as an Assistant Professor at the University of Alberta, Faculty of Nursing and Associate Professor at the University of Northern British Columbia. Since moving to Maine, Kristiina has been appointed as Adjunct Professor of Nursing at the University of Southern Maine.

Kristiina has conducted pioneering empirical research on clinical supervision. She has published scientific articles on such topics as: (1) effects of clinical supervision on quality of care; continuous quality improvement through team supervision; nurse managers' perceptions of promotion of quality management through peer supervision; (2) cost-benefit analysis of team supervision; (3) expert supervisors' views of promoting and inhibiting factors on multi-professional team supervision; (4) team members' perceptions of the effects of multi-professional team supervision; (5) first-line managers' perceptions of the long-term effects of clinical supervision; (6) clinical supervision for nurses in administrative and leadership positions; (7) translating and validating an evaluation instrument for clinical supervision; (8) municipal elected officials'/municipal managers' perceptions of clinical supervision; (9) clinical supervision, burnout and job satisfaction (national study); (10) clinical supervision, burnout and job satisfaction in mental health and psychiatric nurses.

Kristiina is an editorial board member for the *Journal of Nursing Management* and has been an Editor of this journal since January 2008. Kristiina also co-chairs the publication committee of the INDEN (International Network for Doctoral Education in Nursing) newsletter. She is also a member of Sigma Theta Tau and Eastern Nursing Research Society (ERNS)/Membership Board member.

John Fowler PhD, MA, BA, DN, Cert Ed, RGN, RMN, RCNT, RNT trained as a general nurse and then as a psychiatric nurse in Portsmouth, England, in the 1970s and has subsequently been working in nurse education for over 25 years.

He is currently Principal Lecturer at De Montfort University Leicester. Until recently he held a joint appointment as Educational Consultant with Leicester City PCT. John has had a long academic and an applied interest in clinical supervision and in 1998 was one of the first people to publish a handbook on clinical supervision. He has continued to advise and evaluate clinical supervision programmes in the UK. He has published over 50 journal articles/book chapters and edited five textbooks, and is series editor to the Fundamental Aspects of Nursing Series (Quay Books). John is a volunteer tutor with PRIME (Partnerships in International Medical Education) and has had two short placements in Nepal. He is a regular presenter of BBC's Radio Leicester's 'Thought for the Day' and is married with four children.

Nancy Arthur is Professor and Canada Research Chair in Professional Education, Division of Applied Psychology, Faculty of Education, University of Calgary. Nancy's teaching and research interests include multicultural counselling and supervision, career development, and interprofessional practice. Nancy was one of the

Editors and contributing authors

John R. Cutcliffe RMN, RGN, RPN, RN, BSc(Hons)Nrsg, PhD holds the Acadia Professor of Psychiatric and Mental Health Nursing chair at the University of Maine, United States, and a joint appointment at Acadia Psychiatric Hospital; the first and only psychiatric facility in the world to achieve 'Magnet status'. He also holds Adjunct Professor of Nursing positions at the University of Ulster, United Kingdom and the University of Malta. John's clinical background is in nursing, having completed his psychiatric nurse education and then his general nurse education in the United Kingdom. He is an international scholar having worked in universities in four different countries – England, Northern Ireland, Canada and the United States.

John's research interests focus on hope, suicide and clinical supervision and in 2003 he was recognised by the federal government of Canada and cited as one of the top 20 'Research Leaders of Tomorrow' for his research. In 2004, he was nominated for a Canadian Research Chair and was given the highest research rating 'outstanding' from the independent reviewers. He has published extensively – over 150 papers and nine books – and has over $4,000,000 dollars of extra-mural research funding as Primary/Co-Investigator. He is currently working with colleagues from the University of Toronto (Canada), Dublin City University (Ireland) and the University of Ulster (UK) on an international programme of research focusing on suicide in young men.

John's interest in clinical supervision began during his mental health nurse education/training in 1987, where he was fortunate enough to receive supervision during his training. Since then, in whatever the area/speciality of his practice, he has received and/or provided clinical supervision. He has provided supervision to various grades of nurses since 1990, and provided 'train the trainer' clinical supervision training to a wide variety of different health care professional groups and in different parts of the world. He has recently served as the Director of the International Society of Psychiatric Nurses: Education and Research division; he is an Associate Editor for the *International Journal of Mental Health* and an Assistant Editor for the *International Journal of Nursing Studies*; in addition to sitting on the editorial boards of six other health care-focused journals. He retains his interest in clinical work, particularly around care of the clinical supervision, care of the suicidal person, inspiring hope and more broadly in psychiatric nursing. He is married with two children.

principal investigators for a Health Canada-funded study of lateral mentoring and interprofessional practice. Nancy is also a Registered Psychologist.

Kaija Appelqvist-Schmidlechner, MA is a Researcher at the National Institute for Health and Welfare, Finland. Kaija has studied communication science, psychology and sociology at the University of Salzburg, Austria. Since 1999, she has been working as a Researcher, first in the department of nursing science at the University of Tampere in Finland, then in the Research Centre for Social and Health Care at Seinäjoki University of Applied Science and presently in the National Institute for Health and Welfare. Her interest in clinical supervision is directed at evaluation of the effects and facilitative factors of clinical supervision in health care. Furthermore, Kaija has been interested in validating research instruments for clinical supervision and examining the municipal policymakers' views of clinical supervision.

Jenny Bennett, Bob Gardener and **Fiona James**. At the time of writing Bob Gardener, RGN, MA, CPN Cert, IHSM (postgrad cert), was lead professional for mental health nursing, Fiona James, RGN, HV, BN, MSc, was lead professional, health visiting and community health care service, and Jenny Bennett, RGN, was lead professional for community hospital nursing. These three authors are all based at North Derbyshire Community NHS Trust. As a team they have facilitated the implementation of clinical supervision in their disciplines. Part of their work has been to develop a five-year multi-disciplinary strategy for the implementation of clinical supervision across the organisation. They have designed, organised and facilitated clinical supervision awareness training for supervisors and supervisees for various disciplines. At present they all receive clinical supervision and are supervisors for individuals and groups in the Trust.

Ingela Berggren RN, RTN is Senior Lecturer at the Department of Nursing, Health and Culture at University West, Trollhättan, Sweden. Her background is as an intensive care nurse and lecturer in nursing education at basic as well as advanced levels. Her research focuses on the nursing profession, in particular supervision and ethical decision making.

Veronica Bishop PhD, MPhil, RGN, FRSA is Visiting Professor of Nursing at City University, London, and is Editor-in-Chief of the research and development journal, *Journal of Research in Nursing*. She is also a board member of the Hong Kong nurses' journal; for 12 years was a member of the scientific committee for the RCN Research Society and for 11 years served as an executive member of the Florence Nightingale Foundation and a member of its academic panel. Veronica was the national UK lead on clinical supervision. Veronica has worked as a consultant for the WHO in Denmark, India and Romania. She is widely published and has presented keynote speeches at numerous nursing conferences. She has recently been involved with the implementation of clinical supervision in the prison services and remains committed to its effectiveness in supporting staff in the provision of quality care.

Paul Cassedy RMN, Cert Ed, RNT, Dip Humanistic Psychology, MA is a Mental Health Lecturer at the University of Nottingham and teacher to the clinical supervision course in the School of Nursing. As a counsellor, he receives both individual and group supervision. He also provides supervision for health care staff who have a counselling role, and new supervisors within an adult nurse setting.

Michelle Cleary, RN, PhD is Associate Professor (Mental Health Nursing) at the School of Nursing and Midwifery, University of Western Sydney, Australia. Michelle has published over 90 academic papers (many as lead author) and her research areas include clinical innovation, health service evaluation, leadership, nurse education, ethics, outcome measurement, h-index, consumer and carer issues (including stigma), bullying and delivering difficult news. Michelle led an international Cochrane Systematic Review team evaluating psychosocial interventions for people with both severe mental illness and substance misuse. Michelle is also on the editorial board of the *International Journal of Mental Health Nursing*.

James Dooher RMN, MA, FHE Cert, Dip HCR is Principal in Mental Health Nursing at De Montfort University, Leicester. James maintains an active involvement in the practice of clinical supervision through his clinical work. He promotes its further development in both educational and practice settings. James has published widely on mental health issues and is particularly interested in the 'power' relationship. He is currently undertaking further research in this area.

Mike Epling RMN, FETC, Cert Ed (HE/FE) RNT, Dip Ed Counselling, M Ed is Lecturer in Mental Health at the University of Nottingham. Mike is a teacher to the clinical supervision course in the School of Nursing. He is involved in providing supervision to staff within health care settings and counselling settings, as well as providing supervision to groups of supervisors.

Mick Fleming, RMN, MA, BA, YCAP is Lecturer in Mental Health and Programme Leader for the MSc/Postgraduate Diploma in Psychosocial Interventions at the University of the West of Scotland. He has published in the field of psychosocial models of schizophrenia and the evaluation of psychosocial intervention training. His research interests include non-biological models of psychosis, validity of the schizophrenia concept and developments in the training of psychosocial interventions. He is a previous winner of the Foundation of Nursing Studies – Jack Mallabar Award – for his work introducing evidence-based psychosocial interventions into an inpatient mental health unit.

Carlean Gilbert is Associate Professor on the faculty of the School of Social Work, Loyola University Chicago, following 17 years of experience as a pediatric social worker. Her areas of scholarship focus on clinical supervision, health and mental health issues of children and adolescents, the impact of childrens' illnesses on family systems, group therapy, and the role of spirituality and religion in clinical practice. Carlean is editor of *The Clinical Supervisor: An Interdisciplinary Journal of Theory, Research, and Practice* and member of the editorial board of *Social Work in Health Care*. She has been elected to the Case Management Certification Board of the American Case Management Association and Board of Directors of the Society for Social Work Leadership in Health Care. Carlean is a Licensed Clinical Social Worker and a Certified Group Psychotherapist.

Peter Goward RMN, RNT, MSc. At the time of writing Peter was Head of Department, Mental Health and Learning Disability at the University of Sheffield. Peter

is involved in student and peer clinical supervision within undergraduate and postgraduate health-focused programmes. He is also involved in providing supervision for senior trust managers and clinicians within mental health settings.

Helen Halpern MB, BS, FRCGP, MSysPsych, is a general practitioner, family therapist and tutor in supervision skills in London. Helen is interested in applying ideas from systemic family therapy and educational theory to develop a framework for supervision for doctors, dentists and allied healthcare professionals that fits the context of the busy and rapidly-changing world of the National Health Service in the UK. She helps to facilitate courses and workshops for the London Deanery and at the Tavistock Clinic using a questioning approach called Conversations Inviting Change. This work includes bringing supervision skills into training for clinical teachers and appraisers. She also helps to set-up peer supervision groups for continuing professional development and support.

Kerrie Hancox is Co-Director of Clinical Supervision Consultants. In this role she consults to organisations on a range of levels and provides both group and individual clinical supervision. She also works part-time as an Enhanced Crisis and Assessment Clinician in an emergency department. She has been working in psychiatry since 1985 in a wide variety of clinical settings in Australia and overseas. Kerrie has a Bachelor of Nursing and completed her Master in Psychiatric Nursing in 2000. The focus of her research was clinical supervision. Kerrie also has expertise in a range of therapeutic skills including family therapy and gestalt therapy. She also has expertise in organisational dynamics and socioanalysis education. Kerrie was co-developer with Lisa Lynch of Clinical Supervision for Health Care Professionals, and Unlocking the Secret. She remains committed to the importance of quality education for supervisors and supervisees.

Brenda Happell is Professor of Contemporary Nursing, Director of the Centre for Mental Health and Well-being, and Director of the Institute for Health and Social Science Research at CQUniversity Australia. Brenda has a long standing interest in clinical supervision. She is co-author of the book *Clinical Supervision for Nurses* and has co-authored a number of publications on this topic. In her former position as the inaugural Director of the Centre for Psychiatric Nursing Research and Practice, Brenda was responsible for identifying the need for and subsequently overseeing the development of the subject Clinical Supervision for Health Care Professionals and she is currently a member of the Clinical Supervision Taskforce for Queensland Health. She is nationally and internationally recognised for her expertise in nursing, as evidenced by invitations as a visiting scholar and presentations at national and international conferences. Brenda has published prolifically in nursing and related health journals and her work is frequently cited and used to effect practice change. She is the Editor of the *International Journal of Mental Health Nursing* and Associate Editor of *Issues in Mental Health Nursing*, and a member of the Board of Directors of the Australian College of Mental Health Nurses. Brenda is an Honorary Professor at the University of Alberta.

Ann-Kristin Holm Wiebe, **Ingrid Johansson** and **Ingegerd Lindquist** are registered nurses with MA degrees, as well as nurse supervisors. They have many years experience of teaching future and practising nurses about nursing supervision at the Institute of Health and Care Sciences, University of Gothenburg, Sweden.

Their research focus is nursing supervision. The University of Gothenburg has highlighted the importance of supervision of the nursing process in the education of nurses, and in 2008 the above-mentioned nurse supervisors were awarded the University's pedagogical team prize for their work with nursing supervision at the Institute.

Jan Horsfall, PhD, Research Unit, Concord Centre for Mental Health, Sydney South West Area Mental Health Service, Concord Hospital, Sydney.

Alun Charles Jones is a specialist nurse in adult psychotherapy and a UKCP registered psychotherapist at the Betsi Cadwaladr University Health Board, the Department of Psychological Therapies, Wrexham, Wales. Alun is also an adult psychotherapist in the independent sector and has an interest in psychological assessment and support for weight management surgery. Alun has experience of developing liaison psychiatry services. As such, he has competencies concerned with planning psychological interventions for people with physical illness. In past years, areas of specialist practice concerned psychotherapy with the seriously ill, the dying and bereaved, including working with people with cancer, HIV and AIDS and cystic fibrosis in different medical settings. Alun is currently a clinical supervisor to trainee psychotherapists of different disciplines including medicine.

Joe Kellett RMN, RGN, DN (Lond), STD, RNT, BEd (Hons), MSc (Ed Man), PgCert (PSI). At the time of writing Joe was Senior Lecturer at the University of Sheffield. Joe currently provides group supervision to students on the postgraduate Pre-Registration Diploma in Mental Health Nursing Studies. He also provides ongoing clinical supervision to mental health nursing staff at local trusts.

Riina Lemponen MSc has worked as a biostatistician at the Tampere School of Public Health, University of Tampere, Finland for the past ten years. She has participated in a variety of health related studies as a statistical expert. Riina became adept with the clinical supervision research as a part of Kristiina Hyrkäs' and Kaija Appelqvist-Schmidlechner's research initiatives at the University of Tampere. Riina's focus in the project was mainly on analysing and modelling the data.

Lisa Lynch is Director of Child and Adolescent Mental Health and Primary Partnerships at Southern Health and the Co-Director of Clinical Supervision Consultants. She has been involved with clinical supervision, as a supervisor, a supervisee, a manager and an academic, for more than ten years. Lisa was a co-developer of the fully accredited Clinical Supervision for Health Care Professionals course, and the workshop for potential supervisees, Unlocking the Secret, both introduced in Victoria in 2001. These highly successful programmes were amongst the first of their kind. Lisa has recently completed a Master of Nursing by Research; she undertook a study of the implementation of clinical supervision in a mental health service in Victoria. The findings from her work culminated in a model to guide the implementation of clinical supervision within health care settings, now known as the Lynch model. In 2008 Lisa co-authored the popular *Clinical Supervision for Nurses*. This text is a very practical, hands-on guide to understanding and implementing clinical supervision.

David J. Powell is President of the International Center for Health Concerns. In this role he trains worldwide on clinical supervision and addictions. He is author of

Clinical Supervision in Alcohol and Drug Abuse Counseling and over 200 articles. He is on the editorial board of *The Clinical Supervisor* and four other journals. He has trained over 10,000 clinical supervisors in over 80 countries and his three texts on supervision are considered the standard books in the addiction field. He was the Chair of the Treatment Improvement Protocol 52 published by the Substance Abuse Mental Health Services Administration.

Brigid Proctor BA (Oxon), DipSocSci (Edin), CertApplSocStud (LSE) Fellow and Accredited Supervisor, BAC. She has been Director of South West Counselling Course Centre. She has a small private counselling practice, and a large individual and group supervision and supervision training practice. She also does occasional one-off consultancy and training. She has been co-authoring, with Francesca Inskipp, supervision learning materials, including those referenced in her chapter, and is co-author of *Group Supervision: A Guide to Create Practice* (Sage, London 2000).

Shelly Russell-Mayhew is a Registered Psychologist and Associate Professor in the Division of Applied Psychology, Faculty of Education, University of Calgary. Shelly is currently the Co-ordinator for the Master of Counselling (MC) Programme, a course-based masters programme utilising a distributed learning model. In this capacity, she became interested in interprofessional work-place supervision for counselor education and training.

Elisabeth Severinsson RPN, RNT, MCSc, DrPH is Professor and Director of Research at the Centre for Women's, Family and Child Health at Vestfold University College, Tønsberg, Norway. Elisabeth has spent a number of years researching different phenomena in the health care sciences, more specifically nursing and midwifery. She has long experience of the research cultures in the Nordic countries, Australia and Japan. Elisabeth's research interests are wide-ranging and include pre- and postnatal women's health, ethics, as well as clinical and academic supervision. Other international research interests are: research management, research and policy, mental health, public health, nursing education and research problems that are interesting from a methodological perspective. She is the author of more than 190 scientific articles, reports and book chapters as well as several books. Her engagement in international research collaboration is extensive.

Pirjo Sirola-Karvinen MSc, MNSc, BNSc, PHN, RN works as a Senior Specialist at the Finnish Institute of Health (FIOH). Her current work focuses on initiatives regarding a healthy work environment and well-being aiming at sustainable development and changes. Pirjo is also a doctoral student at the Department of Health Policy and Management, Faculty of Social Sciences, University of Eastern Finland, Kuopio. The focus of Pirjo's doctoral thesis is clinical supervision for health care leaders and administrators.

Graham Sloan PhD, BSc (Hons), Diploma in Nursing (London), Post-Graduate Diploma in Cognitive and Behavioural Psychotherapy, RMN, RGN, is a Nurse Consultant in Psychological Therapies, NHS Ayrshire and Arran, holds a joint appointment with the University of the West of Scotland and is a Psychological Therapies Training Co-ordinator with NHS Education for Scotland. He is an accredited psychotherapist, clinical supervisor and trainer (British Association of Behavioural and Cognitive Psychotherapy; International Standards for Interpersonal Psychotherapy). He has extensive experience of supervising psychological therapists and other mental health practitioners and has contributed to the training of a substantial number of clinical supervisors. Graham is the author of *Clinical Supervision in Mental Health Nursing* and has numerous additional scholarly publications on clinical supervision.

Paul Smith RGN, RMN, Dip (NS), Dip (UTR). At the time of writing Paul was a Psychiatric Charge Nurse with Barnsley Community and Priority NHS Trust. Paul has received and provided clinical supervision for the large majority of his nursing career. He is currently developing clinical supervision structures for his team.

Chris Stevenson RMN, BA (Hons), MSc (Dist), PhD, CPsych, is Professor and Chair of Mental Health at Dublin City University and Visiting Professor at the University of Ulster. She has a cumulative grant income of €1,500,000 and her book and paper publications exceed 70. Chris' research interests are suicidality, family systems/therapy, psychotherapy evaluation and clinical supervision, about which she has published consistently over the last decade. She currently teaches MSc/Doctorate Psychotherapy and supervises PhD students in the area of mental health, including clinical supervision.

Liz Williamson and **Gale Harvey**. Liz Williamson RGN, BSc(Hons), Senior Nurse, Surgery, Nottingham City Hospital NHS Trust; Gale Harvey RGN, BSc(Hons), Clinical Leader, Burns Unit. At the time of writing Liz and Gale were responsible for leading, planning and implementing clinical supervision for the Trust. This included a comprehensive in-house training programme, which was devised and delivered by them.

John Wren RMN, RGN, BA (Hons), Cert Ed, PGCE. At the time of writing John was a Lecturer in Mental Health Nursing at the University of Sheffield. He provides clinical supervision to students on the postgraduate Pre-Registration Diploma in Mental Health Nursing studies. He has worked as part of a professional development team to provide a supervision framework for a local trust.

Foreword I

Tony Butterworth

I am particularly pleased to be able to bring some of my own observations to bear at the beginning of this important book.

My career as a clinician, educator and researcher spans forty plus years and during that period I have witnessed significant changes and new approaches in the delivery of care. Nonetheless, several constants have held, and continue to hold true in the delivery of first class health care services. These can be described as:

- the appropriate delivery of thoughtful and well considered care to patients and people who use services;
- care that sustains their dignity and safety; and
- interventions that are evidenced-based and demonstrably useful and finally helping health care organisations to recognise their responsibilities to their employees through supportive employee strategies.

All of these admirable principles require sustained attention and nurture and clinical supervision stands tall amongst the most important of supportive strategies. Sometimes, and somewhat sadly, this is where some organisations can also fall down. I firmly believe that clinical supervision offers focus and support in 'healthy' organisations and it has been one of my great privileges to have worked on the development of clinical supervision as an educator and researcher throughout most of my career. As my energies begin to be directed elsewhere it is so heartening to see others carry forward this important work and no more so than through the descriptions and accounts to be found in this book.

In 1992 my colleagues and I at the University of Manchester in the UK offered the very first published textbook to describe the principles and practice of clinical supervision and mentorship in nursing (Butterworth and Faugier 1992). Since then, the term 'clinical supervision' has entered the language of our profession in a way that was inconceivable those several years ago and this book bears testimony to that significant change. For some practitioners clinical supervision remains words alone. Some organisations have not chosen to provide the necessary expertise and organisational time to develop the necessary platform for clinical supervision, and it is to their great discredit that this is so. A little later in my career my research team and I at the University of Lincoln reviewed the clinical supervision literature (Butterworth *et al.* 2008) in order to determine what progress if any could be seen in an identifiable time period, and through that progress identify the major themes that were emerging from research and practice. Several themes presented themselves,

Although as we suggested there were some rather tired often repetitious discussions in the literature it was clear that some of the most interesting work beginning to emerge (Bradshaw *et al.* 2007) was that of describing the impact of clinical supervision on patient outcomes. This is a worthy next step for exploration and one that finds some expression in this book.

At the time of writing this preface there are emerging constraints on health care funding as the world economies struggle to recover their equilibrium, Health professionals will be asked to work harder, to better effect and show demonstrable outcomes. This agenda can only be properly achieved if health professionals are properly sustained and supported. Clinical supervision offers a vital platform for this necessary work.

I am delighted to see that this new *Routledge Handbook of Clinical Supervision* addresses most if not all of the matters that I raise here. It is likely to sustain its well found reputation established in the original *Fundamental Themes in Clinical Supervision*, as a book of thoughtful reflection, stimulating ideas and reference. This new volume is commendable in both its scope and ambition.

Professor Emeritus Tony Butterworth CBE
Chair, Academy of Nursing, Midwifery and Health Visiting Research (UK)
Manchester, England
June 2010

References

Bradshaw T., Butterworth, T. and Mairs, H. (2007), Does work based clinical supervision during psychosocial education enhance outcomes for mental health nurses and the service users they work with? *Journal of Psychiatric and Mental Health Nursing*, 14(1): 4–12.

Butterworth, T. and Faugier, J. (eds) (1992), *Clinical Supervision and Mentorship in Nursing*, London: Chapman & Hall.

Butterworth, T., Bell, L., Jackson, C. and Pajnkihar, M. (2008), Wicked spell or magic bullet, a review of the clinical supervision literature 2001–2007, *Nurse Education Today*, 28(3): 264–272.

Foreword II

David J. Powell

Much has been written about clinical supervision over the past 30 years, covering various disciplines and perspectives. Despite this body of research and literature, there have been gaps in the books published to date, including my own. This book does an excellent job in filling these gaps and pointing the field in a clear direction for the future.

First, the field of clinical supervision needs further literature, offering updated research activity and findings from various settings, disciplines and especially, different countries. The majority of the literature on the subject has originated from Western countries and not surprisingly reflects a Western perspective. As a result, important questions remain largely unanswered such as: how does one provide clinical supervision in other cultural environments and countries? How does one establish a system of supervision in a different cultural context? Sue and Sue (2007) in *Counseling the Culturally Diverse* write about counselling different cultures. The international, multi-disciplinary journal, *The Clinical Supervisor*, periodically has articles on supervision in different countries. This new book provides a truly international perspective on the most contemporary findings from American, British, Canadian, European, New Zealand and Australian perspectives. If Thomas Friedman (2007) is correct in his acclaimed book *The World is Flat*, this new book's international focus is consistent with globalisation and the global market place of health care delivery.

Second, most of the literature on clinical supervision in North America is from an academic perspective, pre-certified, pre-practice individuals who are in university settings. A 'real-world' perspective is vitally needed. This book provides such a perspective, reviewing the realities of clinical supervision in acute inpatient settings, leadership and governance positions, a National Health Service Community Trust perspective, and a rural health care organisation. The book combines the contributions of scholars, practitioners, and practice developers based in ten different countries.

Third, most books in the field come from a single-discipline perspective: social work, marriage and family counselling, professional counselling or alcohol and drug abuse counselling. Although useful, such a focus is too limiting, as health care delivery systems encompass multiple disciplines and operate as inter-disciplinary entities. This book includes contributions across disciplines, including physicians, psychologists, psychiatric mental health nurses, social workers, palliative care nurses and generic nurses.

Fourth, although the importance of the supervisory alliance and various approaches to supervision have been emphasised in the literature, Cutcliffe *et al.*

bring the latest research to bear on how this alliance affects attitudes, skills and intention of supervisees and supervisors. The book addresses the critical issues of experiential learning, providing an underpinning theoretical perspective on clinical supervision, using solution-focused techniques in clinical supervision, and addressing the key issues related to supervisor training and requirements.

This latter point is critical. As health care agencies undergo difficult financial times and health care reform, justifying the cost of a quality clinical supervision system to management and administrators of these organisations can be a hard sell. Why should we spend money on non-revenue bearing activities, such as training and clinical supervision? The book addresses this issue by exploring the impact of clinical supervision on job satisfaction, burnout and the quality of care. In an outcome-driven health care world, this book shows that the better the clinical supervision, the better patient retention and the quality of care. If you want to sell a system of clinical supervision to management, that's a reasonably cogent argument.

Finally, far too much of the literature in the field is retrospective, looking backward at where we've been rather than looking to the twenty-first century and beyond, the successes, challenges and the road ahead. This book concludes with a dynamic perspective on the future and the role clinical supervision can play in shaping that future.

John Cutcliffe, Kristiina Hyrkäs, and John Fowler appropriately point us in the direction for further writings on subjects such as record keeping, legal issues in clinical supervision, working with special populations (substance abuse), and other international foci (Asia, Africa and South America – populations from which there remains a paucity of research and literature). We look forward to these issues and others being addressed in the future by these and other authors.

John Cutcliffe, Kristiina Hyrkäs, and John Fowler bring outstanding credentials to this book, including vast international and multi-disciplinary perspectives. There are few writings in the field of training and clinical supervision that can offer such a depth of viewpoint. These are highly credible authors, whose work makes a significant contribution to the field.

Today, health care delivery offers many benefits and challenges. Clinical supervision is one of the keys to maintaining and improving the overall quality of care, the professional development of personnel, and patient and staff retention. This book makes a significant contribution to the health care field and the study of clinical supervision. I highly recommend this book to practitioners from all behavioural and health care disciplines.

David J. Powell
President of the International Center for Health Concerns

References

Friedman, T.L. (2007), *The World is Flat*, revised edition, London: Penguin.
Sue, D.W. and Sue, D. (2007), *Counseling the Culturally Diverse*, 5th edn, New York: Wiley & Sons.

Preface

The editors of this book are delighted that we were asked to produce the *Routledge Handbook of Clinical Supervision* and that this provided the opportunity for significantly expanding, enhancing and updating *Fundamental Themes in Clinical Supervision*. The justifications and rationales for writing a book about clinical supervision are just as applicable today as they were when the original book was proposed and subsequently produced. Furthermore, an examination of the extant literature will show that clinical supervision as an international and multi-disciplinary phenomenon may well have grown during the last decade. Our knowledge base focusing on clinical supervision has expanded and perhaps more importantly, deepened. Some disciplines which hitherto have not been associated with clinical supervision have now made (most welcome) substantive contributions to the body of work. Some countries appear to have moved forward with their own clinical supervision agenda; others, very interestingly, have not. As a result, and almost a decade on since *Fundamental Themes in Clinical Supervision*, it seemed that the time was right to move towards producing a new book.

This book retains the features which made *Fundamental Themes in Clinical Supervision* a well-reviewed and highly regarded text and we have added material in the hope that this expands the book's, to borrow a term from Tolkien's parlance, 'applicability'. In addition to reviewing and subsequently updating the material in *Fundamental Themes in Clinical Supervision*, 23 of the 33 are new chapters, many of which are logical progressions and/or developments from chapters included in *Fundamental Themes in Clinical Supervision*. The remaining nine chapters have all been updated and revised. The editors also believe this format and construction of the book will help to provide a sense of continuity, with readers being able to follow the evolution of our knowledge base in certain areas which were covered in *Fundamental Themes in Clinical Supervision* and at the same time, being exposed to new issues, new debates, new developments and new knowledge.

The forewords to this book, generously provided by Professor Tony Butterworth and Dr David Powell, complement that provided by Sarah Mullally, the then Chief Nursing Officer for the United Kingdom for *Fundamental Themes in Clinical Supervision*. Further, given Professor Butterworth's joint editorship of *Fundamental Themes in Clinical Supervision*, we feel this further contributes to a sense of continuity between the two books. And given Dr Powell's international and multi-disciplinary efforts to develop clinical supervision, we feel that this underscores the increasing multi-disciplinary and international interest in the subject. As with *Fundamental Themes in Clinical Supervision*, we welcome feedback, comment and review and hope that such information might inform the production of a new edition in the future.

This book includes all of the outstanding features that made *Fundamental Themes in Clinical Supervision* a success such as:

- Contributions from leading scholars, practitioners and practice developers, each of whom has an established reputation in the substantive area of clinical supervision.
- Chapters representing a broad selection of both new and more familiar (existing) material focused on clinical supervision.
- Considerable breadth – as there are now five discrete yet linked parts in the book (*Fundamental Themes in Clinical Supervision* had four).
- Chapters detailing the most contemporary research activity and findings from various settings, disciplines and countries.
- Contributions from scholars, practitioners and/or practice developers based in ten different countries, thus providing a genuinely international perspective. Such genuinely internationally focused texts are also more in keeping with the increasing shift towards globalisation and the global market place.
- A balance between analytical and descriptive chapters and their associated styles of writing; with a corresponding increase in the width of appeal of potential readers.
- Contributions from a range of disciplines which were not included in *Fundamental Themes in Clinical Supervision*, making this a genuine expansion and development on that earlier book rather than simply updating a few references. These disciplines include clinical supervision contributions from physicians (general practitioners), psychologists, psychiatric/mental health nurses, palliative care nurses, social workers and generic nurses. There is also far more material that focuses on multi-disciplinary and interdisciplinary developments.
- The balance that *Fundamental Themes in Clinical Supervision* had, which should still make it attractive to students, practitioners, educationalists, and researchers.

In putting together the *Routledge Handbook of Clinical Supervision* and recognising and operating within word/space limits, the editors would like to point out that difficult choices had to be made around which issues/developments to include and which not to. The editors wish to emphasise that in no way is our contents list meant to be exhaustive or representative of the only clinical supervision issues that warrant debate. Understandably, the choice of which chapters to include reflect, at least in part, the views, values and to some extent, the interest of the editors. The idiosyncrasies of the editors notwithstanding, we believe the chapters will have currency and meaning for the disciplinary groups currently involved (or engaged) in clinical supervision and for those that are considering this as a future option. The chapters (and their corresponding issues) have been selected, in part: as a result of our communication with the international clinical supervision academe; as a result of searching the extant literature for ongoing issues/developments/debates; as a result of the introduction of some health care policy; and, in part, in an attempt to capture practice, policy, education and research clinical supervision related debates. Accordingly, the chapters might be regarded as a collection of some of the key issues/developments and challenges associated with the substantive area of clinical supervision. Additional issues, developments and challenges that we considered featuring in the book include:

- power and control in clinical supervision;
- clinical supervision for psychiatrists;
- record keeping in clinical supervision;
- clinical supervision contributions from the Far East, Africa and South America;
- legal issues in clinical supervision;
- clinical supervision in doctorally prepared, clinical psychology programmes;
- doctoral level training in clinical supervision;
- magnet hospitals, criteria and clinical supervision;
- clinical supervision for people working with specific populations, groups and/ or problems e.g. alcohol substance misuse.

It is our hope that these and other issues might form the cadre of a new book some time in the future.

Finally, it would be remiss of the editors if they did not point out that these chapters do not constitute the definitive position on any of the issues featured. We acknowledge that debating ongoing issues can (should?) be an iterative process; positions and opinions change as new evidence emerges, as the dominant discourse changes and/or as society's values evolve. The editors hope that this book might be considered as a contribution that adds to our substantive knowledge base of clinical supervision and helps advance our clinical supervision-focused practice, education, policy and research.

John R. Cutcliffe, Kristiina Hyrkäs and John Fowler
December 2009

Stylistic footnote: as with *Fundamental Themes in Clinical Supervision*, the editors have highlighted certain selective sentences, passages or parts of sentences by emphasising these, here, with italics. These selections are not random and to a greater or lesser extent are bound to reflect the particular nuanced views of the editors.

1 Introduction

Global perspectives on fundamental themes in clinical supervision

John R. Cutcliffe, Kristiina Hyrkäs and John Fowler

Why another clinical supervision book?

It is now almost ten years since *Fundamental Themes in Clinical Supervision* (Cutcliffe *et al.* 2001), was written and during these years, clinical supervision (CS) has remained on the radar for those involved in health care practice, education, development and/or education. While it might be argued that attention to CS within academic journal articles may have passed beyond its zenith (arguably this occurred during the 1990s), examination of the extant literature reveals that CS is very much still a matter of high interest. The possible decline in the number of papers notwithstanding, a closer inspection of the extant literature shows a number of interesting things. First, the papers that continue to be published appear to add something new, meaningful and/or significant to the literature (and it would be inaccurate to assert this of the papers produced during the 1990s when there was a great deal of repetition). Second, while it might be said that some of the earlier published work could have 'delved a little deeper' into the substantive issues, the more recent published work appears to do just that. Third, almost no new CS books have emerged during recent years.

As with any longitudinal, evolutionary, cumulative approach to knowledge generation, the existence of earlier work by no means serves to suggest that there is nothing new worth saying; on the contrary, what this actually means is that we have more questions now than perhaps we did before (Toulmin 1967; Popper 1972). A further outcome of interrogating the extant literature is that of the discovery of gaps in our knowledge base. Accordingly, it is perhaps worthy of note that some existing questions do not appear to have been fully debated or resolved and others have yet to be asked. As a result, this book attempts to make a significant (if not seminal) contribution to the extant CS literature by focusing on issues that continue to be of contemporary interest and furthermore by focusing on hitherto under-examined issues.

In addition to the continued widespread interest in CS, there are additional reasons for producing a new book.

First, CS is now much more of a genuine global phenomenon than it was ten years ago. More countries have embraced CS within various practice domains (e.g. see New Zealand, Australia, Canada); more individuals are thus involved in giving/receiving CS, studying CS, introducing CS into policies and practices, and teaching/training CS. The international interest is now far larger than it was ten years ago and yet with this context in mind, few (if any) books have been produced recently that will have the content, international authorship and thus high utility/applicability that this book has.

The ongoing need for CS should also be considered with the context of the evidence-based practice movement which has swept several nations. Those nations and populations who are interested or already engaging in CS thus need to have the most comprehensive, robust empirical evidence upon which to base their practice. This book pulls together numerous key research themes within CS and provides some of the most contemporary findings available. Again, these are in no way limited to one country.

Contemporary issues pertaining to litigation and quality of care still abound (and some would say these have increased during recent years). Mindful of this development and the inescapable link between CS and quality of care/clinical governance, we have included new chapters that specifically focus on these issues. While the original editors touched on this in *Fundamental Themes in Clinical Supervision*, policy and quality matters have moved on, therefore a book that includes chapters on links between CS and these issues is much needed.

Again, with reference to international developments, one of the most compelling developments in recent years is the rise of the Magnet Recognition Program and the associated 'movement'. Perhaps analogous or similar to the Nurse (Practice) Development movement synonymous with the Kings Fund in the 1980s and some United Kingdom universities in the 1990s, Magnet Status is a huge deal right now in the United States. The Magnet Recognition Program was developed to recognise health care organizations that provide excellence in nursing practice. The new Magnet Model emphasises today five domains:

1   transformational leadership
2   structural empowerment
3   exemplary professional practice
4   new knowledge, innovations and improvements
5   empirical outcomes.

We will not belabour the obvious parallels with each of these five domains (and the practices within them) with the nature/rudiments of CS. Bearing in mind that hospitals in the United States are private businesses, many hospitals are aspiring to achieve Magnet Status and with that, an additional element to their marketing strategy for their organisations. As a result, hospitals in the United States that aspire to Magnet Status should, we would argue, consider how embracing CS within their organisation and culture can contribute to their efforts to become (or remain) a Magnet site.

Finally, it needs to be acknowledged that CS has not only spread across nations but it has also spread into disciplines which hitherto had very little or no CS activity. Though we highlighted these possible developments in *Fundamental Themes in Clinical Supervision*, the then possibilities have now become reality to the extent that GPs, palliative care nurses, primary care nurses and others are now engaged in CS. We have accordingly captured the state of the art/practice of CS for these groups by including chapters that specifically focus on these populations. Accordingly, this book not only builds on the strengths of *Fundamental Themes in Clinical Supervision*, it not only updates those still relevant chapters from that book, but it also includes new material to reflect the genuine international nature and the increasingly multi-discipline of CS and does so by bringing together a collection of many of the leading international scholars in this area.

Our experience (and many of the findings detailed in this book) suggest that when people have had some personal experience of CS, they appreciate it, understand it, become aware of its utility, application and worth, and want it. Consequently, rather than a book that is based on theoretical perspectives, this book consists of a collection of chapters from authors each of whom are involved in practice relating to supervision, each of whom have experienced CS; and it has left a lasting impression. Those chapters on education/training have been written by authors who provide education/training (and receive CS) themselves. Those chapters on introducing, implementing or developing CS into an organisation, have been written by authors who have actively engaged in such endeavours (with documented success it should be noted). Those chapters on practicing/experiencing CS have been written by authors who, not surprisingly, practice and experience CS firsthand and thus have their own lived experiences to draw upon. Those chapters that feature contemporary research findings are each based on research conducted by the respective authors. The chapters that catalogue, describe and critique the state of the science of CS in a variety of different countries are each written by experts from the countries and regions represented. It should also be noted that these different sections lend themselves (arguably) to a different style of writing; accordingly some have a more academic sense or 'flavour' than others.

The structure of the book

After the first two chapters set the scene (so to speak) and provide some background and context to CS, Part I of the text is concerned with education, training and approaches to CS. Consequently, Chapter 3 examines the how and the why of Brigid Proctor's Supervision Alliance model, and looks at some of the open learning methods of training in CS. Chapter 4 makes the case for training/equipping student practitioners to become competent supervisees rather than supervisors, and suggests a possible structure for such education/training. Chapter 5 looks at experiential learning as a theoretical underpinning to CS and includes some pragmatic suggestions as to how one can assess, identify and address issues that sometimes lead to malfunctioning in CS. Chapter 6 features the development and delivery of a diploma-level CS training course at the University of Nottingham. Chapter 7 examines the hitherto under-examined matter of training requirements for competent CS. Chapter 8 focuses on CS through a post-modernist lens and Chapter 9 offers the original idea of adopting a solution-focused approach to CS.

Part II of the text is concerned with the introduction, implementation and development of CS into practice, policies and into health care organisations. Therefore, Chapter 10 examines the relationship between clinical supervision and clinical governance and draws them together with a convergence model. Chapter 11 outlines how a group of practitioners (lead professionals) facilitated the widespread implementation and development of CS within a National Health Service Community NHS Trust. Chapter 12 provides a summary of the literature review of CS, ten years on from the review of CS literature commissioned by the UKCC (now the Nursing and Midwifery Council). Chapter 13 focuses on a recent effort to introduce CS within a large National Health Service acute care trust. Chapter 14 presents a number of descriptive accounts of how CS is working in one geographical area in the United Kingdom, including a number of case studies which provide very different pictures of how the essential elements of CS were adapted to the needs of each specific environment. And Chapter 15 describes an innovative and systematic approach to introducing CS in a rural health care organisation in Australia.

Part III of the text is concerned with the actual practice and lived experiences of CS within different health care professions (disciplines) and specialisms. Consequently, Chapter 16 leads with a focus on the experiences of a Community Mental Health nurse. Chapter 17 looks at CS for nurses working in palliative care settings. Chapter 18 features the experiences of general practitioners (physicians) in the United Kingdom who receive and participate in CS. Chapter 19 explores the practice of cross-discipline group supervision and Chapter 20 features the cultural realities of CS in an Australian acute inpatient setting. Chapter 21 concludes this part by examining CS supervision for nurse educationalists and sets this practice within the context of a post graduate psychiatric/mental health nursing course.

Part IV is a collection of research reports and empirical studies which constitute some of the contemporary (and international) research activity that examines aspects of CS. Accordingly, Chapter 22 draws on recent extensive research from Scandinavia and in other parts of Europe. Chapter 23 describes an empirical study which sought to explore relationships between CS, burnout and job satisfaction. Chapter 24 features a research study that examined the under-explored issue of multi-disciplinary attitudes towards CS in the United Kingdom, whereas Chapter 25 reports on the findings of a qualitative study that used a focus group method to evaluate the experience of receiving CS. Chapter 26 focuses on research findings pertaining to CS for those who occupy administrative and leadership positions and Chapter 27 considers the argument and evidence for using case studies as one means of producing qualitative evaluative data; and it reports findings from a series of case studies which produced evidence regarding personal, professional and practice developments enhancements that ensued as a result of participating in CS.

Part V of the text is concerned with presenting international perspectives on, and experiences of, CS and seeks to provide the reader with an understanding of the state of the science regarding CS in these featured countries. Therefore, Chapter 28 reports on the state of the science of CS in Australia and New Zealand. Chapter 29 reports on the state of the science of CS in Europe. Chapter 30 shifts our emphasis across the Atlantic Ocean and reports on the state of the science of CS in the United States and Chapter 31 on the state of the science of CS in Canada. Chapter 32 rounds off this part and takes a slightly different slant and offers up some key comparisons between European and North American conceptualisations of CS. The book concludes by considering: where do we go from here? Consequently, Chapter 33, on the future of CS, highlights some key issues/debates that arguably need to be resolved; highlights important policy, practice, education and research concerns and offers the editors' view on what could be addressed during the next decade.

The editors' position on clinical supervision

As with the editors of *Fundamental Themes in Clinical Supervision*, the editors of this new book share the view that there is no one single correct or 'best' way to carry out

CS. However, any activity is based on certain implicit or explicit assumptions. Rather than give yet another definition of CS, we want to spell out some of those assumptions, of what we think it is or is not in our considered opinion. The contributors to this book are all talking about the kind of CS that fits within these parameters. In no particular order of priority, the editors posit that these parameters indicate clinical supervision is necessarily:

- supportive;
- safe, because of clear, negotiated agreements by all parties with regard to the extent and limits of confidentiality;
- centred on developing best practice for service users;
- brave, because practitioners are encouraged to talk about the realities of their practice;
- a chance to talk about difficult areas of work in an environment where the person attempts to understand;
- an opportunity to ventilate emotion without comeback;
- the opportunity to deal with material and issues that practitioners may have been carrying for many years (the chance to talk about issues which cannot easily be talked about elsewhere and which may have been previously unexplored);
- not to be confused with or amalgamated with managerial supervision;
- not to be confused with or amalgamated with personal therapy/counselling;
- regular;
- protected time;
- offered equally to all practitioners;
- involves a committed relationship (from both parties);
- separate and distinct from preceptorship or mentorship;
- a facilitative relationship;
- challenging;
- an invitation to be self-monitoring and self-accountable;
- at times hard work and at others enjoyable;
- involves learning to be reflective and becoming a reflective practitioner;
- an activity that continues throughout one's working life.

We would argue that, ultimately, CS has to be concerned with benefiting service users as well as health care practitioners. The truth of the matter is that we are all potential clients or users of health care. Additionally, each of us has, in some way, paid for such care and it is entirely understandable that when we are to be recipients of health care, we would all want the best care possible for ourselves and our significant others. We posit that this 'best care possible' can only be delivered by the front line staff, who are competent enough and healthy enough. We believe that engaging in CS has the potential to help bring about precisely that scenario. It can help keep practitioners become and remain competent and healthy enough to provide this best care possible. Unless CS ultimately does have an influence on the care provided, it ceases to be what it was designed to be and becomes something of a rather narcissistic, self-absorbed activity for staff or yet another (unwanted) managerial monitoring tool.

There is an increasing requirement for staff who are engaged in helping relationships within health care to be accountable for their actions. However, the mechanisms for encouraging, nurturing and monitoring this accountability remain vague and somewhat immature in their conceptual development. At the same time there is an ongoing requirement for such individuals to re-register as competent practitioners. Inextricably linked with one's eligibility for re-registration is the need to demonstrate a commitment to continuous and ongoing professional development and, at the same time, a degree of individual accountability (Cutcliffe and Forster 2010, in press). In order to operate as a competent, ethical and safe practitioner, one first needs to be accountable to oneself and then accountable to another. It is the belief of the editors (and the authors in this book) that CS provides one mechanism whereby these processes can be achieved.

What should you gain from this book?

Having identified that this book offers the reader something different from other books on CS, the reader ought to gain something different from reading it. So what should the reader be able to gain as a result of reading this book?

Perhaps you should first ask yourself: what do I want to know about CS?

Then, if you are interested in becoming a supervisor (or supervisee), you should turn to Part I, on education, and there you will discover what type of training/education is available, what options you can pursue and at what academic level. If you are interested in implementing/developing CS in practice and/or in your organisation, you should examine Part II and can then see some options of the ways this can be brought about, and identify some of the hurdles to the introduction of CS. If you are interested in the practice of CS you should look to Part III on practice and become aware of what practice is occurring, how practitioners are experiencing CS and how it might be of benefit to them. If you are interested in research, then you should examine Part IV and can then determine what are the next logical questions to be asked in CS, where the current knowledge base is and where future research should be focused. And if you are seeking a greater sense of this global phenomenon that you might logically begin with the final part of this book, on the international state of the science.

It is the editors' opinion that this book identifies some of the real benefits of receiving CS and this evidence has been obtained from real experiences. The evidence has been provided by practitioners who share the difficulties, constraints and dilemmas that many hard-pressed and busy health care practitioners experience. The writing does not come from a collection of academics who live in world far from the realities of clinical practice. As a result, the editors view this book as a 'carrot' book, rather than another 'stick' book. It provides the reader with some hope, something to encourage them, rather than adding to the already stifling load of 'shoulds and oughts' that practitioners bear. It demonstrates, as a result of the international chapters, how different countries interpret CS within their national context(s). It is thus interesting and illuminating to see different perspectives; and such perspectives might make practitioners, educationalists, managers/administrators, policymakers and researchers think about CS in a different way. It shows that in the substantive area of CS, there is evidence to suggest that several countries now occupy an influential potential, and thus there may well be something that we can all learn from other countries. Finally, it sets CS in context within a multidisciplinary context and reflects that whilst CS may have been available for decades in certain nations, its potential to support staff, to help them become more individually accountable and to improve client care has not yet been fully realised.

Consequently, the ending of this chapter in *Fundamental Themes in Clinical Supervision* remains as salient and relevant today as it did at the end of the twentieth century. To borrow an expression that arises from contemporary parlance: CS has come far, but there is still a long way to go.

References

Cutcliffe, J.R. and Forster, S. (in press), Guest editorial. Professional registration bodies: international variation in the protection of the public, *International Journal of Nursing Studies* (accepted for publication October 2009).

Popper, K.R. (1972), *Objective Knowledge: An Evolutionary Approach*, Oxford: Clarendon Press.

Toulmin, S.E. (1967), The evolutionary development of natural science, *American Scientist*, 55(4): 456–471.

2 Clinical supervision
Origins, overviews and rudiments

John Fowler and John R. Cutcliffe

This chapter explores the origins of clinical supervision and proposes reasons why it was adopted into the profession at that particular time in history, questioning whether clinical supervision is just another fad that has entered the nursing language and culture. Undoubtedly the nursing profession is prone to fashions and fads and at times it is difficult to differentiate what is useful and what is a whim. The chapter then examines the conceptual overlap of similar terms such as mentoring and preceptorship and identifies some key features of clinical supervision.

We believe that this is an important chapter for managers, clinicians and educators. Whatever role we play in the profession it is important to understand the why and how of our supporting structures. At its worst, clinical supervision has the potential to be a time-consuming negative experience but at its best, clinical supervision has the potential to galvanise and motivate individuals and teams and to be a significant part in the quality assurance process. So what is it? Where did it come from? And is it here to stay?

Introduction

Many years ago, in the US, Peplau (1927) identified that nurses had a need for clinical supervision. She talked implicitly about reflective practice as part of clinical supervision, stating that the staff nurse should come prepared with notes or verbatim data and that the supervisee should do most of the talking. The aim of the supervisor was to try to perceive the interactions in the context of the situation and to suggest alternative modes of responding. There appears little else in the nursing literature from this time that identifies anything that resembles Peplau's original concept of supervision as a formal meeting with a supervisor in which a supervisee comes with reflective notes and the supervisor's main role is not to lecture, but to ask questions and suggest alternative perspectives.

Although the idea of senior nurses directing junior nurses in their clinical work has been in existence since the days of Florence Nightingale, the practice of clinical supervision was not formally debated in the UK until the late 1980s. One of the early formal definitions of clinical supervision appearing in the UK literature was from the Department of Health in a document entitled *A Vision for the Future – The Nursing, Midwifery and Health Visiting Contribution to Health and Health Care* (Department of Health 1993). The document was endorsed by the Secretary of State for Health, the Chief Executive of the National Health Service Executive and the Chief Nursing Officer. It was an important and influential document. The 'vision' contained within the document drew upon a number of major political, professional and health policy documents of the time. Twelve key targets were set, the tenth of which related specifically to clinical supervision, which was defined as

> a formal process of professional support and learning which enables individual practitioners to develop knowledge and competence, assume responsibility for their own practice and enhance consumer protection and safety of care in complex clinical situations.
>
> (Department of Health 1993: S.3.27, p. 15)

Professor Bishop, who was lead Nursing Officer at the DOH for clinical supervision when subsequently writing about the background of clinical supervision (Bishop 1998), indicates that this high visibility political drive to introduce formal clinical supervision into the nursing profession was driven by *'a number of concerns about supervision and support of safe, accountable practice'* Bishop 1998: 1), this concern being fuelled by a high profile inquiry into the unlawful killing of a number of children by the nurse Beverly Allitt (Clothier Report: Department of Health 1994). *(Professor Bishop has contributed a chapter for this book examining clinical supervision and clinical governance – see Chapter 10.)* Bishop states that it was no coincidence that on the day that the Clothier Report was published there was also a Department of Health commissioned paper distributed to the NHS and professional bodies on clinical supervision (Faugier and Butterworth 1993). Bishop points out that although this may appear to be a political 'sop for bad publicity' it was actually a genuine move from within the nursing profession to support the development of high quality care. Anecdotally it has been suggested that senior nurses of that time used the political momentum generated from the negative publicity relating to the Beverly Allitt inquiry to move the concept of clinical supervision from the professional nursing agenda to the central government's policymaking agenda.

So why did clinical supervision become such an important topic in the early 1990s? Why did it attract such strong professional and political backing at that specific time in the development of the nursing profession?

Undoubtedly the move from the professional agenda to the political one was strongly facilitated by the national publicity of the Allitt inquiry as described above. But why was clinical supervision already on the professional agenda at a national level and why was it welcomed by clinical nurses at all levels of the profession? There are a number of factors which seem relevant to this question:

1   In the middle of the 1970s nursing began moving away from a task-orientated system of care to one where patients' care was planned and delivered in a 'holistic' way, 'the nursing process', with one nurse assessing, planning and delivering the care for a small group of patients. This reinforced the role of the nurse as an increasingly individual practitioner in their own right. Previously the custom in task-orientated care had been for the senior nurse, the 'ward sister', to list the care for each patient, often in a routine way. She then grouped the tasks for all the patients and then allocated the tasks to one of the staff in the team. e.g. the staff nurse would give out medication, the junior nurse would empty bed pans and keep the sluice clean, the less junior nurse would wash patients etc. with each group of tasks being allocated to a person with the appropriate skill level. Towards the end of each shift the ward sister would do her rounds of the

patients and inspect the various tasks that had been performed. Thus there previously existed a system whereby a senior and experienced nurse assessed her patients, planned their care, allocated different aspects of that care to appropriately trained personnel and then monitored their performance. In terms of nursing care this was an efficient 'factory line' production that had quality assurance built in. Built into this way of working was the apprenticeship model of training and support. As the junior nurse mastered the bed pans and sluice, they then progressed to washing patients and then to doing simple dressings, etc. Central to both task-orientated care and the apprenticeship system was the ward sister, not uncommonly caricatured as a 'motherly dragon'. As both these systems evolved into individualised care and an educational philosophy replaced the apprenticeship one, then the underpinning supervision and quality assurance provided by the hierarchical structures began to weaken and become lost.

2   Accountability began to move from the hierarchical structures embodied in the ward sister and medical consultant to the individual nurse. This was demonstrated by the development in the UK of the *Code of Professional Conduct* (UKCC 1992) which made individual nurses accountable for their own actions.

3   At the same time as these organisational and philosophical nursing approaches were changing, cost effectiveness, and efficiency savings became prominent topics on the health care agendas. Additionally, the nurses working week gradually reduced from 48 hours to 37.5 to fit in with national trends and European working regulations. The effects of this are typified by the loss of the handover period. The handover period was the overlap of the morning shift with the afternoon shift and the afternoon shift with the night shift. It was not uncommon for the shift patterns to resemble the following: morning shift 7 am–4 pm, the afternoon shift 12 noon–9 pm and the night shift 8 pm–8 am. Typically the afternoon saw a four hour overlap between morning and afternoon shifts. This allowed for staff to have a lunch break and also gave two or three hours during which training, support and supervision took place. The senior nurse would teach the less senior one dressings, drug actions etc. Many of the elements now recognised as clinical supervision occurred during these overlap periods. With the drive for cost efficiency combined with the reduction of the working week, these overlap periods were seen as a waste of resources. Shift patterns gradually changed reducing the overlap periods resulting in a 15 minute overlap in most clinical areas. *Thus traditional organisational systems of support, development and supervision were fast disappearing from the established working patterns for most nurses.*

4   The 1980s also saw nursing developing as an independent profession in its own right. Individual nurses were taking on far more specialist and independent roles. This culminated in 2006 (NMC 2006a) with suitably qualified nurses being eligible to become independent prescribers in the UK.

5   The final significant factor in the health care system at this time was the vast development in medicine with far more invasive treatments. Patients were undergoing intensive treatments and chemotherapy; life-saving operations and subsequent intensive care nursing become common place. Patients on the wards were far more acutely ill, but were in hospital for much shorter times. The days of recovering patients taking the tea trolley around the ward were long gone. Thus the work of the nurse was becoming far more intense, patients were far more ill and the turnover of patients much greater.

The effects of these social, political, health and professional developments in the mid-1970s through to the late 1980s resulted in the gradual erosion of well established support and supervision structures coupled with the increase in the severity of patients' conditions and volume and intensity of work. Additionally accountability at an individual level became established within the profession. By the late 1980s senior nurses were recognising the role of the nurse had changed and was continuing to change. However, the traditional support and supervision structures were no longer in existence or appropriate for the developing role. Thus a formalised structure of support and supervision which gave assurance of customer protection began to appear as a clinical need on the agenda of a number of senior nurses in the profession. The concept of clinical supervision was born.

Supervision as an umbrella term

There are a number of terms used in the nursing language that have aspects of supervision as part of their core concept. The terms mentorship, preceptorship and clinical supervision and reflective practice are used in the everyday language of the clinical nurse (Burnard 1990; Maggs 1994; Fowler 2005). Some people appear to use them interchangeably, acknowledging that there probably is a difference between the various terms, but not being sure quite what that difference is. Core to

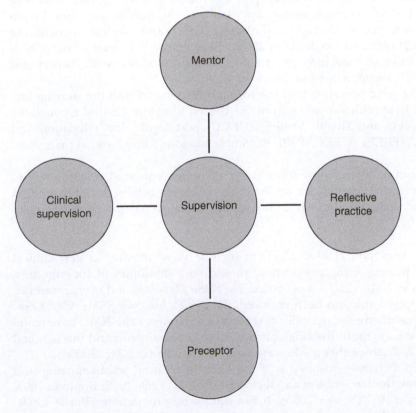

Figure 2.1 Four common terms found in the nursing literature and their relationship to/with clinical supervision.

most of these terms is the concept of supervision. Barber and Norman (1987) provided one of the earlier definitions of supervision within the nursing profession as:
*"an interpersonal process where a skilled practitioner helps a less skilled or experienced practi-
tioner to achieve professional abilities appropriate to his role. At the same time they are offered
counsel and support".* There are four terms that have appeared in the nursing literature and culture that fulfil in some way this initial definition of supervision and have
a relationship to or with it. These are:

- preceptorship
- mentoring
- reflective practice
- clinical supervision.

Preceptorship

Peutz (1985) differentiates preceptorship from mentoring in that it has a more
active teaching and supervision role, and this general differentiation between mentoring and preceptorship is true across continents. However even the term preceptorship has different interpretations in the US and UK. In America the term is used
to describe the support, teaching and direction that student nurses receive while on
clinical placement. Thus in the US preceptorship includes: teaching (Williams *et al.*
1993), learning contracts (Andrusyszyn and Maltby 1993), developing clinical competence and confidence (Myrick and Barrett 1994) and clinical socialisation
(Ouellet 1993; Dibert and Goldenberg 1995). In addition, it is used to describe a
general orientation and teaching programme for new or junior staff (Dibert and
Goldenberg 1995; Dusmohamed and Guscott 1998).

In the UK the term preceptorship was formally introduced into the nursing language in 1990. Its specific use arose from the United Kingdom Central Council for
Nursing, Midwifery and Health Visiting (UKCC) post-registration education and
practice project (PREP) (UKCC 1990). Recommendations 1 and 2 stated that:

> There should be a period of support for all newly registered practitioners to
> consolidate the competencies or learning outcomes achieved at registration
> (4.4). A preceptor should provide the support for each newly registered practi-
> tioner (4.10).

This was later developed (UKCC 1993) to include those moving to new clinical
areas, and the preceptorship programme should be a minimum of four months.
More recently the NMC (2006) has revised *The PREP Handbook* and overt reference
to the term preceptorship has been removed. *The PREP Handbook* (NMC 2006) now
defines the requirements for periodic re-registration. However the NMC have maintained their commitment to the original concept of preceptorship and this is noted
in one of their A–Z advice sheets – Preceptorship (NMC 2006c, NMC 2006d).

Preceptorship for newly qualified staff has been introduced within nursing in a
fairly consistent in the UK (Ashton and Richardson 1992; Gately 1992; Brennan 1993;
Burke 1994; Skyte 1997, Fowler 2005). It is a short-lived programme (Burke 1994),
with the focus on the acquisition of knowledge and skills designed specifically to
enable the newly registered nurse to work safely and effectively in a new environment.

There is an emphasis on assessing this nurse's individual needs (Ashton and Richardson 1992), with instruction and support, rather than emphasising a one-to-one relationship common to the mentor literature (Brennan 1993). Once the period of preceptorship has finished the registered nurse is subject to whatever staff development and support processes are available in their place of employment.

Mentoring

Mentoring is a frequently used term both within and outside nursing. It is often used in everyday nursing conversation but appears to mean different things to different people. As with the term preceptorship, mentoring has different interpretations in the US and in the UK:

> Finding a definition of mentorship is not difficult. The problem lies in selecting one from the many available and widely contrasting definitions.
>
> (Earnshaw 1995: 274)

Many of the reviews of mentoring within the nursing profession make reference to the historical derivation of the term 'mentor' from Homer's Odyssey, in which Odysseus entrusts the upbringing of his son Telemachus to his trusted advisor and friend Mentor (Donovan 1990; Earnshaw 1995). This model has been adopted quite widely by the general business world as a relationship in which a more experienced person nurtures a junior person as they either enter a job or take on a new role (May 1982; Hagerty 1986). The use of mentoring has also become increasingly common in schools where it tends to be called a 'buddy system' when using senior students to support and orientate new students or 'mentoring' if adults from outside the school are paired with students who have specific needs.

American nurses tend to see mentoring in a fairly traditional way as a relatively long-term relationship between an experienced practitioner and a protégé (Peutz 1985). Darling's (1984) work from the US on mentoring identifies three main aspects of the mentoring role. Firstly one who 'inspires' the mentee with a 'vision' of what to aim for, secondly as an 'investor', someone who believes in the mentee and communicates that belief, and finally as 'supporter', the mentor providing encouragement and reassurance, thus developing confidence.

In the UK, mentoring within nursing has two usages. As with the American interpretation it has a general meaning within management circles of a relationship between an experienced person and a protégé. This tends to be an informal and ad hoc relationship seen mainly in the more senior management levels of nursing (Burnard 1990; Maggs 1994; Butterworth 1998). Here, the term is not well defined and tends to have a wide usage. It ranges from a committed and intense relationship, focusing on personal and professional development of the mentee, to a more general and ad hoc meeting.

The second and more formal use of the term mentor within the UK is now well established as the relationship between the qualified nurse who oversees a student nurse whilst on placement. The assessment of student nursing competence and proficiency must be completed by a mentor who is a first-level registered nurse who has undergone further preparation to fulfil the role of mentor, this includes teaching, supporting and acting as the formal assessor.

Originally the English National Board (ENB) (1989) who then regulated nurse education in England, gave the role of mentor prominence by stipulating that each student nurse should have a mentor throughout the clinical placements of their training (ENB 1989, 1993). It defined this as someone who would, by example, facilitate, guide and support the learner in the development of new skills, new behaviours and new attitudes. There was a separate and more experienced person who undertook the assessing of students (ENB 1993). Later, the ENB altered the focus regarding the supervision of students. They combined the assessor and mentor roles into one mentor role, which was to take on the full responsibility for the teaching, assessing and support of the student (ENB/DoH 2001). In 2002 the ENB ceased to exist and the Nursing and Midwifery Council (NMC) took over the responsibility for setting training and assessment standards. However, the role and function of the mentor as supervisor and assessor has remained central for student supervision standards (NMC 2002).

The NMC (2008) currently defines a mentor as

> a registrant who, following successful completion of an NMC approved mentor preparation programme, has achieved the knowledge, skills and competence required.
>
> (NMC 2008)

The NMC also introduced the term 'sign off mentor' as a role in assessment of pre-registration nursing for students who are on final placements or for post-registration students who are on specialist practice programmes leading to a registrable or recordable award (NMC 2008). For most nurse training curricula, the mentor is a clinically-based nurse, who oversees the student for the time that they are learning in their clinical area, normally 4–12 weeks. This means that the student will have a number of different mentors throughout their pre-registration period – one for each clinical placement and 10–15 throughout their three years of preparation. There are only rare examples where the same mentor is attached to a pre-registration student for all or most of their training (Morris *et al.* 1988).

Reflective practice

Reflection underpins much of the practice of preceptorship, mentoring and clinical supervision. The work on reflection by Argyris and Schön (1974) has influenced a number of practice-based professions. Schön (1987, 1991) identifies two types of reflection: reflection-on-action and reflection-in-action. Reflection-on-action, as the title suggests, occurs after the experience has occurred and can be recognised in nurse education settings and in clinical supervision (McCaugherty 1991, Fowler 2006); with the mentor or supervisor being a key figure in helping the student to reflect on practice. Reflection-in-action occurs while the practice is being undertaken and, according to Schön, has the potential to directly influence decisions and practice outcomes.

The general move to develop a more questioning profession was being articulated to some extent by the emphasis on reflection on practice. Most reviews of reflective practice acknowledge the stages of reflection (e.g. Mezirow 1981; Schön 1991; Johns 1993; Fowler 2006) and the difficulty of undertaking reflection in isolation (Johns 1993). Reflective practice was welcomed within the nursing profession (Snowball *et al.* 1994; Marrow *et al.* 1997; Johns 1997) as a way to integrate theory and practice.

Atkins and Murphy (1993) state that reflection must involve the self and must lead to a changed perspective. This is echoed by Snowball *et al.* (1994: 1235):

> It is clear in the literature that the involvement of self is a crucial element of the reflective process.

Atkins and Murphy (1993) state that for reflection to occur the individual needs to be minimally defensive and be willing to work in collaboration with others. While this openness and willingness to 'expose the self' is appropriate for some staff, it is an exercise that many people find difficult to accomplish without guidance from a skilled person. The clinical supervision relationship offered an opportunity for reflection on clinical practice under the guidance of a more experienced clinician. In this relationship the practice of reflection and the role of clinical supervision come together. *Prior to the early 1990s, implementation of reflective practice had been predominantly with student nurses. It was seen as a valuable tool by others, but required a structure that was not present in any systematic way within the general nursing profession. Clinical supervision offered an infrastructure for reflection-on-practice for all registered nursing staff.*

Clinical supervision

As discussed in the early part of this chapter, in 1993, the Department of Health NHS Management Executive (DOH 1993) published a strategic document, *A Vision for the Future*. It was the first time that the term clinical supervision had been used in a way that implied the introduction of a systematic structure. The document (paragraph 3.27) described clinical supervision in broad terms that included: development, individual responsibility, consumer protection, self-assessment and reflection. This has been supported by the NMC whose most recent guidance is in the form of an information sheet (NMC 2006b) with the aims of clinical supervision as:

- identify solutions to problems;
- increase understanding of professional issues;
- improve standards of patient care;
- further develop their skills and knowledge;
- enhance their understanding of their own practice.

Models of supervision

In the early 1990s, the number of accounts describing how clinical supervision could work proliferated in the literature. Different models of clinical supervision began to emerge. At the more humanistic end of the spectrum, Faugier (1992) described a growth and support model. Initially this emphasises the relationship between the individuals, then, using the interactions within the relationship, it focuses on the role of the supervisor to facilitate both educational and personal growth for the supervisee. This relationship must also, according to Faugier, provide support for the developing clinical autonomy of the supervisee. Faugier describes many of the humanistic qualities associated with such growth and support, e.g. generosity, openness, humanity, sensitivity and trust. Chambers and Long (1995) identify a similar facilitative model of growth and support based on the relationship between the supervisor and supervisee. These approaches have their roots in a humanistic school of counselling (Farrington 1995), with its focus on self-awareness and personal growth.

From a more behaviourist perspective, Nicklin (1995) argued that tangible outcomes are required from clinical supervision. He proposed that clinical supervision should analyse issues and problems, clarify goals and identify 'strategies for goal attainment and establish an appropriate plan of action'. The focus was on the outcomes rather than the process. Nicklin (1997) developed these ideas into a six-stage process of supervision. It includes practice analysis, problem identification, objective-setting, planning, implementation action and evaluation. Nicklin (1995) states that the process of clinical supervision should complement other managerial processes and that clinical supervision should not develop as a vehicle for diluting or fragmenting managerial responsibility. This 'outcome' approach, with its focus on problem identification and problem-solving, has its roots in a behavioural school of psychology (Farrington 1995).

Principles of clinical supervision

People's experiences of clinical supervision vary widely. Three principles, however, appear to be core (Fowler 1996):

1   At least two people meeting together for the purpose of clinical supervision.
2   Reflection is used to focus upon clinical practice.
3   Meetings are structured and organised.

A short article by Proctor (1986) writing about youth work, identified three components of supervision as: normative (standard setting), formative (development) and restorative (support). These were quickly adopted by the nursing profession as key elements in the clinical supervision literature (Bishop 1998).

These three components have stood the test of time with the purpose and function of clinical supervision encompassing one or a combination of the following:

•   a learning process
•   a supportive process
•   a monitoring process.

The literature on clinical supervision in nursing is quite vast, most of it written in the last 20 years. A simple 'Google' search on 'clinical supervision in nursing' reveals 548,000 hits. If you spent two minutes reading each paper, it would take you over two years to read everything and that would be two years without sleep, nutrition or anything else. The rest of this book draws upon some of the most noted authors and authorities on clinical supervision and attempts to condense those two years of reading for you, into this one authoritative text.

References

Andrusyszyn, M. and Maltby, H. (1993), Building on strengths through preceptorship, *Nurse Education Today*, 13(4): 277–281.

Argyris, C. and Schön, D. (1974), *Theory in Practice*, San Francisco: Jossey Bass.

Ashton, P. and Richardson, G. (1992), Preceptorship and PREP, *British Journal of Nursing*, 1(3): 143–146.

Atkins, S. and Murphy, K. (1993), Reflection: a review of the literature, *Journal of Advanced Nursing*, 18(8): 1188–1192.

Barber, P. and Norman, I. (1987), Mental health nursing: skills in supervision, *Nursing Times*, 83(2): 56–57.

Bishop, V. (1998), *Clinical Supervision in Practice*, London: Macmillan.

Brennan, A. (1993), Preceptorship: is it a workable concept? *Nursing Standard*, 7(52): 34–36.

Burke, L. (1994), Preceptorship and post registration nurse education, *Nurse Education Today*, 14(1): 60–66.

Burnard, P. (1990), The student experience: adult learning and mentorship revisited, *Nurse Education Today*, 10(4): 349–354.

Butterworth, A. (1998), Clinical supervision as an emerging idea in nursing, in T. Butterworth, J. Faugier and P. Burnard (eds), *Clinical Supervision and Mentorship in Nursing*, Cheltenham: Stanley Thornes.

Chambers, M. and Long, A. (1995), Supportive clinical supervision: a crucible for personal and professional change, *Journal of Psychiatric and Mental Health Nursing*, 2(5): 311–316.

Darling, L. (1984), What do nurses want in a mentor? *The Journal of Nursing Administration*, 14(10): 42–44.

Department of Health, Clothier Report (1994), *The Allitt Inquiry. Independent inquiry relating to deaths and injuries on the childrens ward at Grantham and Kesteven General Hospital during the period February to April 1991*, London: HMSO.

Department of Health, NHS Management Executive (1993), *A Vision for the Future: The Nursing, Midwifery and Health Visiting Contribution to Health and Health Care*, London: HSMO.

Dibert, C. and Goldenberg, D. (1995), Preceptors' perceptions of benefits, rewards, supports and commitment to the preceptor role, *Journal of Advanced Nursing*, 21(6): 1144–1151.

Donovan, J. (1990), The concept and role of mentor, *Nurse Education Today*, 10(4): 294–298.

Dusmohamed, H. and Guscott, A. (1998), Preceptorship: a model to empower nurses in rural health settings, *Continuing Nurse Education*, 29(4): 154–160.

Earnshaw, G. (1995), Mentorship: the students' views, *Nurse Education Today*, 15(4): 274–279.

ENB (1989), *Preparation of Teachers, Practitioners/Teachers, Mentors and Supervisors in the Context of Project 2000*, London: English National Board for Nursing, Midwifery and Health Visiting.

ENB (1993), *Regulations and Guidelines for the Approval of Institutions and Courses*, London: English National Board for Nursing, Midwifery and Health Visiting.

ENB/Department of Health (2001), *Preparation of Mentors and Teachers: A New Framework of Guidance*, London: English National Board for Nursing, Midwifery and Health Visiting/ Department of Health.

Farrington, A. (1995), Models of clinical supervision, *British Journal of Nursing*, 4(15): 876–878.

Faugier, J. (1992), The supervisory relationship, in A. Butterworth and J. Faugier (eds) *Clinical Supervision and Mentorship in Nursing*, London: Chapman & Hall.

Faugier J. and Butterworth, A. (1993), *Clinical Supervision: A Position Paper*, Manchester: School of Nursing Studies, University of Manchester.

Fowler, J. (1996), The organization of clinical supervision within the nursing profession, *Journal of Advanced Nursing*, 23(3): 471–478.

Fowler, J. (ed.) (1998), *The Handbook of Clinical Supervision: Your Questions Answered*, Salisbury: Quay Books, Mark Allen Publications.

Fowler, J. (ed.) (2005), *Staff Nurse Survival Guide*, Salisbury: Quay Books, Mark Allen Publications.

Fowler, J. (2006), *The Use of Experiential Learning within Nurse Education*, unpublished PhD thesis, Leicester: DeMontfort University.

Gately, E. (1992), PREPP: from novice to expert, *British Journal of Nursing*, 1(2): 88–91.

Hagerty, B. (1986), A second look at mentors, *Nursing Outlook*, 34(1): 16–24.

Johns, C. (1993), Professional supervision, *Journal of Nursing Management*, 1(1): 9–18.

Johns, C. (1997), Reflective practice and clinical supervision – Part 1: the reflective turn, *European Nurse*, 2(2): 87–97.

McCaugherty, D. (1991), The use of a teaching model to promote reflection and the experiential integration of theory and practice in first-year student nurses: an action research study, *Journal of Advanced Nursing*, 16(5): 534–543.

Maggs, C. (1994), Mentorship in nursing and midwifery education: issues for research, *Nurse Education Today*, 14(1): 22–29.

Marrow, C., Macauley, D. and Crumbie, A. (1997), Promoting reflective practice through structured clinical supervision, *Journal of Nursing Management*, 5(2): 77–82.

May, K.M., Meleis, A.I. and Winstead-Fry, P. (1982), Mentorship for scholarliness: opportunities and dilemmas, *Nursing Outlook*, 30(1): 22–28.

Mezirow, J. (1981), A critical theory of adult learning and education, *Adult Education*, 32(1): 3–24.

Morris, N., John, G. and Keen, T. (1988), Mentors: learning the ropes, *Nursing Times*, 84(46): 24–27.

Myrick, F. and Barrett, C. (1994), Selecting clinical preceptors for basic baccalaureate nursing students, *Journal of Advanced Nursing*, 19(1): 194–198.

Nicklin, P. (1995), Super supervision, *Nursing Management*, 2(5): 24–25.

Nicklin, P. (1997), A practice centred model of clinical supervision, *Nursing Times*, 93(46): 52–54.

NMC (2002), *Standards for the preparation of teachers of nurses, midwives and specialist community public health nurses*, Standards 06.04, London: Nursing and Midwifery Council.

NMC (2006), *The PREP Handbook*, Standards 03.06, London: Nursing and Midwifery Council.

NMC (2006a), *Standards of proficiency for nurse and midwife prescribers*, Standards 06.06, London: Nursing and Midwifery Council.

NMC (2006b), *Advice Sheet – Clinical Supervision*, Nursing and Midwifery Council, London.

NMC (2006c), *Preceptorship Guidelines* Circular 21/2006 SAT/gl 3 October 2006, London: Nursing and Midwifery Council.

NMC (2006d), *Advice Sheet – Preceptorship*, London: Nursing and Midwifery Council.

NMC (2008), *Standards to Support Learning and Assessment in Practice – NMC Standards for Mentors, Practice Teachers and Teachers*, London: Nursing and Midwifery Council.

Ouellet, L. (1993), Relationship of a preceptorship experience to the views about nursing as a profession, *Nurse Education Today*, 13(1): 16–23.

Peplau, H. (1927), *The Goals of our Life and the Paths that Lead to It: Writings of H Peplau and selected articles*, Schlesinger Library, Radcliffe College, Cambridge, MA. No 84-M107 H Peplau Archives, carton 8, volume 264, cited in A. O'Toole and S. Welts (eds) *Hildegard Peplau Selected Works: Interpersonal Theory in Nursing* (1994), London: Macmillan.

Peutz, B. (1985), Learning the ropes from a mentor, *Nursing Success Today*, 2(6): 11–13.

Proctor, B. (1986), Supervision: a cooperative exercise in accountability, in M. Marken and M. Payne (eds), *Enabling and Ensuring*, Leicester: National Youth Bureau for Education in Youth and Community Work.

Schön, D. (1987), *Educating the Reflective Practitioner*, San Francisco: Jossey Bass.

Schön, D. (1991), *The Reflective Practitioner*, Aldershot: The Academic Publishing Group.

Skyte, S. (1997), PREP the key to safe practice and upholding standards, *Nursing Times Learning Curve, Nursing Times*, 1(10): 2–3.

Snowball, J., Ross, K. and Murphy, K. (1994), Illuminating dissertation supervision through reflection, *Journal of Advanced Nursing,* 19(6): 1234–1240.

UKCC (1990), *The Report of the Post-Registration Education and Practice Project (PREP),* London: United Kingdom Central Council for Nursing, Midwifery and Health Visiting.

UKCC (1992), *Code of Professional Conduct,* London: United Kingdom Central Council for Nursing, Midwifery and Health Visiting.

UKCC (1993), *The Councils Position Concerning a Period of Support and Preceptorship,* Registrar's letter 1/1993 Annexe One, London: United Kingdom Central Council for Nursing, Midwifery and Health Visiting.

Williams, J., Baker, G., Clark, B. *et al.* (1993), Collaborative preceptor training: a creative approach in tough times, *Journal of Continuing Education in Nursing,* 24(4): 153–157.

Part I

Education, training and approaches to clinical supervision

3 Training for the supervision alliance
Attitude, skills and intention

Brigid Proctor

This chapter focuses on the 'supervision alliance model'. It was originally presented in *Fundamental Themes in Clinical Supervision* (Proctor 2001: 25–46) and in this book we offer an edited version of the chapter. It now offers a brief description of the key components of the model, and then explores the training process the author uses and the open learning structure. Brigid Proctor's model is perhaps the most commonly used clinical supervision model within health care. It is based on very important and seminal works and is, therefore, a classic and timeless model. For those interested in the development of the model, its antecedents and a detailed discussion of its foundational elements, it is well worthwhile to refer to the author's exposition in *Fundamental Themes in Clinical Supervision*.

We believe that this is an important chapter for any practitioner interested in clinical supervision. Because the model has been very popular, not all representations of it are fair or accurate. It is then, very interesting to note that Brigid herself highlights that the principal function of her model is its supportive function. Effective supervision requires a supportive underpinning as the foundation upon which the formative and normative aspects of supervision are built.

A model geared to practice

Practitioners – of supervision and health care – need support and help in 'seeking virtue and embracing wisdom' in a complex and multi-cultural world. One way they can get this is by being offered regular space to reflect on their moment-to-moment practice. The picture in Figure 3.1 sketches the outline of the supervision alliance model transposed into health care settings. *Editors' comment: These values and assumptions have been discussed in detail in* Fundamental Themes in Clinical Supervision *(Proctor 2001: 25–46).*

Contracts and agreements

The overall contract

The model emphasises that clinical supervision always involves more than two stakeholders. All have a right to be respected in the process of clinical supervision. However, the central figures are, first, the recipient of the supervision – the practitioner. In the world out there, he or she is the channel through which the service is offered – the public face of the service and a person in his or her own right.

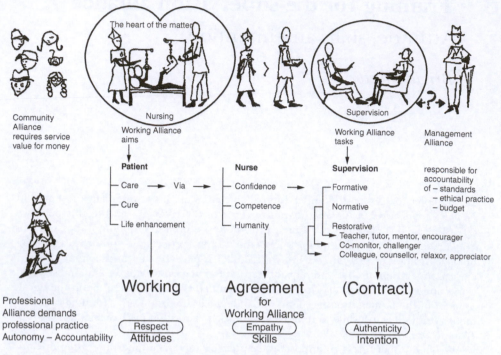

The heart of the matter

Community Alliance requires service value for money

Nursing
Working Alliance aims

Supervision
Working Alliance tasks

Management Alliance

Patient		**Nurse**	**Supervision**	responsible for accountability of – standards
– Care	→ Via →	– Confidence →	– Formative	– ethical practice
– Cure		– Competence	– Normative	– budget
– Life enhancement		– Humanity	– Restorative	

Teacher, tutor, mentor, encourager
Co-monitor, challenger
Colleague, counsellor, relaxor, appreciator

Working   Agreement   (Contract)
for
Working Alliance

Professional Alliance demands professional practice
Autonomy – Accountability

Respect
Attitudes

Empathy
Skills

Authenticity
Intention

Figure 3.1 Supervision: alliance towards reflective practice.

Box 3.1 Values and assumptions of the Supervision Alliance Model

It assumes that practitioners are usually keen to work well, and to be self-monitoring, if they are brought to professional maturity in a learning environment which sufficiently values, supports and challenges them.

It values the ability to reflect on experience and practice as a major resource for life and learning.

It presumes that reflective practice can be learned – taught even – but that learners require a trusting and safe environment if they are to share their experience and practice honestly with themselves or others.

It views supervision as a co-operative enterprise between colleagues – who may (or may not) be unevenly matched in work experience or age, but who share a common humanity and common professional interests, ethics and, often, ideals.

Second, there is the supervisor who is responsible for creating a climate and a relationship in which the practitioner can reflect on his or her practice within clear boundaries of freedom and responsibility.

Those clear boundaries are first set by the contract that the employer makes with the supervisor and practitioner as to the purpose and manner of clinical supervision in a particular context. This will necessarily be bounded by guidelines or codes regarding wider professional ethics and practice.

The working agreement

Within the overall contract, I suggest that a working agreement for a particular supervision alliance is made between supervisor and practitioner. At one level, its clarification and negotiation is practical, identifying such key matters as responsibilities and roles, contextual factors, administrative arrangements, supervisor's methods of working in supervision, practitioner's developmental needs and learning goals, preferred learning styles, and supervisor and practitioner resources. At another level, it is a shared process of clarification and negotiation that begins to establish the degree of trust, safety or wariness there may be in this relationship and to shape a suitable working climate.

A working relationship

The contract and the working agreement are not seen as bureaucratic devices, but as a means of establishing sufficient safety and challenge. The overall contract signals continuing accountability to the other stakeholders in the supervision enterprise – this is both opportunity and responsibility to mature in practice and offer a better service. The working agreement signals the co-operative nature of the enterprise and the complementary roles of each party. The process of discussing and establishing the alliance is the vehicle through which an intentional and unique relationship is initiated between this particular practitioner and this particular supervisor, in this particular context.

Tasks and tension of clinical supervision

This brings us to the best known feature of the model – the complementary but sometimes contradictory tasks of clinical supervision – normative, formative and restorative. In health care contexts, the constituent tasks of supervision should probably be transposed.

- *Clinical supervision will be a major opportunity for professional and, hopefully, personal refreshment so the restorative task in these stressful times should, I think, be placed first. If supervision is not experienced as restorative, the other tasks will not be well done.*
- Second, the opportunity to become increasingly reflective on practice, and to learn from one's own experience and the experience of another qualifies clinical supervision as a uniquely formative process.
- Whereas in counselling contexts supervision may be the major forum of professional accountability, in most health settings there will be other places where account is rendered. Nevertheless, there will necessarily be self-monitoring elements to the work, for the practitioner. At best, clinical supervision is the safe enough setting where he or she can share and talk about practice and ethical dilemmas without jeopardising him- or herself.

The supervisor has responsibility for making clear his or her own criteria of good practice, and comparing that with the practitioner's perspective. She/he may nevertheless have to decide to take things further if they consider or suspect that the practitioner continues to practice unwisely or unethically. So, for both practitioner and supervisor, clinical supervision will always be a forum where normative issues are addressed and engaged with and the supervisor may, very occasionally, become a whistle-blower (see Cutcliffe *et al.* 1998a, 1998b).

By whatever means clinical supervision is distinguished and detached from formal manage-rial assessment procedures, this element of monitoring will be present and both practitioner and supervisor will need to recognise the tension between the restorative and the normative tasks. In training, most supervisors and supervisees find it difficult to develop the ability to manage this tension skilfully and with integrity within a single role relationship.

Role flexibility

Each task carries attendant informal roles, which will be reciprocal for practitioner and supervisor. It can be helpful for both to recognise this, because it allows them to 'play' at relating flexibly and appropriately to the task they are engaged in at any one time. Figure 3.1 suggests a number of complementary roles, and we have already seen that aspects of the 'preceptor-initiate' and the 'mentor-evolving practitioner' dialogue may also find a place in supervision (Morton-Cooper and Palmer 2000).

However, the overall role responsibilities are those of supervisor and supervisee (or practitioner-in-supervision) as negotiated in the working agreement for the supervision. Any settling down into a single set of roles (for instance, taking only restorative roles or falling regularly into a teacher-learner dyad) will not be fulfilling the working agreement.

Attitudes

Attitudes are the outward expression of what we value and understand. We engage in tasks with certain attitudes towards them, based on the values we consciously or unawarely espouse, and also on the understanding we have about them. A supervisor who uses this model needs to understand the underlying values of working in alliance (as opposed to hierarchically) and be prepared, at least, to test these values out in his attitude to the task. For instance, he needs to believe that agreements are co-operative, and act on that. He has to assume that the practitioner he is supervising has good will to her work, at least until he has clear evidence to the contrary. He has to understand that clarity of roles and responsibilities is a safeguard against oppressive supervisor (or supervisee) behaviour. He has to 'act in' to the understanding that this is a human relationship between two (or more) adult practitioners, rather than, say, a pedagogic relationship between master and pupil. A human relationship implies that either party may feel, and be, vulnerable within the relationship from time to time, so attitudes towards vulnerability need to be accepting and helpful, for the well-being of both participants and for the furtherance of the task of supervision.

The practitioner coming for supervision, in turn, has to develop certain attitudes to the task if she is to make good use of her opportunity for reflection and learning. These attitudes may be unfamiliar and countercultural. The title 'supervisor' has strong hierarchical connotations. A practitioner new to this kind of clinical supervision may have well-founded scepticism of being apparently trusted and valued as an equal contributor. The first initiation in clinical supervision will be crucial in allowing practitioners to get a feel for the potential of this unfamiliar process.

Interpersonal communication and reflective skill

These are examples of implications of the model's values for appropriate attitudes. But even if supervisor and supervisee identify with those values and have a similar understanding of the tasks they are engaged in, their lack of skill in communicating in this rather unusual interpersonal arena may still defeat their intentions. Attitudes are what the 'receiver' sees, hears and imagines, not necessarily what the 'protagonist' intends or imagines. So the final strand to this model is the spelling out of specific jobs which need to be done within the overall tasks and the micro-skills which the supervisor and practitioner need to have at their disposal if they are to do 'this supervision alliance stuff' well.

Both parties need the skills which go with his or her job. For the supervisor, there are the jobs and skills of:

- *climate building*, through setting up a physical environment which is welcoming, inviting information, listening without prior judgment or prejudice, checking what has been heard, sharing appropriate information, gauging the degree of appropriate formality/informality for this practitioner, licensing lightness and humour;
- *clarifying and negotiating the contract and working agreement*, through the key skills of clear *purpose stating* ('we/you must') and *preference stating* ('you/we may') as well as listening, clarifying, and checking shared understanding;
- *furthering the supervision process*; using all of the above skills, plus
- *challenging* in an authoritative (as opposed to authoritarian) manner; *giving and receiving feedback* – both evaluative and non-evaluative; *acknowledging and respecting experiences and feelings*: for instance, distress, vulnerability, confusion, anger, shame, guilt, remorse, pride, pleasure; *co-managing agreements* within boundaries – time management, reviews, administrative responsibilities.

For the supervisee, there are also jobs and accompanying skills to be developed. Consisting of ability to reflect and skill in communicating, these include:

- *preparing* for supervision, including log-keeping; identifying puzzling, interesting or upsetting experiences which could benefit from reflection; setting priorities;
- *presenting issues* in a way that makes them accessible and lively to herself and to her supervisor and is economical of time;
- *setting* and monitoring learning aims;
- increasingly *being open* to the supervisor's perspectives, and being able to discriminate what is useful;
- being *open to feedback*, and learning to identify if it is useful, and if necessary, to ask for no more at the moment;
- *giving feedback* to the supervisor, both spontaneously at the time when some response is helpful or confusing; and in a more considered way, at reviews.

The range and flexibility of communication asked for by this model is quite formidable when spelled out in this way. Either or both parties may already be skilled in this sort of relationship and process and everyone will have a range of transferable assets. However, in such a time-limited situation, which by its nature needs to

feel unhurried and to offer space for reflection, acquiring unselfconscious competence takes time, attention and openness to feedback.

Box 3.2 Supervision skills for helping practitioners reflect, learn and change

This framework for the Helping Process is adapted from the work of Gerard Egan
(1994). It is based on the systematic processes of *Exploration, Deeper Understanding,
Action* – usually though not necessarily in that order. It is a useful compilation of
helping skills derived from a wide range of sources which can be used flexibly. There
are other frameworks – e.g. the 6 Category Intervention Model, Heron (1990) – which
can be used in its place within the wider model.

Exploration

- Listening empathically
- Reflecting back what has been heard about the experience being described, in its
  subjective and its objective aspects
- Clarifying, paraphrasing and summarising what has been heard

Deeper Understanding

- Enabling the storyteller to focus in a way that makes for increased understanding
- Exploring and developing the story through, for instance:
  – open-ended questioning
  – awareness-raising enquiry – thinking, feeling, sensation, imagining etc.
  – deeper level empathy – testing hunches
  – making connections
  – offering alternative perspectives
  – informing
  – challenging
  – confronting.

Action

- Enabling appropriate action through, for instance:
  – envisaging outcomes
  – exploring options
  – cost-benefit analysis
  – rehearsing
  – considering unintended consequences
  – goal setting
  – action planning.

The training process

Training is a slightly misleading word. The task is 'to assist practitioners to use the
reflective opportunity of clinical supervision' or 'to assist the formation of clinical
supervisors'. It is not 'about' supervision, but about learning 'how to do it well'.
Clinical supervision is a process which has no set procedures or regimen like many

practical disciplines. It depends for its success on the attitudes, qualities and inter-personal skill of the participants.

How educators assist participants to develop supervision skill, in usually very limited time, will depend on the particular skill, experience and qualities that they bring and the resources and experience that course participants bring. The guidelines and methods offered here are those which my colleagues and I use and adapt for differing course formats and participants. Box 3.3 outlines those guidelines and methods.

The training experience

Excellent working alliances between more and less experienced workers are still relatively rare in work settings that are systematically hierarchical. This is not because workers and managers, or other senior colleagues, are inherently incapable of working co-operatively. Rather, the culture trains us in role behaviour which is appropriate to hierarchy, and can appear to punish us if we experiment with more co-operative relating. If clinical supervision is to be welcomed rather than mistrusted, these residual attitudes have to be counteracted.

So I conclude that the experience of the supervision course will be the major learning medium.

Box 3.3 Guidelines and methods for facilitating the development of supervisors and practitioner/supervisees

We seek to:

- Offer a *training experience* which consciously models co-operative working on tasks, values, attitudes and skills.
- Make *careful working agreements* for the course and respect them; and spend time on creating a culture of participation, safety and challenge.
- Offer opportunities for *progressive development* – that is, first offer participants good clinical supervision (or audio/videotaped examples) and encourage them to practice attitudes and skills for *using* supervision well; subsequently offer opportunities for developing the abilities for supervising.
- For those who necessarily start at 'supervisor' level, we still *begin* with the skills for using supervision.
- Encourage preparation through *Open Learning Materials*. These include:
  - simple and graphic theoretical frameworks
  - audio or video examples of the process and skills of supervision, acting as a trailer for the subsequent course
  - simple and inviting self-awareness exercises which can help participants realise that they will be expected to develop self-awareness and self-management.
- Offer opportunities *to learn by experience and by doing*, so courses – even one day courses – will include:
  - experiential exercises, to help people know from inside what the theory is talking about; attitude and skills modelling; and practice with feedback
  - skills modelling allows for people to see for themselves what is being talked about; practising with feedback in a safe-enough setting develops skill and self awareness.

Careful working agreements

As in supervision, safety is created by clear and open statements of set parameters and honest negotiation of what is negotiable. Overall course aims, content and any assessment methods and criteria, the extent of the staff members' responsibility and the members' responsibilities for their own learning, and the limits of staff confidentiality, can be stated ahead of time. This is the direct equivalent of the clinical supervision *contract*.

The *working agreement* is paralleled by inviting participants to share and then write up the kinds of ground rules they would like in order to make this a learning forum which would be both safe and risk-taking enough for them. Special needs are identified, and participants told that they will be invited to join in experiential exercises. They are also told that they can choose not to join in these and this will be honoured. They will be offered alternative 'observer' tasks, which again they have choice about taking. Time is given to set and share their own personal learning aims for the course. These aims may be shared publicly on flip chart, or shared only with a partner or small group. Either way, time is allowed for re-visiting the aims along the way and at the end of the course.

As with the clinical supervision alliance, this process serves a practical purpose while it also allows the rapid building of a culture and relationship suitable for this group to work well.

Progressive development

Learning about *using* supervision is always the first step in becoming a supervisor within the supervision alliance model. We have found that informed and skilled supervisees can work well even if their supervisor is new to the role or feels less than expert. Supervisors who have experienced good supervision have already done much of the crucial learning they need in order to offer fruitful working alliances (Cutcliffe and Proctor 1998a, 1998b) and have increased awareness of the potential vulnerability of the supervisee role.

Open learning materials

Editors' comment: In *Fundamental Themes in Clinical Supervision,* Proctor (2001: 25–46) suggested using open learning materials such as those created and produced for counsellors (Inskipp and Proctor 1993, 1995, 2nd edition revised 2009). They consist of short blocks of information; self-management, self-awareness and practice exercises; and extensive audiotaped (now on CD) illustrations and discussions.

Subsequently, those materials have been revised and re-edited and the authors have also produced two DVDs and an accompanying booklet, Creative Group Supervision (University of Wales, Newport).

Experiential and creative exercises

Creative exercises are those that invite participants to engage senses rather than just words. The object is to help people access what they 'know', which they had not realized. So, for instance, we often ask participants to create the supervision alliance model (as depicted in Figure 3.1) as kind of sociogram. The method is described in Box 3.4.

Box 3.4 Experiential portrayal of the Supervision Alliance Model

Having made name cards for all the characters and words in the picture (see Figure 3.1) we invite participants in turn to take a card, starting with the patient (or client), and to take up a position in the centre of the room. Moving through supervisor, professional manager, Trust manager, GNC, to positions representing the working alliance, the contract, normative, formative and restorative tasks – and so on (depending on available numbers, of course.) until all who choose to join in have a position. When all are in their chosen place, they speak for that role and reflect on what they realise when standing in that position. The exercise sounds complicated, but in practice is simple to set up.

It is invariably surprising, enlightening and humbling to hear the various insights.

Box 3.5 Experiential and creative activities

Exploring resources

Mull over your network of colleagues, friends, family, supervisor, other professionals etc. and identify and write down who or what could meet the needs listed.

1 Sharing your work in confidence;
2 Getting feedback/guidance;
3 Developing professional skills, ideas, information;
4 Letting off steam if you are angry, discouraged, fed-up;
5 Acknowledging feelings of distress, pleasure, failure etc.;
6 Feeling valued by those you count as colleagues;
7 Widening your horizons;
8 Increasing your physical, emotional or spiritual wellbeing.

(*There follows some suggestions, including dog/cat, your local community organisations, yoga, political activity*)
• Which needs do you consider well enough met at the moment?
• Which of them are, or might appropriately, be met in supervision?
• Which need some topping up?
• How might you do this?
• Which are not at all well met?
• How might you meet them within your available resources?
• Have you other professional needs?
(*These questions can also be used in a kind of musical questions exercise to break the ice near the start of a course. Participants mill around and when the music stops, speak about one of the questions with their nearest neighbour for half a minute. Then the music starts again and at the next stop, the next question is discussed. It invariably produces quite a buzz.*)

Adapted from Inskipp and Proctor (1995, 2nd ed. 2009)

Attitude and skills practice with feedback

Since one of the most difficult learnings for beginning supervisors seems to be managing formative, restorative and normative tasks within the same alliance and relationship, recognising what it takes, behaviourally and emotionally, to challenge authoritatively while remaining respectful and empathic is a first step. Developing verbal range and accuracy for communicating differing intentions follows from that. Instant feedback, about the impact on the receiver of the way chosen, or better still, on oneself when hearing or seeing video or audio recordings – is invaluable.

Participants who are learning to be supervisors need to have seen and heard a variety of supervisory interventions which illustrate specific micro-skills either on the course or in pre-course materials. When they recognise what is expected, they can go on to find ways of using those interventions in their own style and manner.

Feedback skills are some of the first that need modelling and playing with. Giving and receiving feedback and ground rules for making feedback useful are essential for both supervisee and supervisor in the working alliance and they are also a requisite for fruitful skills learning on the course.

Doing supervision

To enable participants to develop their version of a helping process in supervision, we set up structured exercises for practicing particular responses. Since supervising puts pressures on the supervisor to find solutions, we focus on reminding people about the skills of reflecting, paraphrasing and summarising what is being talked about, the exploration phase, before moving into focusing and action. It is this that encourages the practitioner to 'hear' what she is saying and begin to ponder and reflect.

Focusing

We have developed ways of thinking about and practising a variety of focus points to aid deeper understanding in the supervision process. These are based on the process model of Hawkins and Shohet (1989). However, I believe that a framework for focusing in settings in which practitioners are not solely, or predominantly, concerned with interpersonal issues needs to be developed. For instance, at any particular time, would it be helpful to focus on the practical aspects of a situation, on issues of responsibility, on interpersonal dilemmas, on the practitioner's feelings or thinking at the time, or on the buttons which the issue had pressed for her? Without an awareness of the range of possible foci, supervisors tend to become routine in the areas they focus on or the factors or perspectives they ignore.

Having noticed the range of possible foci, it is also important to raise awareness about *how* focus is determined. Experienced practitioners, when developing as supervisors, tend to feel it is their responsibility to identify and pick a focus for the supervisee. However, the alliance model entails reminding them that this need not – often should not – be the case. Needs will differ with the developmental stage of the practitioner, but increasingly supervisees should be able to respond to an offer of choice of focus points, and often themselves determine where the appropriate focus lies. If, in training to use supervision, a framework of possible foci is given to them, they will quickly become more self-directing.

Action

Skills for encouraging *action planning* can also be taught specifically before being incorporated in supervision practice.

Practicing 'doing supervision'

To enable participants to juggle with the responsibilities of setting up working agreements, 'doing supervision', monitoring learning aims and reviewing, we encourage practice for real with a partner or in threes. Where time is limited, live peer practice between course sessions can be taped and used for identifying particular skills or tracking the course of a specific piece of supervision work. The tape can also include feedback and comments from the supervisee and observer, if there is one.

Changes that are to do with the way we are with other people can be uncomfortably close to the bone if they call into question our sense of self. For experienced practitioners, especially, changing may mean acknowledging shortcomings of which they were previously unconscious. Self-conscious incompetence is very painful. That is why it is so important to allow for free choice on a course and why time is well spent in helping people identify what is in it for them in learning to become a competent supervisee or supervisor. This means acknowledging and accepting reluctance, incomprehension and resentment.

However, like supervisors, educators and trainers are also in an advocacy relationship for the off-scene stakeholders – employers; professional colleagues; and, most particularly, patients, clients, or whatever. While accepting and understanding reluctance, they also have a responsibility to speak for the obligation to offer our best service. Becoming competent at offering and using opportunities to reflect on practice can be both personally and professionally rewarding.

In summary

This supervision alliance model spells out aspirations and tensions which will be inherent in non-hierarchical (or co-operative) supervision, wherever it is practiced. The training programme outlined is extensive. It can be offered in progressive modules which need to be adapted for specific contexts. Experience suggests that the learning opportunity offered is of use in many settings other than clinical supervision.

For some trainers, and some participants, aspects of it might be quite alien and unhelpful. However, any training which results in the good use and provision of the kind of clinical supervision advocated in this book will necessarily have to address, in some way, appropriate attitudes and skills, and offer frameworks which make clear the intentions behind the complex task of clinical supervision.

References

Cutcliffe, J.R. and Proctor, B. (1998a), An alternative approach to clinical supervision: Part One, *British Journal of Nursing*, 7(5): 280–285.

Cutcliffe, J.R. and Proctor, B. (1998b), An alternative approach to clinical supervision: Part Two, *British Journal of Nursing* 7(6): 344–350.

Cutcliffe, J.R., Epling, M., Cassedy, P., McGregor, J., Plant, N. and Butterworth, T. (1998a), Ethical dilemmas in clinical supervision 1: need for guidelines, *British Journal of Nursing*, 7(15),pp. 920–923.

Cutcliffe, J.R., Epling, M., Cassedy, P., McGregor, J., Plant, N. and Butterworth, T. (1998b), Ethical dilemmas in clinical supervision 2: need for guidelines, *British Journal of Nursing*, 7(16): 978–982.

Egan, G. (1994), *The Skilled Helper*, 4th edn, Pacific Grove, CA: Brookes/Cole.

Hawkins, P. and Shohet, R. (1989), *Supervision in the Helping Professions*, Buckingham: Open University Press.

Heron, J. (1990), *Helping the Client*, London: Sage.

Inskipp, F. and Proctor, B. (1st ed. 1993, 2nd ed. Revised 2009), *The Art, Craft and Tasks of Counselling Supervision Part 1: Making the Most of Supervision*. Twickenham: Cascade Publications, p. 184.

Inskipp, F. and Proctor, B. (1st ed. 1995, 2nd ed. 2009), *The Art, Craft and Tasks of Counselling Supervision Part 2: Becoming a Supervisor*, Twickenham: Cascade Publications.

Morton-Cooper, A. and Palmer, A. (2000), *Mentoring, Preceptorship, and Clinical Supervision*, Oxford: Blackwell Science.

Proctor, B. (2001), Training for the supervision alliance attitude, skills and intention, in J.R. Cutcliffe, T. Butterworth and B. Proctor (eds), *Fundamental Themes in Clinical Supervision*, London: Routledge, pp. 25–46.

4   An alternative training approach in clinical supervision

John R. Cutcliffe

This chapter focuses on training practitioners to become supervisees rather than supervisors. It examines the drawbacks to training practitioners to become supervisors and some of the principal problems that are facing the widespread introduction of clinical supervision in nursing practice. It then provides an argument that illustrates the advantages of training practitioners to become supervisees. It suggests a possible structure for this training and considers ways that it could be evaluated.

The editors feel that students, trainees and learners as aspirant health care practitioners, should be exposed to the practice and theory of clinical supervision early on in their education/training. Once such foundations are in place, they serve as the building blocks upon which more sophisticated and advanced clinical supervision practices can be built. The editors also believe that early exposure to high quality clinical supervision will engender in the practitioner a desire to continue receiving and participating in clinical supervision throughout their career.

This chapter is based on the papers that were originally published in the *British Journal of Nursing* in 1998:

Cutcliffe, J.R. and Proctor, B. An alternative approach to clinical supervision: Part One, *British Journal of Nursing*, 7(5): 280–285.

Cutcliffe, J.R. and Proctor, B. An alternative approach to clinical supervision: Part Two, *British Journal of Nursing* 7(6): 344–350.

Introduction and background

Since its relatively broad introduction into health care in the United Kingdom in the late 1980s and early 1990s, clinical supervision (CS) has remained as an important issue within the National Health Service (NHS) (Cutcliffe and Burns 1998). The argument for formalised support mechanisms for nurses in the form of clinical supervision was pioneered by Professor Tony Butterworth in the early 1990s (Butterworth 1991, 1992). Additionally reported work from other professions was beginning to influence thinking in nursing (Butterworth *et al.* 1996) and supervision models from counselling and psychotherapy were starting to be incorporated into nursing practice (Proctor 1986; Hawkins and Shohet 1989). Subsequent to these developments, according to Bishop (1994a) the significant factors to emerge from the United Kingdom Central Council (now the Nursing and Midwifery Council, NMC) *Code of Professional Conduct* (UKCC 1992a) and *The Scope of Professional Practice* (UKCC 1992b) were the individual's increased accountability combined with the demise of traditional support systems, which make clinical supervision essential.

Furthermore, the findings of the Allitt enquiry (Clothier *et al.* 1994) emphasised the need for safe and accountable practice. Clinical supervision within nursing was then endorsed by the Chief Nursing Officer of the Department of Health (1994) who considered it to be fundamental to safeguarding standards, the development of expertise and the delivery of quality care.

Subsequent to these endorsements, the growth of the knowledge base, evidence base and associated policy literature has developed over the last two decades (and in various countries) to the extent that, for some, CS is now regarded as a core professional competency (see for example, Falender *et al.* 2004). For others, CS is seen as necessary for ethical practice and practitioner/client safety/well-being (British Association for Counselling and Psychotherapy 2007; Kilminster and Jolly 2007; United Kingdom Council for Psychotherapy 2008).

Reported benefits

The evidence-base of CS, while still in a stage of relative infancy, has grown significantly over the decade or so. What were previously thought of, or more accurately described as, *alleged* benefits, can now be described as *reported benefits or outcomes.* Some of these key benefits are outlined in Box 4.1.

Box 4.1 Reported benefits of clinical supervision

- Increased feelings of support and feelings of personal well being (Butterworth *et al.* 1996; Hyrkäs 2005).
- Increased knowledge and awareness of possible solutions to clinical problems (Arvidsson *et al.* 2000).
- Increased confidence, decreased incidence of emotional strain and burnout (Hallberg and Norberg 1993; Berg and Hallberg 1999).
- Higher staff morale and satisfaction leading to a decrease in staff sickness/absence, increased staff satisfaction (Butterworth *et al.* 1996; Begat *et al.* 2005).
- Increased participation in reflective practice (Fowler 1998; Jarrett and Johns 2005).
- Increased self-awareness (Cutcliffe and Epling 1997; Severinsson 2001).
- Improved patient/client outcomes (McKee and Black 1992; Gennis and Gennis 1993; Sox *et al.* 1998).

It can be argued that ongoing attempts to investigate these reported benefits continue to centre around the three components suggested by Proctor (1986), these being normative (organisational, professional ethics and quality control), restorative (support for staff) and formative (education and development). Relatively early findings from Butterworth *et al.*'s (1997) multi-site study, which explored several questions of clinical supervision, provided some evidence to suggest that receiving clinical supervision benefits the recipient, in particular in the realms of reducing emotional exhaustion and depersonalisation. Furthermore, early qualitative and anecdotal evidence was produced which suggested clinical supervision can improve client care (Paunonen 1991; Booth 1992; Timpson 1996; Cutcliffe and Burns 1998). As the studies listed in Box 4.1 indicate, our evidence base since these early studies has increased dramatically to the extent that the findings from these preliminary studies has been confirmed by more recent studies and additional narrative evidence.

The training/education of clinical supervisors

Examination of the well-developed literature that focuses on the introduction of CS into practice and/or the training/education/preparation of supervisors indicates that there is no one singular method of implementation, or indeed one approach to training/education. After their review of CS in four mental health professions in Australia, Spence *et al.* (2001) arrived at the same conclusion; arguing that little information exists on what might be the most effective ways of training/educating supervisors. A similar position was asserted by Fleming *et al.* (1996) regarding CS in the United States, where they advocated for additional research into the specification, measurement and training of supervisory skills. It is noteworthy that these two international perspectives share the same commonality of much of the European CS literature on this issue: namely that, a) it would be disingenuous to claim that a consensus exists on what the composition of CS education/training should look like, and b) issues of training/education centre around equipping and enabling individuals to become supervisors not supervisees. While this approach has benefits, it also has major drawbacks which warrant further consideration.

The drawbacks of training/educating nurses to be supervisors

CS has a specific and separate skill set; while some of the interpersonal skills utilised in CS may be transferable from nursing, psychotherapy or counselling training/education, CS encompasses far more than basic interpersonal skills and has its own unique set of skills. Consequently, while there is no consensus on what the specific composition of CS training/education should be, there is a consensus that there is a clear need for specific clinical supervision training (see for example, Milne 1998). Yet there are no standardised minimum quality indicators or competencies and no widely accepted definition of what constitutes CS training/education. Within Butterworth *et al.*'s (1997: 17) multi-site study it is reported that the respondent sites had offered a wide variety of training opportunities: 'Courses and training ranged from 6.5 days to 1 day, most commonly 2–3 days.' This cross-sectional view of CS clinical supervision education/training reflects the experience of the author. During the last 20 years and more, the author has encountered, through contact with self-governing (NHS) trusts, higher education institutions and individuals who offer clinical supervision education/training privately, a wide range of practices and desired outcomes, all under the general heading of CS training/education. Yet the diversity in the quality of the training may well have a detrimental affect on the quality of supervision provided; a view shared by Hoffman (1994). Cutcliffe (1997) argued that there is a need to examine if a correlation exists between the quality or intensity of CS training/education and the extent of positive outcomes/benefits (for both practitioners and clients). The author postulates that if a nurse receives insufficient or inappropriate training/education in supervision, then the quality of the supervision they provide is unlikely to be capable of producing measurable change in the supervisees' overall well-being or improvements in the care they provide.

However, enabling all potential supervisors to attend high quality supervision training/education presents many logistical problems. It is likely to be relatively lengthy and expensive when compared to the other options, such as in-service training. Smith (1995) reported that a director of patient care and nursing estimated that it would cost around £100,000 to implement CS based on the calculation that each nurse in her hospital would receive two hours of supervision per month. It is unclear whether or not these calculations take into account the cost of training/educating the nurses to become supervisors, so this could be considered as a conservative estimate. Admittedly, a counter-argument exists that suggests £100,000 is not really very much as, at that time, it represented the cost of employing an NHS trust chief executive for a year (Smith 1995). This problem is exacerbated if Regional Health Authorities do not provide additional funding to pay for the training/education and/or pay for additional nurses to ensure the clinical areas are staffed adequately while the training/education occurs. Furthermore as we operate in a climate where economics play an ever increasing role in determining the strategic planning of health care delivery units, the real and reasonable position of these organisations is to say we cannot afford to release large numbers of staff to undertake extensive, intensive and expensive training/education courses.

Problems with implementing clinical supervision in nursing

In addition to the absence of a plausible economic option for NHS trusts, the culture of the NHS does not yet have the infrastructure necessary for the widespread uptake of CS. Some of the problems relate to the limited understanding of CS practice; how can managers be expected to facilitate the equipping of nurses to the necessary extent if the nurses themselves do not have this understanding? Fowler (1996: 382) supported this argument suggesting,

> Nursing and health visiting does not, at yet, have a culture of clinical supervision for qualified nurses.... If we have little or no experience of being supervised ourselves, how do we clinically supervise others?

Smith (1995) stated that feedback from the National Health Service Executive conference on CS upheld this viewpoint. Conference participants argued that a cultural shift was necessary in order to move the CS agenda into the whole organisation, and that crucially, CS may be needed but it also has to be wanted. Bishop's (1994b) survey of nurse's attitudes towards CS indicated that only 0.2 per cent of the *Nursing Times'* estimated readership responded to the questionnaire. While workload pressure and slow circulation rates may account for some of this very low response rate, a distinct

---

Box 4.2 Reasons for resisting clinical supervision within nursing

- A tradition and culture that discourages the public expression of emotion (Menzies Lyth 1959).
- The perception of CS as yet another management monitoring tool (Yegdich 1999).
- The perception of supervision as a form of personal therapy (Bond and Holland 1998).
- Perceptions that the nurses don't have sufficient time/resources to be able to engage in CS (Cleary and Freeman 2005).
- A continuing lack of clarity regarding the purpose of supervision (Lyth 2000).
- Resistance itself is an unavoidable component of the process of change (Wilkin *et al.* 1997).

lack of interest in CS also be considered as a reason (Bishop 1994b). This ambiva-lence has been detected elsewhere (see for example, Cleary and Freeman 2005). Furthermore less than half of Bishop's sample (46 per cent) had CS up and running. It remains the case that there are many nurses who do not want CS at this time. Such resistance has many reasons for its existence and these are described in Box 4.2.

The author argues that when considering the resistance to CS there is a crucial point that needs attention: and that is the apparent, continuing, lack of clarity regarding the purpose of CS in nursing. Examination of the extant literature highlights (at least) two perspectives on the purpose of CS. One view posits CS as an opportunity for a more experienced nurse to monitor, educate and support a less experienced nurse in how they 'do' tech-nical skills. Practising CS this way requires all supervisors to be more expert in the par-ticular speciality of nursing than the supervisee. Alternatively, there is another view that posits CS as an opportunity to help and support nurses reflect on their dilemmas, difficulties and successes, and to explore how they reacted to, solved or achieved them. This view posits CS as a forum for considering the personal, interpersonal and practical aspects of care so as to develop and maintain nurses who are skilled and reflective practitioners. This situation creates the need for supervisors to be effective at supporting nurses in self-monitoring, identifying difficulties in practice and finding the proper place to make good the deficit, not necessarily to be more expert in the particular nursing speciality. This pivotal difference is seldom spelled out in the nursing literature and consequently it is not surprising that a sense of confusion exists for many nurses. Confusion concerning the purpose appears to create a resistance to CS as some nurses appear to be unsure what they are entering into.

The author has stated previously that, despite this resistance, some trusts and educational institutions have made real progress in the implementation of CS and such endeavours should be applauded. If these efforts are combined with systematic review and action research that produces additional evidence supporting the link between receiving supervision and improved client care/positive outcomes for staff, then this resistance may begin to decline. However, such change will take time and may be somewhat parochial. The author argues that while such implementation should be encouraged, what is needed is a radical shift in the emphasis of training/educating nurses in the practice of CS. An alternative approach is needed; one that features training nurses to be supervisees.

Alternative approaches to training/education in clinical supervision

It is interesting to note that feedback from the National Health Service Executive con-ference on CS (Smith 1995) argued that training was necessary but that creating special courses should be avoided; this is a somewhat counterintuitive argument to put forward. Logic and reason would seem to indicate that if CS has a specific skill set then it would appear to denote the need for specific training/education in order to acquire and develop the said skill set. It has been argued that all nurses should become familiar with the theory and practice of CS and it should be a part of every nurse's career, then there may be merit in examining how other common training requirements for nurses have been met. However, if there is resistance to offering stand-alone specific CS training/education courses, and yet simultaneously a need for all nurses to be conversant with CS, then perhaps we might consider the view of the NHSE supports the argument for providing standardised training; a training that could be available to all nurses.

All qualified nurses share a commonality in that they undertake a period of education before qualifying. Given that there is an identified need for some form of education/training for CS and that all nurses have a common experience prior to becoming qualified, the logical solution to this problem is to incorporate CS education/training into pre-registration nurse education programmes/courses. The crucial difference of this education/training however is that student nurses would be prepared to *be supervisees and not supervisors*. This approach has many advantages, which will be discussed later; however, it also addresses the problems identified in the preceding paragraph, in that this form of CS education/training reduces the need for lengthy and costly post-registration CS courses. The author is not suggesting that preparing student nurses to be supervisees removes the need for post-registration education/training, but a common foundation could establish the framework on which their future CS knowledge and experience can be built. It sets in place, for the future, cohorts of new practitioners who can use CS well, even if the supervisors are limited in their knowledge and experience. Additionally, it would provide fertile foundations upon which any additional education/training as a supervisor can be based; consequently new supervisors can build on their training and experience as 'good' supervisees rather than starting from scratch.

Perhaps what this approach would do most is change the climate from the bottom upwards. While it does not meet the training/education needs of those nurses who are already qualified, it reduces the amount of time that future nurses would spend in post-registration supervision training since they would already possess a basic understanding and experience of CS. Consequently, post-registration education/training in CS would be shorter, thus saving a great deal of money. Additionally the supervisee training would be relatively straightforward to standardise so that each nurse education centre provides at least the same minimum quality, thus in part helping to address the problem of the wide diversity evident in current supervision training/education.

Training/educating student nurses to be supervisees

Advantages of supervisee training/education

In addition to the substantial reduction in training costs, and the possible standardisation of supervisee training, this approach brings additional advantages. These are listed in Box 4.3 and then discussed in more detail.

Box 4.3 Advantages of nurses being supervisees

1   The creation of greater equality and intentionality in the working alliance.
2   The increased awareness and understanding that supervision is something for the supervisee.
3   The sharing and agreeing of values, ground rules, terms and aims between the supervisee/supervisor and the organisation.
4   A sense of comradeship between peers, a greater sense of team cohesion a counteraction to a culture of divide and rule.
5   The development of basic intrapersonal skills (e.g. reflecting on practice, choosing issues, asking for and using help appropriately) in a less personally threatening forum.

The creation of greater equality and intentionality in the working alliance

Clinicians' resistance to supervision includes justifiable concerns that it is another management monitoring tool (Wilkin *et al.* 1997; Yegdich 1999; Cutcliffe and Hyrkäs 2006) and consequently the 'locus of control' remains very much with the supervisor. If students are equipped to become supervisees, they are placed in an empowered position. The awareness and experience of the supervision process during their training/education could enable them to realise they are not 'done unto' during CS; there is more equity in the distribution of power. Hawkins and Shohet (1989) suggested that evaluation within supervision is a two-way, reciprocal process where both parties have the opportunity to give and receive open, honest, constructive feedback. Inskipp and Proctor (1989) argued that there is a joint responsibility for the supervision, and thus supervisees need to be active in seeking the right sort of CS for themselves. If subsequent supervision moves away inadvertently from support, development, growth and education and becomes custodial, punitive or disabling, the students' knowledge and experience of the process could enable them to deal with this more effectively and seek help in bringing the CS back within the defined boundaries. The intentionality is increased in that both supervisor and supervisee are aware of the reasons for their time together. Hawkins and Shohet (1989) pointed out that this intentionality helps supervisees become more proactive in gaining the support they need. Thus the CS becomes a shared responsibility, a purposeful, deliberate, conscious act of support, education and development aimed at facilitating client care and it ceases to be an ambiguous and amorphous concept.

The increased awareness and understanding that clinical supervision is something for the supervisee

The current introduction of CS may well be viewed by nurses as yet another imposition from nursing hierarchies. If CS is seen as serving the organisation, not the client or the clinician, then it is understandable that resistance exists. In order for this resistance to be counteracted nurses need to discover that CS is primarily for them and their clients, not something for the supervisor, and certainly not something primarily designed as a tool for the management of the organisation. By making supervisee training an integral component of nurse education, students would be acclimatised to the experience of CS and encounter the benefits for themselves. This argument is supported by Bishop (1994b) who reported that 98 per cent of nurses who had previously participated in peer review expected to benefit from CS. There appears to be a phenomenon whereby the experience of receiving high quality CS rapidly removes miscomprehensions, anxieties and resistance. Fowler's 1995 study also corroborates this argument. He examined post-registration nursing students' perceptions of the elements of good CS and suggested that a key finding was that

> all students wanted to see evidence of supervisors putting themselves out and helping the student build on their knowledge base.
>
> (Fowler 1995: 37)

Students who had experienced CS felt it was for them, and wished to see evidence of this in the behaviour of the supervisor. While the sample size in this study

(50 students from two courses) represents only a fraction of the population of nursing students, it provides a valuable insight into the lived world of students. This increased awareness that exposure to CS generates also addresses the issue raised in the first part of this chapter, that of confusion concerning the purpose of CS and the subsequent resistance this confusion creates.

Ritter *et al.* (1996) described a model of CS provided to undergraduate general nursing students who undertook clinical placements on psychiatric wards. The model incorporates Schön's (1984, 1987) work on reflective practice and coaching whereby each student is helped to identify and articulate his/her own experience on his or her own behalf and in his or her own way: in other words it makes attempts to be supervisee led. Ritter *et al.* (1996: 155) stated:

> the model of clinical supervision enables students to choose to demonstrate their understanding by turning up to the supervision with something quite different from what the supervisor asked for.

The students who became self-directed in their supervision appear to have grasped that it is for them. While this model appears to be a move towards training/educating supervisees as it has an element of being supervisee led, it is still driven and guided by the supervisor. It is only when the supervisee has some understanding of the process and structure of the CS that it becomes more completely supervisee led and consequently that supervisees acknowledge that supervision is for them. It is worth wondering how much more would the students benefit from this CS if they began their placement already equipped with an understanding of what CS is for and what it is to be a supervisee.

The sharing and agreeing of values, ground rules, terms and aims between the supervisee/supervisor and the organisation

If all student nurses are provided with the same supervisee education/training then this can create a commonality in the perception of the roles and tasks of supervision and how these can be distinguished from similar roles and tasks. If one looks at the terminology used in different countries to describe the same (or very similar) process, then it becomes clear that the term CS has yet to be universally distinguished by practitioners from preceptorship, mentorship, clinical instruction, individual performance review or personal therapy. Therefore while students may be unclear about the values, ground rules and terms of CS prior to receiving it, participation in the practice of receiving CS (of being a supervisee) can help to clarify their understanding of terminology, perhaps to move the nursing academe towards a more shared CS nomenclature. Once more, the value of providing students with experience of being a supervisee during nurse preparation is illustrated. Supervisee training exposes the student to the process of negotiating ground rules, and the need for this explicit contracting is identified by Proctor (1988) who has argued that if supervision is to become and remain a co-operative experience which allows real rather than token accountability, a clear, if not actually tough working arrangement, needs to be negotiated. Additionally an awareness of the aims of CS is increased. The student can start to appreciate how CS can contribute to client, clinician and organisational need as a result of the increased self awareness that CS can bring (Cutcliffe and Epling 1997). When given supervisee training the students can begin to appreciate their need for development and, importantly, the personal responsibility they have for their own development. The student can begin to see how CS affects the way they deliver care and consequently, the quality of care they provide. Similarly, such improvements in care will probably be part of the organisation's philosophy and/or strategy and thus both student and managers can see how the aims of CS can also contribute to meeting the organisation's needs.

A sense of comradeship between peers, a greater sense of team cohesion a counteraction to a culture of divide and rule

It is reasonable to suggest that traditionally nurses have been encouraged to contain their emotions and keep a lid on things (Menzies Lyth 1959). The classic phrase from Menzies Lyth's study of 'nurses crying in the sluice room' having just dealt with yet another emotional traumatic interpersonal situation, perhaps serves as a meaningful example of this behaviour. Such repression can only bring about a sense of isolation and inadequacy; especially if the nurse believes that her peers regard her as someone who cannot cope because she weeps or lets of steam. Faugier (1992: 27) also pointed out that nursing has a system loaded against the development of continued learning, fuelled by 'the threat of losing position or face before junior or untrained members of staff'.

For continuing learning to emerge from reflective practice, a culture of safety and honesty needs to be systematically developed. Supervisee training could begin to eradicate debilitating and restrictive attitudes. What better way to begin to change the culture than by introducing students to the practice of reflection, of being open, of being able to recognise and express the impact of emotionally charged experiences, all of which are encouraged within well set up CS. The increase in self-awareness brought about by participating in CS (Faugier 1992; Cutcliffe and Epling 1997) enables supervisees to realise when they need to express emotion and obtain support and, importantly, that such processes are healthy; furthermore, that such processes are an integral component of each nurses' professional life. It encourages them to realise that 'mistakes' are usually opportunities rather than marks of failure. The sense of a shared experience, of participating in a common, widespread phenomenon, creates a collective sense of cohesion. Additionally the support experienced in CS enables the nurse to think 'I am cared for by these people, I am not on my own, I belong to this team.'

The development of basic intrapersonal skills (e.g. reflecting on practice, choosing issues, asking for and using help appropriately) in a less personally threatening forum

Training/educating students to be supervisees creates an environment where the student will need to enter into reflective practice, self-examination of learning needs and to practise being assertive. Yet all this can occur in a forum where there is no punitive presence, since the underpinning essence of CS is support. Students who experience this support in supervisee training/education, and conceptualise that, in order to support, one needs to listen actively and empathise (Jones and Cutcliffe 2009) become arguably more capable of providing support. Butterworth (1992) hypothesised that a student who is trained in a learning environment which encourages active listening, empathy and support will lead to qualified nurses who foster similar therapeutic exchanges between nurses and patients. This argument is supported by Cassedy and Cutcliffe (1998) who reasoned that students need to experience in counselling training the kind of empathy, genuineness and respect for their own personhood which the author wants them to be offering clients. This entire training/education ideology of nurturing qualities is captured by Connor (1994: 37) who stated:

> Qualities are not developed by just practising skills or writing essays. They develop through the sum total of the learning experience and they are more likely to develop if there is intentionality in the learning process through ongoing structural experiences of reflection, reviewing and objective setting.

A suggested structure of supervisee training in nurse education

One possible structure for this training is as follows.

Year One: Teaching provided on the theories of supervision; examine definitions of supervision and delineation from related concepts; models and formats of supervision; a historical overview of its inception; how the processes of reflection and self-examination are interwoven with supervision; roles of supervisees/supervisors; ground rules and boundaries; the process of contracting; giving and receiving feedback; ethical issues in supervision and examination of the current evidence base for CS.

Year Two: Following early clinical placements students would have a minimum of one hour per month of CS sessions, using material they have recorded in their personal learning journals. The particular format of this CS (i.e. one-to-one, group) would be determined partly by the human resources available, and partly by the number of students on each course. In addition to the benefits of receiving the supervision, at the end of each module, placement or term, feedback could be given to the student on their use of supervision. How evident was it that the student participated in the roles, responsibilities and expectations of a supervisee? Have they taken responsibility for the actions, reflections and learnings? Did they appreciate and act on their own need for support?

Following this the student would complete a case study which would include his/her participation in CS and how he/she found this experience. The student would need to illustrate his/her active participation in CS and how this influenced his/her client care and personal/professional development. This would include a written piece of work, but could also include audio or videotaped sessions of the student's practice.

Problems with preparing students to be supervisees

This alternative approach to education/training in CS is not without problems. One argument against the idea centres around the issue that this process will have to be experiential, with students using material from their clinical practice as a source of learning (Schön 1984). However, since students are at an early stage of their preparation, they may have insufficient critical incidents or clinical material to bring to the clinical supervision session. Clinical supervision would have limited relevance until the student has some clinical practice. Another problem might be that students at this early stage in nurse education/training are too inexperienced to have an awareness of what they do not know or what they need to know. Individuals would only gain an awareness of their deficits once they have faced clinical situations and found themselves lacking. There is also the issue that trained supervisees could produce feelings of anxiety and disempowerment in their supervisor. Such new practitioners will be able to use supervision well and will not require such highly trained supervisors. However, being faced with a supervisee who knows more about the process of supervision may be unnerving. Supervisors may well be anxious that they are unable to deal with the issues the supervisee raises.

In reply to these arguments, there is a case for first educating/training the student in the theory of supervision and then exposing them to the process. In the same way that students are taught the theory of interpersonal communication skills prior to these skills being utilised or applied in a clinical environment. Therefore the experiential component of this education/training would only commence after a student has been on a clinical placement. As the student accrues more experience they will access more material that can be brought into the supervision. Yet the theory would already equip them with reasons why the processes that occur in supervision are necessary. The possible anxieties and feelings of disempowerment for a new supervisor are not exclusive to those individuals providing supervision to trained supervisees. The same feelings could well be present for any supervisor as Hawkins and Shohet (1989: 33) declared: 'Suddenly becoming, or being asked to be a supervisor can be both exhilarating and daunting.'

Additionally, if supervisors are equipped with information about the supervisees' education/training, it can both inform and challenge their existing supervision practice. Another problem would be incorporating this education/training into an already cramped pre-registration nurse training curriculum. While the author acknowledges this issue, he still feels the need to construct the argument for including education/training to become a supervisee at this early stage in each nurse's training. Indeed, he would argue that this could perhaps replace redundant or less valuable curricula content. The specific content of nursing programme curricula can then be debated widely, and the argument this chapter puts forward could then be included in those debates.

Evaluating supervisee training in nurse education

Butterworth *et al.* (1996) highlighted that initial attempts to evaluate CS centre around the three components suggested by Proctor (1986), these being: normative (organisational and quality control), restorative (support for staff) and formative (education and development), and they provide a format for this evaluation (Butterworth *et al.* 1997). It would be logical for evaluation of supervisee education/ training to follow a similar format. However, the author feels that evaluation in the normative category needs to be refined to ensure that the distinction between the supervisors' and supervisees' responsibility for overall normative development is clarified. This category needs to reflect their shared responsibility for learning, the internalising of professional ethics and standards of practice, and their shared responsibility for learning and developing competent practice. Crucially comparisons would have to be made between a control group of students who receive no supervisee training and a group of students who do receive supervision training, measured in terms of Butterworth's multi-centre study.

Normative

Quantitative research into this component would centre on audit data concerned with rates of student sickness/absence and student satisfaction levels. In particular, do students find they are more satisfied with their nurse preparation if they have supervisee training? Qualitative data could include supervisee lived experiences of the education/training. Additionally, in their case study (see above) students would be required to cite an instance where supervision has helped them with an issue of evaluating good practice or making an ethical decision, thus addressing the shared normative responsibility in supervision.

Restorative

Quantitative research into this component would centre around measurement of student stress levels, sick time, coping levels questionnaires and burnout inventories. In particular, how supported and listened to do students feel on a course that provides supervisee education/training? How does being on a clinical placement and receiving CS education/training compare to being on a placement that does not have this? i.e. does the education/training make it easier for the student to meet other educational criteria? Qualitative data would include identifying what being supported and listened to felt like on a course providing CS education/training, i.e. how does the education/training for CS increase the students' confidence, well-being and creativity in a way that contributes to them meeting other educational and practice criteria?

Formative

Research into this area would centre around evaluating observed performance, perhaps in the form of audio tape records, video tape records, or observations of clinical practice. This method of evaluation has already been used on Thorn training courses. This could also include the case study assignment which could provide qualitative evidence of the benefits of receiving supervisee training, i.e. comparisons between students' experiences of clinical problems and how these were addressed. In addition, in the case study, trainees would be expected to include particular incidences of how supervision had affected subsequent understanding and practice.

Conclusion

Clinical supervision is considered to be fundamental to safeguarding standards, to the development of expertise and to the delivery of quality care and it is reasonable to say it is here to stay. It reportedly brings significant benefits to clients and clinicians, and recent research has produced both quantitative and qualitative evidence that supports this argument. Many organisations have made widespread attempts to introduce CS into practice, with most developments being concerned with equipping clinicians to be supervisors not supervisees. This presents several logistical and financial problems, and currently neither the infra-structure nor culture are in place throughout nursing that would facilitate its widespread and effective uptake. However, an alternative method of tackling this problem would be to include supervisee education/training within the Common Foundation Programme component of diploma nurse education and in within the first two years of undergraduate nurse education. Training/educating student nurses to be supervisees has several alleged advantages. These are:

- a substantial reduction in training costs and time;
- a possible standardisation of training/education curricula;
- the creation of greater equality and intentionality in the working alliance,
- the increased awareness and understanding in the student that supervision is something for them;
- the sharing of values, ground rules, terms and aims between the supervisee/ supervisor and the organisation;
- a sense of comradeship between peers in a culture that is often described as having a sense of divide and rule, and a greater sense of team cohesion; and
- the development of basic intrapersonal skills (e.g. reflecting on practice, choosing issues, asking for and using help appropriately) in a less personally threatening forum.

An educational model would include both theoretical and experiential components with the theory preceding the experience, thus addressing some of the arguments raised against supervisee training. Evaluation of this education/training would be carried out using a format similar to that used by Butterworth *et al.* (1997) when they evaluated the impact of receiving CS. Finally, the idea of supervisee training is supported by Butterworth (1992: 12) who states:

> Introduction to a process of clinical supervision should begin in professional training and education, and continue thereafter as an integral part of professional development.

References

Arvidsson, B., Lofgren, H. and Frilund, B. (2000), Psychiatric nurses' conceptions of how group supervision in nursing care influences their professional competences, *Journal of Nursing Management*, 8(3): 175–185.

Begat, I., Ellefsen, B. and Seversinsson, E. (2005), Nurses' satisfaction with their work environment and the outcomes of clinical nursing supervision on nurses' experiences of well-being – a Norwegian study, *Journal of Nursing Management* 13(3): 221–230.

Berg, A. and Hallberg, I.R. (1999), Effects of systematic clinical supervision on psychiatric nurses' sense of coherence, creativity, work-related strain, job satisfaction and view of the effects of clinical supervision: a pre-post test design, *Journal of Psychiatric and Mental Health Nursing*, 6(5): 371–381.

Bishop, V. (1994a), Developmental support: for an accountable profession, *Nursing Times*, 90(11), pp. 392–394.

Bishop, V. (1994b), Clinical supervision questionnaire, *Nursing Times*, 90(48): 40–42.

Bond, M. and Holland, S. (1998), *Skills of Clinical Supervision for Nurses*, Oxford: Open University Press.

Booth, K. (1992), Providing support and reducing stress: a review of the literature, in T. Butterworth and J. Faugier (eds), *Clinical Supervision and Mentorship in Nursing*, London: Chapman & Hall.

British Association for Counselling and Psychotherapy (2007), *Ethical Framework for Good Practice in Counselling and Psychotherapy*, Lutterworth: BACP.

Butterworth, T. (1991), Setting our professional house in order, in J. Salvage (ed.), *Working for Change in Primary Health Care*, London: King's Fund Centre.

Butterworth, T. (1992), Clinical supervision as an emerging idea in nursing, in T. Butterworth and J. Faugier (eds), *Clinical Supervision and Mentorship in Nursing*, London: Chapman & Hall.

Butterworth, T., Bishop, V. and Carson, J. (1996), First steps towards evaluating clinical supervision in nursing and health visiting: I: Theory, policy and practice development, a review, *Journal of Clinical Nursing*, 5(2): 127–132.

Butterworth, T., Carson, J., White, E., Jeacock, J., Clements, A. and Bishop, V. (1997), *It is Good to Talk. Clinical Supervision and Mentorship. An Evaluation Study in England and Scotland*, Manchester: The School of Nursing, Midwifery and Health Visiting, The University of Manchester.

Cassedy, P. and Cutcliffe, J.R. (1998), Empathy, students and the problems of genuineness, *Mental Health Practice*, 1(9): 28–33.

Cleary, M. and Freeman, A. (2005), The cultural realities of clinical supervision in an acute inpatient mental health setting, *Issues in Mental Health Nursing*, 26(5): 489–506.

Clothier, C., MacDonald, C. and Shaw, D. (1994), *Independent Inquiry into Deaths and Injuries on the Children's Ward at Grantham and Kesteven General Hospital during the period February to April 1991* (Allitt Inquiry), London: HMSO.

Connor, M. (1994), *Training the Counsellor: An Integrative Model*, London: Routledge.

Cutcliffe, J.R. (1997), Evaluating the success of clinical supervision, *British Journal of Nursing*, 6(13): 725.

Cutcliffe, J.R. and Burns, J. (1998), Personal, professional and practice development: clinical supervision, *British Journal of Nursing*, 7(21): 1318–1322.

Cutcliffe, J.R. and Epling, M. (1997), An exploration of the use of John Heron's confronting interventions in clinical supervision: case studies from practice, *Psychiatric Care*, 4(4): 174–180.

Cutcliffe J.R. and Hyrkäs, K. (2006), Multidisciplinary attitudinal positions regarding clinical supervision: a cross-sectional study, *Journal of Nursing Management*, 14(8): 617–627.

Department of Health (1994), CNO Letter 94(5) *Clinical Supervision for the Nursing and Health Visiting Professions*, London: HMSO.

Falender, C., Cornish, J.A.E., Goodyear, R., Hatcher, R., Kaslow, N.J., Leventhal, G. *et al.* (2004), Defining competencies in psychology supervision: a consensus statement, *Journal of Clinical Psychology*, 60(7): 771–785.

Faugier, J. (1992), The supervisory relationship, in T. Butterworth and J. Faugier (eds), *Clinical Supervision and Mentorship in Nursing*, London: Chapman & Hall.

Fleming, R.K., Oliver, J.R. and Bolton, D.M. (1996), Training supervisors to train staff: A case study in a human service organization, *Journal of Organizational Behavior Management*, 16(1): 3–25.

Fowler, J. (1995), Nurses' perceptions of the elements of good supervision, *Nursing Times*, 91(22): 33–37.

Fowler, J. (1996), Clinical supervision: what do you do after saying hello? *British Journal of Nursing*, 5(6): 382–385.

Fowler, J. (1998), Evaluating the efficacy of reflective practice within the context of clinical supervision, *Journal of Advanced Nursing*, 27(2): 379–382.

Gennis, V.M. and Gennis, M.A. (1993), Supervision in the outpatient clinic: effects on teaching and patient care, *Journal of General Internal Medicine*, 8(7): 378–380.

Hallberg, I.R. and Norberg, A. (1993), Strain among nurses and their emotional reactions during 1 year of systematic clinical supervision combined with the implementation on individualized care in dementia nursing, *Journal of Advanced Nursing*, 18(12): 1860–1875.

Hawkins, P. and Shohet, R. (1989), *Supervision in the Helping Professions*, Milton Keynes: Open University Press.

Hoffman, L.W. (1994), The training of psychotherapy supervisors: a barren scape, *Psychotherapy in Private Practice*, 13(1): 23–42.

Hyrkäs, K. (2005), Clinical supervision, burn out, and job satisfaction among mental health nurses and psychiatric nurses in Finland, *Issues in Mental Health Nursing*, 26(5): 531–556.

Inskipp, F. and Proctor, B. (1989), *Skills for Supervisees and Skills for Supervisors*, audiotapes, St. Leonards: Alexia Publications.

Jarrett, L. and Johns, C. (2005), Constructing the reflexive narrative, in C. Johns and D. Freshwater (eds), *Transforming Nursing Through Reflective Practice*, 2nd edn, Oxford: Blackwell.

Jones, A. and Cutcliffe, J.R. (2009), Listening as a method of addressing psychological distress, *Journal of Nursing Management*, 17(3): 352–358.

Kilminster, S.M. and Jolly, B.C. (2000), Effective supervision in clinical practice settings: A literature review, *Medical Education*, 34(10): 827–840.

Lyth, G.M. (2000), Clinical supervision: a concept analysis, *Journal of Advanced Nursing*, 31(3): 722–729.

McKee, M. and Black, N. (1992), Does the current use of junior doctors in the United Kingdom affect the quality of medical care? *Social Science and Medicine*, 34(5): 549–558.

Menzies Lyth, I. (1959), The functions of social systems as a defence against anxiety: A report on a study of the nursing service of a general hospital, *Human Relations*, 13: 95–121.

Milne, D. (1998), Clinical supervision: time to reconstruct or to retrench? *Clinical Psychology and Psychotherapy*, 5(3): 199–203.

Paunonen, N. (1991), Changes initiated by a nursing supervision programme: an analysis based on log-linear models, *Journal of Advanced Nursing*, 16(8): 982–986.

Proctor, B. (1986), Supervision: a co-operative exercise in accountability, in M. Marken and M. Payne (eds), *Enabling and Ensuring*, Leicester: National Youth Bureau and Council for Education and Training in Youth and Community Work.

Proctor, B. (1988), *Supervision: A Working Alliance*, videotape training manual, St. Leonards: Alexia Publications.

Ritter, S., Norman, I.J., Rentoul, L. and Bodley, D. (1996), A model of clinical supervision for nurses undertaking short placements in mental health care settings, *Journal of Clinical Nursing*, 5(3): 149–158.

Schön, D.A. (1984), *The Reflective Practitioner*, New York: Basic Books.

Schön, D.A. (1987), *Educating the Reflective Practitioner: Towards a New Design for Teaching and Learning in the Profession*, New York: Basic Books.

Severinsson, E.I. (2001), Confirmation, meaning and self-awareness as core concepts of the nursing supervision model, *Nursing Ethics*, 8(1): 36–44.

Smith, J.P. (1995), Clinical supervision: conference by the NHSE, *Journal of Advanced Nursing*, 21(5): 1029–1031.

Sox, C.M., Burstin, H.R., Orav, E.J., Conn, A., Setnik, G., Rucker, D.W., Dasse, P. and Brennan, T.A. (1998), The effect of supervision of residents on quality of care in five university-affiliated emergency departments, *Academic Medicine*, 73(7): 776–782.

Spence, S.H., Wilson, J., Kavanagh, D., Strong, J. and Worrall, L. (2001), Clinical supervision in four mental health professions: a review of the evidence, *Behaviour Change*, 18(3): 135–155.

Timpson, J. (1996), Clinical supervision: a plea for 'pit head time' in cancer nursing, *European Journal of Cancer Care*, 5(1): 43–52.

UKCC (1992a), *Code of Professional Conduct for the Nurse, Midwife and Health Visitor*, London: United Kingdom Central Council for Nursing, Midwifery and Health Visiting.

50   *J.R. Cutcliffe*

UKCC (1992b), *The Scope of Professional Practice*, London: United Kingdom Central Council for Nursing, Midwifery and Health Visiting.

United Kingdom Council for Psychotherapy (2008), *Standards for Education and Training: The Minimum Core Criteria for Psychotherapy with Adults*, SETS Document Number 1PwA, London: UKCP.

Wilkin, P., Bowers, L. and Monk, J. (1997), Clinical supervision: managing the resistance, *Nursing Times*, 93(8): 48–49.

Yegdich, T. (1999), Clinical supervision and managerial supervision: some historical and conceptual considerations, *Journal of Advanced Nursing*, 30(5): 1195–1204.

5 Experiential learning

An underpinning theoretical perspective for clinical supervision

John Fowler

This chapter explores the theoretical framework of experiential learning, highlighting its congruence with the principles associated with clinical supervision. There has currently been little theoretical explanation as to how and why clinical supervision is so effective, when it works: but conversely and all too frequently often fails to take hold and be effective. Why do some people believe the experience to be so valuable, whilst others find it a waste of time? By examining how experiential learning works and can be maximised the author gives a number of pertinent insights into the workings of clinical supervision.

We believe that a greater understanding of this underpinning theory allows us to explain the variations in experiences and outcomes of clinical supervision. Application of these principles offers practical approaches to maximising the effectiveness of clinical supervision both at an individual and strategic level.

Introduction

It has been acknowledged from the early days of the literature on clinical supervision, that it is an umbrella term (Butterworth and Faugier 1992) and encompasses a number of models and perspectives. Central to most of the literature is the concept that clinical supervision is a professional relationship in which the supervisee reflects on experience (NMC 2008). The body of literature on reflection is vast in its own right, with Chris Johns (1993) being a key figure in originally highlighting the relationship of reflection and clinical supervision. He states that reflection can exist outside of clinical supervision, but believes that clinical supervision cannot exist without reflection being an integral part.

Anyone who has been practically involved in clinical supervision either as a supervisee or a supervisor will realise that considerable learning occurs which is out of proportion to any direct input of teaching. In fact I would argue that didactic 'teaching' should be avoided if at all possible. Teaching has its place in the preceptorship relationship (see Chapter 2) either of a student or a newly qualified health care professional, but only a minor place in a clinical supervision relationship. *Once we begin to understand why and how clinical supervision works, we can maximise on its use, both as practitioners and strategic managers.*

The underpinning theories on which clinical supervision embeds itself are the educational theories and in particular, experiential learning. The following sections describe the development of the educational theories and any congruence with the underpinning principles of clinical supervision.

Background to educational theories

In the early twentieth century a reductionist view of human behaviour dominated the academic field of psychology and education. Classical conditioning (Pavlov 1927) and operant conditioning (Skinner 1951) were the stimulus response theories that dominated educational thinking in the first half of the century. They made the assumption that what happened inside the brain could not be observed, therefore what was important was what went into the brain, the 'stimulus' and what came out, the 'response'. As experimental observations became more sophisticated, particularly in the area of perception (Piaget 1929) it became apparent that stimulus response theories could not explain some of the experimental findings. The view was developing that the brain was not just a passive recipient to be filled up, but was somehow actively involved in the learning process. In the 1960s and 1970s, the traditional reductionist view was being displaced by a more complex non-reductionist view. Collectively these were categorised as cognitive theories in that they acknowledged the active part that the brain plays in the learning process. Different theorists identified different areas of the cognitive process: developmental stages (Piaget 1929), meaningful connections (Ausbel, Novak and Hanesian 1978), self-motivation and discovery (Brunner 1979), memory (Gagne 1977). At a similar time other theorists were stressing the importance of role models in the learning process (Bandura 1969) which led to another perspective on learning, the social learning theorists. In addition a more general humanistic perspective emphasised the importance of individuals taking control of their own learning (Maslow 1954).

Whilst cognitive, social learning and humanistic theorist all acknowledged the importance of experience in the process of learning (Kelly 1997) none could formulate an adequate theory as to its function within learning, apart from being a source of stimuli. *There was recognition that these existing learning theories were missing some of the more profound truths of learning in terms of the knowledge that is gained in non-institutional settings, in particular the knowledge that is gained from experience.*

In the early 1980s the concept of 'experiential learning' became an acknowledged term within education (Warner Weil and McGill 1989, Hobbs 1987). Mezirow (1981, 1991) and Freire (1972) stressed that at the heart of all learning lies the way we process experience, in particular, our critical reflection of experience. Kolb (1984) introduced what has now become a well-established 'experiential learning cycle'. Experiential learning initially acknowledged the non-institutional aspect of learning and offered a more pragmatic approach to learning. In subsequent years a plethora of literature appeared under the heading of experiential learning, each having a slightly different perspective on the nature of experiential learning. This critical reflection of experience is also common to our understanding and expectations of clinical supervision. *Thus it is within this holistic theoretical concept of experiential learning – which has at its heart 'experience', the underpinning working of clinical supervision – has congruence.* So what is experiential learning?

Component nature of experiential learning

Boud and Pascoe (1978) identified three important characteristics of experiential learning: first, the student was fully involved with the learning, second, that it was the quality of the experience rather than the location of the experience that was important and, finally, that the learner had control over the experience. Murgatroyd (1982) put forward four components that are a little more explicit than Boud and Pascoe's characteristics. First, the person was aware of the processes that were taking place which enabled learning to occur. Second, a reflective experience allowed the person to relate past, present and future together. Third, the 'what and how' of what was being learnt was personally significant to the learner. Fourth, there was involvement of the whole self: body, thoughts, feelings, actions – not just the mind. These four components were reinforced and expanded upon by Woolfe (1992) who identified what he termed concrete propositions of experiential learning: the experience of the individual, who actively participates, with the locus of control shifting from the teacher to the learner, resulting in the participant being responsible for their own learning. These propositions fit quite congruently with any such analysis of clinical supervision.

All of these 'component' perspectives have a similar approach; they try and identify what it is about experiential learning that makes it different from other styles of learning. They identify the importance of the learning experience, the holistic involvement of the learner, the importance of reflection and that the locus of control moves from the teacher to the learner. It is apparent that these components apply equally to clinical supervision.

Cyclical nature of experiential learning

Other authors concentrate on the stages that occur within the experiential learning process. The most famous of these approaches is that of Kolb (1984) with his four-stage learning cycle, however there are a number of other models with different numbers of intervening stages, varying from one to eight. All of these theorists make the assumption that experience alone is not enough to initiate learning, it needs to be 'packaged' in at least one other activity. The number of supposedly relevant activities usually relates to the number of stages in the learning cycle. A one-stage model is typified by the famous Confucius quotation of 450 BC

> Tell me, and I will forget
> Show me, and I may remember
> Involve me, and I will understand.

A two-stage model is one often seen in 'outward bound' philosophies and training programmes (Neill 2004). This is the combination of experiences and time for reflection on what was happening. A three-stage model which builds on from this is that of: experience, reflection, followed by 'plan'. This can be seen in the work of Greenaway (2002). The four-stage model is that of Kolb (1984) which brings together the concrete experience, reflective observation, abstract conceptualisation followed by active experimentation, with a particular emphasis on the active experimentation leading back into the concrete experience, and so on. There are a number of five-stage models: Joplin (1981), focus–action–support–feedback–debriefing; Kelly (1997), encounter–(dis)confirmation–revision–anticipation–investment, each of which takes a different organisational approach to the learning cycle and each appearing to be more prescriptive in its application to learning. A six-stage model of Priest (1990) experience–induce–generalise–deduce–apply–

evaluate, takes the basic four-stage model and breaks down the reflective stage into induce–generalise–deduce.

This cyclical analysis of experiential learning is also a valid approach to the practice of clinical supervision and particularly brings in the reflective element which is seen to be central in most of the literature on clinical supervision. *Clinical supervision is cyclical in nature, it is about an ongoing relationship which brings past experiences into the present and then into the future.*

What is experiential learning?

In 1938, Dewey who was probably one of the most significant and influential educators of his time, founded an educational movement based, at least in part, on the concept of, 'experience plus reflection equals learning'. This was the foundation of what came to be termed 'progressive education' in that it challenged the traditional teacher-centred system of the time. Despite the somewhat mixed reception and criticism that progressive education received over the years, the concept of experience plus reflection equalling learning, has become well established in educational literature (Jarvis 2004). It is here that the origins of experiential learning can be seen, with Dewey's recognition of the importance of experience and reflection in learning.

In subsequent years a plethora of literature and practices have developed, based on the ideas within this apparently simple concept of combining experience and reflection. Moon (2004), commenting on the large number of different definitions that have appeared in the literature regarding experiential learning, concluded that any unifying definition is complicated by the fact that that experiential learning is at least in part a constructed term. McGill and Warner Weil (1989: 248) attempted to provide a definition that incorporated a wide range of interpretations:

> the process whereby people engage in direct encounter, then purposefully reflect upon, validate, transform, give personal meaning to and seek to integrate their different ways of knowing. Experiential learning therefore enables the discovery of possibilities that may not be evident from direct experience alone.

You can begin to appreciate the common themes and components between experiential learning and how it underpins the structure, process and outcomes associated with clinical supervision. In an attempt to develop a conceptual understanding of experiential learning, Boud *et al.* (2000) developed five propositions concerning experiential learning. They identified that:

> experience is the foundation of and stimulus for learning in which learners actively learn
> - in a holistic way
> - which is socially and culturally constructed and is
> - influenced by the socio, emotional context in which it occurs.

They claim that the outcome of experiential learning has the potential to result in self-growth, ranging from individual to communities. Thus the application and subsequent implications of experiential learning appear far more widespread and profound than might be conjured by the relatively simple Deweyian concept of 'experience plus reflection equals learning' (Dewey 1938). In particular, how can experiential learning proponents claim its effects on social action and strategic changes?

From a Frierian and Illichian perspective (Freire 1972; Illich 1971) the focus that experiential learning puts on an individual's experience rather than the learning institutions (and hence the government or state) is highly significant. For when the locus of control of what is learnt lies with the individual or, as in clinical supervision, the supervisee, then the potential for the challenge of social norms become a reality; a bottom-up rather than a top-down change agent. These are considerable claims not only for 'learning' in its everyday sense, but for social action as a result of experiential learning. *Thus in clinical supervision if the locus of control remains with the supervisee, then the potential for such bottom-up change and all its implications becomes a reality, and the phrase which is not an uncommon expression in some people's experiences of clinical supervision, of it being a* 'life changing' *experience, is better understood.* But is the combination of experience and reflection really that powerful?

Dewey discusses the nature of the experience, stressing that it not just any experience that has the potential for learning; it is in Dewey's terms the *quality* of the experience that provides a measure of its educational significance. Quality is described by Dewey as a union of the 'continuity', which he describes as the bringing together of the before and after of the experience on events and the 'interaction' of the internal and external factors of the experience. Thus experience is not just a simple matter of exposure to an event; there is an element of the experience needing to become internalised and positioned in relation to existing knowledge and experiences. This has important implications for clinical supervision, it begins to explain why some people's experiences and associated outcomes of clinical supervision are relatively limited and for others they are more significant. It also points a way as to the role of the supervisor in facilitating this internalisation and positioning of experiences by the supervisee.

Reflection is the other factor in Dewey's equation of 'experience plus reflection equals learning'. Whilst Dewey acknowledged the significance of reflection, the focus within his writings was on the experience and how to harness its potential. Reflection appeared to Dewey to be a natural process that occurs in periods of quietness whilst focusing on the activity:

> There should be brief intervals of quiet reflection provided for even the young. But they are periods of genuine reflection only when they follow times of more overt action and are used to organise what has been gained in the periods of activity.
>
> (Dewey 1938: 63)

In the 1980s and 1990s there appeared a considerable volume of literature on the subject of reflection as a subject in its own right (Schön 1983; Mezirow 1998; Moon 1999) however with the exception of Moon (2004: 81) little connection was made to the earlier work of reflection within the context of experiential learning. Kolb (1984) believes that learning comes about by the 'grasping' of experience, what he terms 'prehension' and the subsequent 'transformation' of that experience. Initially this is by 'reflective observation' to make sense of and organise the experience and subsequently via active experimentation. Kolb proposes that the two dimensions of 'prehension' and 'transformation' each contain dialectically opposed adaptive orientations and it is the resolution of the conflict between these orientations that results in learning. The 'grasping' or 'prehension' dimension is at one extreme that of a concrete experience and at the other an abstract comprehension. Thus reflection, for Kolb, is far from the passive 'quietness' suggested by Dewy. It is an active transformational process seeking to resolve internal conflict between the two intersecting continuums. Kolb represents these ideas pictorially by the use of his learning cycle and much of the reworking and application of Kolb's idea focuses on the cyclical nature of the interactions, and often misses the internal dynamic forces relating to the dialectically opposed adaptive orientations.

Another dimension to the experience–reflection interaction is added by Steinaker and Bell (1979) particularly to the experience factor in the equation. Steinaker and Bell developed the idea of a taxonomy of experiential learning in which the learner becomes increasingly immersed in the learning experience, moving from exposure through participation, identification, internalisation and finally dissemination. Whereas other authors depict experience as a single all or nothing event, Steinaker and Bell envisage a taxonomy or ongoing and deepening involvement with the experience. They see their work as complementing the cognitive (Bloom *et al.* 1964), affective (Krathwohl *et al.* 1968) and psychomotor (Harrow 1972; Simpson 1966) taxonomies, acting as a gestalt, bringing together and synthesising the various categories, arguing that experiential learning is about the total experience.

Steinaker and Bell add two important factors to the meaning of experiential learning that are particularly relevant to its application to clinical supervision. First is the gestalt or holistic perspective, the bringing together of knowledge, skills and attitudes. Second is the idea that an experience happens at different and progressive levels. Whereas Dewey and Kolb in particular acknowledge the cyclical and ongoing nature of the experience and the fact that what is learnt is fed back into the experience, which is again reflected upon; they do not seem to acknowledge the taxonomy perspective of different levels of deepening experience as do Steinaker and Bell.

Reflection, for Steinaker and Bell (1979), has a particular significance at the identification stage, rather than a continuous process. This is an interesting perspective which adds a quantitative dimension to the nature and act of reflection and its application to clinical supervision. A number of authors in the 1990s began to distinguish between levels of depth in reflection (Hatton and Smith 1995; Moon 2004). However, they seemed to make the assumption that 'no' reflection is associated with 'surface learning' whilst 'critical reflection' is associated with 'deep learning'. They do not seem to acknowledge that the stage or level of reflection may be associated with the level of exposure to the experience. In essence, there may be an inappropriate time for reflection and an appropriate time. This has interesting ramifications for clinical supervision in that the supervisor really needs to be able to appreciate quite where the supervisee is in relation to the way they use reflection, realising that the approach that works for one supervisee will not necessarily transfer to another.

For Steinaker and Bell (1979) it is at the identification stage that the learner begins to reflect and internalise what they are learning and it begins to become part of their own values, rather than an external skill or aspect of knowledge that they are mimicking. The author's own research on clinical supervision and its relationship to reflection would support this idea of reflection not being a continuous process and in particular some learners appeared reluctant to enter into a supervision relationship which required reflection (Fowler and Chevannes 1998).

The outcomes of experiential learning appear to be diverse, ranging from the acquisition of a new skill or personal development through to social consciousness raising. However at the heart of experiential learning lies the Deweyian concept that it is the combination of experience plus reflection that results in learning. Thus the core principle of clinical supervision, that of reflection upon experience under the guidance of a skilled practitioner (NMC 2008), fits congruently with those of experiential learning.

Clinical supervision and its relationship to experiential learning

Experiential learning is a philosophy of learning which encompasses the traditional learning theories but emphasises that the source of the learning material can be from experience, as opposed to the more traditional view of classrooms and lectures (Fowler 2008). In terms of a learning theory, it is not a reductionist theory as none of the literature attempts to identify what specific bit of the experience it is that stimulates learning, nor of how the brain processes it. It is, however, a learning theory which is holistic in nature – which the author has defined as:

> Experiential learning is the learning which results from the coming together of experience, of a certain quality, with meaningful reflection.

> (Fowler 2006: 40)

It is this underpinning of clinical supervision with these core concepts of experiential learning that begin to explain its theoretical basis. A simple representation of this is shown in Figure 5.1.

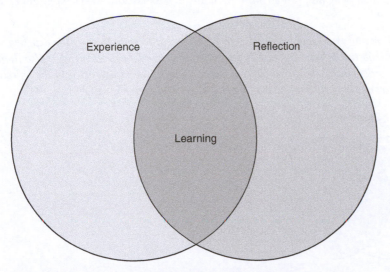

Figure 5.1 Experiential learning underpinning clinical supervision.

Clinical supervision is a vehicle for the bringing together of experience and reflection.

If the notion of the quality of experience and meaningful reflection, are added to the diagram using the criteria particularly relevant to clinical supervision, e.g. the degree of involvement of the supervisee with the experience, the subject relevance of the experience, whether the experience is task- or patient- centred and the tools used to aid reflection, the student's activity and the planned or ad hoc nature of the reflection (Fowler 2003, 2006, 2006a), then the diagram becomes more complex, as in Figure 5.2.

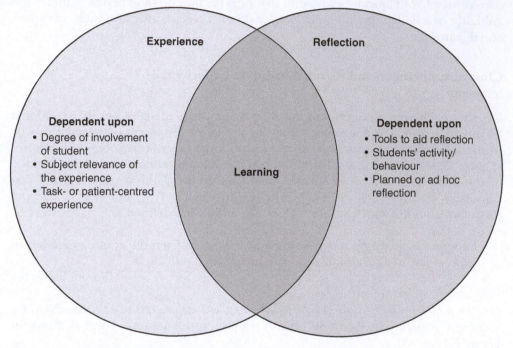

Figure 5.2 Experiential learning underpinning clinical supervision with experience and reflection.

Experiential learning is dependent upon both experience and reflection. If the experience is of limited quality and the reflection is also limited then the experiential learning is also limited (represented as smaller circles). Thus in clinical supervision, if the experience and the reflection is limited, the outcomes of clinical supervision are also limited. See Figure 5.3.

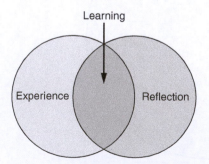

Figure 5.3 Limited experiential learning/clinical supervision.

Similarly, if the person's experience is of good quality, but the reflection is limited, then the learning/supervision will also be limited. See Figure 5.4.

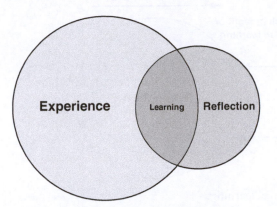

Figure 5.4 Limited reflection in experiential learning supervision.

Likewise, if the person reflects in a meaningful way, but the experience is limited, then learning/supervision will be limited. See Figure 5.5.

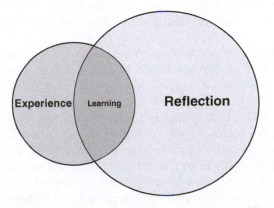

Figure 5.5 Limited experience in experiential learning/supervision.

It is not just the presence of experience and reflection, but the meaningful interaction or overlap of the two. This bringing together or interaction requires energy. Factors that provide this energy or facilitate the interaction will enhance learning, one of which is clinical supervision.

A prediction that can be made from this model concerns not only what promotes the interaction of experience and reflection e.g. clinical supervision, but what may prevent the interaction e.g. barriers to interaction. It is hypothesised that barriers may prevent the interaction of experience and reflection, keeping them separated, thus reducing the experiential learning. See Figure 5.6.

Factors which prevent or are barriers to learning can be seen as those which prevent the experience and reflection interacting. Thus, the experience may be happening, and the person has the ability and prompts for reflection to occur, but the two are not brought together.

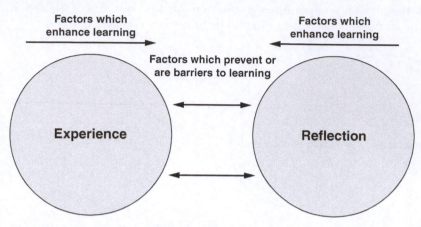

Figure 5.6 Factors influencing experiential learning.

Barriers to experiential learning/clinical supervision

- *Competing priorities in the mind of the nurse.* In the clinical area, a nurse may have arranged a clinical supervision session with her supervisor, but time constraints, busy-ness of the ward or complexity of her clinical workload may drain the energy that would otherwise be used to bring reflection and experience together.
- *Internal energy is drained* possibly due to personal or social problems. The inter-action of experience and reflection requires internal, personal energy. Unlike rote learning and simple absorption of knowledge, experiential learning requires the students' holistic involvement (Boud and Pascoe 1982) and this requires personal energy. Likewise clinical supervision requires this holistic involvement of the supervisee. For some people, at some points in their lives, all of their personal energy is required to function at a survival level. There are obvious overlaps here with Maslow's hierarchy of needs and self actualisa-tion (Maslow 1954, 1968). Thus, anything which drains this internal energy will act as a barrier to the person bringing together experience and reflection.
- *Active resistance* on the part of the person to bring together the experience and the reflection. Many subjects within nursing practice are not emotionally neutral. Examples of these are: reactions to death, dying and pain; the needs of different cultures, racism, spiritual beliefs; etc. If a person has strong fun-damentalist beliefs or preconceptions on a subject, then they may be unwill-ing to reflect upon an experience that may be outside their belief structure. This is not an uncommon experience for a supervisor to meet in a supervisee: at times there seems to be an active blocking of exploration and moving forward. The energy that is required to enhance the interaction of experience and reflection is redirected to inhibit the interaction reducing the person's ability to learn from new experiences. This is a complex psychological argu-ment which is not the subject of this chapter, but is worthy of further exploration.

Coaching, clinical supervision and experiential learning

It is hypothesised that the breaking down of any of these barriers would enable experience and reflection to interact and thus enhance learning. It is proposed that this is a far more interventionist form of teaching than the facilitation mode normally found within the clinical supervision relationship, of encouraging the coming together of reflection and experience. It is this barrier-breaking or interventionist mode that forms the teaching principles used by coaches and can form part of a mentoring relationship. A coach seeks to refocus the person's priorities, re-motivate when necessary, and break down any resistance to learning (Thomas 1995).

Final thought

This chapter has provided an overview of experiential learning and its theoretical underpinning of clinical supervision. It proposes that a central feature of clinical supervision is the bringing together of experience of a certain quality with meaningful reflection. Factors that enhance the interaction of experience and reflection are those commonly associated with those facilitated in clinical supervision. At the more interventionist end of the continuum are factors which break down the barriers which prevent interaction of experience and reflection, and those are the techniques more commonly associated with coaches and personal trainers. This is an interesting proposition arising from the experiential learning framework developed within this chapter, as it provides a theoretical basis for a relationship between the facilitation of learning, coaching and clinical supervision.

References

Ausubel, D., Novak, I. and Hanesian, E. (1978), *Educational Psychology: A Cognitive View*, New York: Holt, Rinehart & Winston.

Bandura, A. (1969), *Principles of Behaviour Modification*, New York: Holt, Rinehart & Winston.

Bloom, B., Englehart, M., Furst, E., Hill, W. and Krathwohl, D. (1964), *A Handbook of Educational Objectives: The Cognitive Domain*, New York: David McKay.

Boud, D. and Pascoe, J. (1978), *Experience-Based Learning: Developments in Australian Post-Secondary Education*, Sydney: Australian Consortium on Experiential Education.

Boud, D., Cohen, R. and Walker, D. (2000), Understanding learning from experience, in Boud, Cohen and Walker (eds), *Using Experience for Learning*, Milton Keynes: Society for Research into Higher Education/Open University Press.

Brunner, J. (1979), *On Knowing*, Cambridge, MA: Belknap/Harvard University Press.

Butterworth, A. and Faugier, J. (eds) (1992), *Clinical Supervision and Mentoring in Nursing*, London: Chapman & Hall.

Dewey, J. (1938), *Experience and Education*, reprinted in 1963 in Kappa Delta PI Lecture Series, Collier-Macmillan Books, London.

Fowler, J. (2003), Supporting staff in giving high quality care, in S. Hinchliff, S. Norman and J. Schober (eds), *Nursing Practice and Health Care*, London: Arnold Press.

Fowler, J. (2006), *The Use of Experiential Learning within Nurse Education*, unpublished PhD thesis, Leicester: De Montfort University.

Fowler, J. (2006a), Nurse consultations: implementing the learning plan, in A. Hastings and S. Redsell (eds), *The Good Consultation Guide for Nurses*, London: Radcliff.

Fowler, J. (2008), Experiential learning and its facilitation, *Nurse Education Today*, 28(4): 427–433.

Fowler, J. and Chevannes, M. (1998), Evaluating the efficacy of reflective practice within the context of clinical supervision, *Journal of Advanced Nursing*, 27(2): 379–382.

Freire, P. (1972), *Pedagogy of the Oppressed*, Harmondsworth: Penguin.

Gagne, R. (1977), *The Conditions of Learning*, New York: Holt, Rinehart & Winston.

Greenway, R. (2002), *Experiential Learning Articles and Critiques of David Kolb's Theory*, online, available at: www.reviewing.co.uk/research/experiential.learning.htm [accessed 24 May 2010].

Harrow, A. (1972), *Taxonomy of Psychomotor Domain: A Guide for Developing Behavioural Objectives*, New York: David McKay.

Hatton, N. and Smith, D. (1995), Reflection in teacher education: towards definition and implementation, *Teacher and Teacher Education*, 11(1): 33–49.

Hobbs, T. (1987), *Running Workshops*, London: Croom Helm.

Illich, I. (1971), *Deschooling Society*, London: Calser and Buyars.

Jarvis, P. (2004), *Adult Education and Lifelong Learning*, 3rd edn, London: Routledge Falmer.

Johns, C. (1993), Professional supervision, *Journal of Nursing Management*, 1(1): 9–18.

Joplin, L. (1981), On Defining Experiential Education, *Journal of Experiential Education*, 4(1): 17–20.

Kelly, C. (1997), David Kolb, the theory of experiential learning and ESL, *The Internet TESL Journal*, III(9), online, available at: http://iteslj.org/Articles/Kelly-Experiential [accessed 17 November 2009].

Kolb, D. (1984), *Experiential Learning: Experience as the Source of Learning and Development*, Upper Saddle River, NJ: Prentice Hall.

Krathwohol, D., Bloom, B. and Masia, B. (1968), *A Handbook of Educational Objectives: The Affective Domain*, New York: David McKay.

McGill, I. and Warner Weil, S. (1989), Continuing the dialogue: new possibilities for experiential learning, in Warner Weil and McGill (eds), *Making Sense of Experiential Learning*.

Maslow, A. (1954), *Motivation and Personality*, New York: Harper and Row.

Maslow, A. (1968), *Towards a Psychology of Being*, 2nd edn, New York: D. Van Nostrand Company.

Mezirow, J. (1981), A critical theory of adult learning and education, *Adult Education*, 32(1): 3–24.

Mezirow, J. (1991), *Transformative Dimensions of Adult Learning*, San Francisco: Jossey Bass.

Mezirow, J. (1998), On critical reflection, *Adult Education Quarterly*, 48(3): 185–199.

Moon, J. (1999), *Reflection in Learning and Professional Development*, London: Kogan Page.

Moon, J. (2004), *A Handbook of Reflective and Experiential Learning: Theory and Practice*, London: Routledge Falmer.

Murgatroyd, S. (1982), Experiential learning and the person in pursuit of psychology, *British Psychological Society Education*, (6)2: 112–118.

Neill, J. (2004), *Experiential Learning Cycles: Overview of 9 Experiential Learning Cycle Models*, online, available at: www.wilderdom.com/experiential/ExperientialLearningCycle.htm [accessed 20 November 2009].

NMC (2008), *Clinical Supervision Advice Sheet*, online, available at: www.nmc-uk.org/aArticle.aspx?ArticleID=2765 [accessed 28 October 2009].

Pavlov I. (1927), *Conditioned Reflexes*, New York: Oxford University Press.

Piaget, J. (1929), *The Child's Conception of the World*, London: Routledge & Kegan Paul.

Priest, S. (1990), Everything you always wanted to know about judgement, but were afraid to ask, *Journal of Adventure Education and Outdoor Leadership*, 7(3): 5–12.

Schön, D. (1983), *The Reflective Practitioner*, San Francisco: Jossey Bass.

Skinner, B. (1951), How to teach animals, *Scientific American*, 185(6): 26–29.

Simpson, E. (1966), *The Classification of Educational Objectives, Psychomotor Domain*, Champaign-Urbana, IL: University of Illinois Press.

Steinaker, N. and Bell, R. (1979), *The Experiential Taxonomy*, New York: Academic Press.

Thomas, A. (1995), *Coaching for Staff Development*, Leicester: British Psychological Society.

Warner Weil, S. and McGill, I. (1989), *Making Sense of Experiential Learning*, Milton Keynes: Society for Research into Higher Education, Open University Press.

Woolfe, R. (1992), Experiential learning in workshops, in T. Hobbs, *Experiential Training*, London: Tavistock/Routledge.

6 Clinical supervision

Visions from the classroom

Mike Epling and Paul Cassedy

This chapter focuses on the development and delivery of a clinical supervision training course at Nottingham University. It provides a brief background to the course, looks at methods of assessment on the course, and then the developmental nature of the training is emphasised. The chapter then uses data obtained from evaluation of the course to highlight emerging issues. Three key issues arising are: issues of confidentiality; theoretical orientation of the supervisor/supervisee; and, the status of the supervisor in relation to the supervisee.

Aspirant clinical supervisors (and supervisees) often state that they would prefer a supervisor (or to be supervised) by a practitioner who is from the same discipline. These preferences appear to be grounded in context that, only another person from the same discipline would understand what it is like to operate in that discipline, and that this person needs to be more 'expert' than the supervisee. However, an alternative argument, supported by a growing body of evidence, posits that viewing the supervisor as 'the expert' or 'more expert' in the supervisee's discipline can impede an exploratory and reflective style of supervision, one in which supervisees are helped to find their own answers and solutions (where they exist). We would reiterate that there is no one perfect way to organise and conduct supervision. Nevertheless, we would encourage aspirant supervisors/supervisees to consider the cogent argument made in this chapter when choosing a supervisor.

Introduction

This chapter will concentrate on the development and delivery of a clinical supervision course, run by the authors at the School of Nursing within the University of Nottingham. An examination of data which emerged from experiential group-work teaching sessions in the classroom on the clinical supervision course will be discussed; this highlights aspects of teaching and learning and raises issues that learners bring to the course. Initial ideas were to devise a programme with the intention of providing a supervision course which would complement a counselling course as the recognised need for supervision in counselling is well documented (Page and Wosket 1994). However, examination of the literature (Hawkins and Shohet 1989; Butterworth and Faugier 1992) pointed out that the concept of clinical supervision was clearly located in the helping professions. Clinical supervision was no longer the exclusive activity of those primarily offering psychological interventions. The emphasis of the course developments embraced this notion of clinical supervision training and education being offered to a much wider audience. The length of training in clinical supervision is a debatable point; this needs negotiation between purchaser and provider and raises the issue of what are the essential components and elements required by the supervisee and supervisors. There is a danger that prospective supervisors could be offered too little training and that lengthy courses could be superfluous to requirements (Power 1999).

It is the authors' experience that unless purchasers recognise the need for well-trained staff they may be offered either nothing to prepare for this role or minimal guidance and support. Some students report that they are providing supervision with no previous training whilst others receiving supervision comment that their supervisors have equally received no formal training for the role of supervisor. We have found that over the period of the course, these practitioners often engage in a critical examination of their previous experience, which results in a redefinition of the role of supervision. The two modules 'Making the Most of Supervision' and 'On Becoming a Supervisor' are titles which were adopted from the work of Inskipp and Proctor (1993, 1995) as the authors considered these to reflect the nature and pro-gression of the course. The first module is designed to enhance the knowledge and understanding of clinical supervision from a supervisee's perspective on the premise that developing skills and qualities of the supervisee will make the unity, intention and purpose of supervision more therapeutic. Building on the principles of the first module, the second module is aimed at those practitioners who are providing or anticipate providing clinical supervision for others.

Course assessment

The assessment of the course is in two parts, which aims to reflect the general course content of each of the two modules. Schön (1987) called for a new way of assessing learning and to achieve this suggested that assessment might have two interrelated components: first, some assessment of the art of skilful 'doing' and second, an assessment of theory underpinning this skilful doing.

Part one: Making the Most of Supervision, encourages a critical analytical review of clinical supervision in a 4,000 word written assignment. Most students focus on the theoretical frameworks and operational/organisational issues of clinical supervision, placing this in the context of their own practice and often examining issues such as implementing supervision and resistance to it. The focus of this assignment is flexi-ble enough to meet the individual's needs and concerns about clinical supervision.

Part two: On Becoming a Supervisor is a 2,000 word reflective analysis of the stu-dents' video or taperecorded clinical supervision session of themselves in the role of a supervisor, the emphasis being that the recorded session provides a means for ana-lysing the supervisory alliance. It is not an assessment of the performance of the actual clinical supervision session. This analysis encourages students to reflect on and punctuate the clinical supervision session utilising a framework such as Heron's (1990) six category intervention analysis for examining the interpersonal aspects of the supervisory relationship within the context of Proctor's (1986) normative, form-ative and restorative framework for supervision.

Developmental model for clinical supervision training

Developmental models of supervision have become the mainstream of supervision thinking, the focus of how supervisees and supervisors change and develop as they enter into and gain experience. Moving towards increased competence through a series of stages can provide reference points for the individual as well as the education provider. Consideration of these stages may help to externalise what is being experienced intuitively. There are many developmental models of supervision mostly taken from the fields of counselling and psychotherapy (Russell *et al.* 1984).

However they do not appear to translate wholly to the nursing profession which is more diverse in its range of helping interventions. Supervision may be one of only a few safety nets for the counsellor to explore and discuss their work whereas nursing has a greater variety of managerial systems to monitor practice. However a developmental model is still a useful aid for the beginning supervisor, which can map out the processes and frameworks which encompass function and process of supervision. In terms of education this can be viewed as the themes and content of the course and the process of learning, which are translations of the aims and learning outcomes at levels of competence. Most students are at the 'beginner supervisee' stage. (See Figure 6.1, the learning and development model of training, in relation to receiving and providing supervision.) They have developed skills through practice which are transferable, such as basic communication, listening and attending

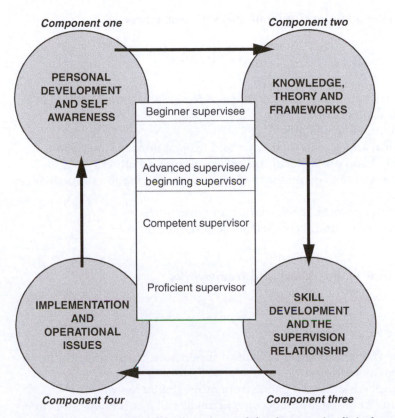

Figure 6.1 A training model for learning and development in clinical supervision.

skills but still need to further develop the specific skills of supervision to understand and facilitate reflective practice in others. In order to understand the purpose of supervision students need to critically examine various models and theoretical frameworks and the qualities of interpersonal relationships, which can enhance a meaningful and effective supervisory alliance.

By the end of the programme, participants will have more of an in-depth understanding of clinical supervision and enhanced competence to implement and practice. In order to achieve this, the authors have developed a training model that has four essential components and can be viewed as a learning cycle that is experiential (Connor 1994).

Whilst the programme is designed to move through the four components in sequence they are however integrated and revisited within the cycle of learning. The student is at the heart of the model and may enter the course with different levels of experience. The aim of the course is to develop learners to a competent level, analogous to Benner's (1984) work on *Novice to Expert.* Depending on the previous experience of the learner, certain course components may become more of a focus. For example some learners may have developed competent interpersonal skills and be providing supervision but have little understanding of the theories and frameworks which may enhance the effectiveness of supervision. See Figure 6.1.

Component one: personal development and self-awareness

Learning objectives

Learners will be able to:

- explore and clarify attitudes, values and beliefs for greater awareness and effectiveness in clinical supervision;
- develop core therapeutic qualities;
- be aware of ethical and professional issues and expectations in supervision;
- develop a personal and professional code of standards and ethics;
- facilitate reflection in self and others through active participation in supervision practice groups;
- gain confidence in appropriate self-sharing and disclosure;
- review and ensure own clinical competence and standards.

Component two: knowledge, theory and frameworks

Learning objectives

Learners will be able to:

- critically analyse the development of clinical supervision in nursing and its recommended implementation;
- define clinical supervision and separate from other similar activities;
- develop a working knowledge and become familiar with a core model for supervision: Normative, Formative and Restorative (Proctor 1986);

- become aware of other models for supervision and reflection. (Kolb 1984; Hawkins and Shohet 1989; Johns 1994; Faugier 1992);
- become aware of group processes and dynamics that occur in group supervision.

Component three: skill development and the supervision relationship

Learning objectives

Learners will be able to:

- develop a climate for an effective supervisory alliance and therapeutic process;
- develop skills of immediacy and the giving and receiving of feedback;
- learn, develop and apply a variety of therapeutic techniques and interventions consistent with the principles of supervision with individuals and groups;
- identify personal strengths and limitations in relation to skills and interventions;
- maintain a balance of support and challenge;
- regularly reflect upon supervision practice and experience supervision through active participation in supervision practice groups;
- develop confidence as both a supervisee and supervisor;
- develop the internal supervisor.

Component four: implementation and operational issues

Learning objectives

Learners will be able to:

- set up contracts for supervision in the work setting;
- be aware of the rights and responsibilities of both supervisee and supervisor;
- be aware of responsibilities to the organisation;
- critically analyse different modes of supervision and apply to own work setting such as group, individual or peer supervision;
- consider the appropriate environment, time and frequency for effective supervision and apply to own work setting;
- review and evaluate the effectiveness of the supervisory alliance;
- develop an awareness of the importance of research in the field of supervision.

Developmental levels

Beginner supervisee

- recognises own need for personal and professional development;
- overcomes resistance to seeking out clinical supervision;
- understands the definitions and purpose of supervision;
- is confident in the ability to recognise the benefits of supervision provided;
- develops reflective skills;
- *is open to self-disclosure through increased self-awareness.*

Advanced supervisee/beginning supervisor

- needs to develop the skills of encouraging reflection in others;
- recognises the need to provide support in the development of others;
- is open to constructive feedback and challenges;
- *develops challenging skills and immediacy;*
- overcomes anxieties of being in a position of responsibility;
- is able to identify and own personal strengths and limitations.

Competent supervisor

- is congruent and able to trust in self;
- recognises changes to own practice and benefits to patients and clients;
- receives and continues own supervision;
- is flexible in meeting supervisee needs;
- transfers inter/intra personal and professional skills of helping into the supervisory relationship;
- maintains, holds and organises structures and boundaries of supervision in groups and individually;
- is able to work more holistically, more egalitarian, less reliant on status differential;
- is less prescriptive and informative, more facilitative and explorative, promoting growth and challenge;
- is confident to facilitate group supervision;
- is aware of parallel process, transference/counter-transference;
- is able to make accurate, reliable observations and interpretations of supervisees' work.

Proficient supervisor

- can work creatively with group dynamics;
- is confident supervising other disciplines within the profession;
- accepts supervision as a major part of clinical role;
- implements and utilises supervisory structures which impact on organisational systems as well as individuals;
- is able to work with issues of transference and parallel process;
- has a sense of competence in own speciality and practice integrating a range of therapeutic skills providing clinical supervision for others;
- continues own professional development and lifelong learning;
- is aware of specific needs and agendas in relation to culture, gender and sexual orientation;
- is recognised and respected for role as a supervisor;
- utilises research and systematic enquiry to enhance supervision.

Teaching process and principles

The authors encourage students to participate in experiential learning (Kolb 1984) as part of the overall strategy to develop self-awareness (Cutcliffe and Epling 1997).

To increase participation in reflective practice as suggested by Hawkins and Shohet (1989), the principles of adult student-centred learning (Rogers 1983) underpin the learning process.

The authors attempt to model and parallel the supervision working alliance in the classroom reflecting the interactional framework of the normative, formative and restorative functions of supervision as suggested by Proctor (1986).

It is intended that the quality of the teaching will parallel a climate of high support and high challenge creating an atmosphere of immediacy and self-disclosure (Connor 1994) while an empathic understanding is communicated (Cassedy and Cutcliffe 1998). At every opportunity the authors facilitate the training in a style that would parallel the skills of running a clinical supervision group. Our approaches to training have been largely adopted and adapted from the material of Bond and Holland (1998). Sessions begin with a 'settling stage' enabling learners to feel welcomed and relaxed.

Ground rules are established not only for group collaboration but also for maintaining boundaries. Students agree to avoid going back into the content of personal work during breaks and we agree to timekeeping. Settling is also about clarifying the aims and objectives of the session and establishing the order of the content. Whilst there is lecture time and information giving we endeavour to deliver these as workshops or small group discussions to enable the 'energising phase'.

Challenge and feedback are introduced early in the course as it is the authors' belief that you need to set out your stall from the onset of how you intend to work and the style of learning which will ensue: this creates respect and understanding. We are attempting to create a live experience for the students, emulating a climate of effective supervision either as a giver or receiver, as the overall aim is to establish a working alliance. Activities, sessions and days are ended by the 'completing stage' of the process. Here we attempt to tie up loose ends, give students an opportunity to debrief, clarify outcomes or set goals for themselves, reflect on issues raised and summarise the content.

Developing skills in clinical supervision

Supervision practice groups are an integral part of the course, which provides an opportunity for students to participate in clinical supervision practice during the second module of the course for one and a half hours of the teaching day per week. Students are given the opportunity to select and divide themselves into small groups of threes or fours in which supervision will be practised. The initial process encourages members to consider the varied aspects of selecting a supervisor, such as orientation, expertise and trust to mention a few. This process parallels the possibilities of selection of supervisors in practice; where possible the authors would endorse the principle of choosing a supervisor based upon the consideration of the overall aims of clinical supervision. Students are encouraged to utilise either audio or videotape during the sessions to provide an opportunity for further reflective analysis of the supervisory alliance. Dreyfus and Dreyfus (1980) suggest that skills development should be embedded in actual clinical situations. To this end, the learners are encouraged to bring real aspects of practice to the supervision practice groups. This enhances the development and practice of the skills of receiving and providing clinical supervision. The authors demonstrate live supervision with volunteers from the group in an attempt to model a session. This provides an opportunity for critique and feedback utilising the frameworks the group have explored. It is our intention to provide an example of the learning process which can be transferred into their practice groups, rather than a performance to emulate.

Whilst in closed groups, working on a supervision issue, other group members will provide observed critical feedback; the opportunity to experience and facilitate group supervision is also possible. One of the difficulties in utilising this approach to learning is the student's perception of experiential learning; the psychology of interpersonal relationships may feel alien and unfamiliar to some nurses depending on their previous experience and background.

The nature of clinical supervision inevitably raises the need to focus on human relationships. We remind students that this is not counselling, but it focuses on self-development with the intention to raising self-awareness in order to understand the supervisory alliance. Learning needs to feel accessible to all disciplines; it needs to be non-threatening yet challenging. The gentle introduction of experiential learning early in the course encouraging student participation helps to facilitate an atmosphere whereby students feel more comfortable with this approach to learning. Students evaluations have consistently valued the opportunity to practice supervision and whilst the use of recording equipment is initially anxiety provoking, overcoming this is outweighed by the benefits of practice and feedback.

Group supervision

Whilst approaches and models for clinical supervision will vary according to a wide range of factors, the authors have encountered many instances of students reporting that it is the intention of their employers to develop clinical supervision in groups. Most students accessing the course are from general nursing backgrounds and have limited experience and or education in group work approaches. Students undertaking the clinical supervision course are therefore exposed to the concepts of group dynamics in order to develop a better understanding of group processes and to aid the critical analysis of the pros and cons of group supervision as suggested by Inskipp and Proctor (1995). To meet the needs of students embarking on the rather arduous task of group supervision the authors have included sessions in the course which encompass the participation in and examination of group dynamics, processes and tasks.

Issues emerging from the classroom

Data has emerged from classroom activities that were originally planned to focus on group work processes and dynamics in relation to clinical supervision. This became a small-scale study, which highlighted several important factors which students brought to the course.

What emerged and was striking was the concordant and consistent level of agreement across the different cohorts in relation to some of the statements ranked. The information was extracted from a seventeen-statement ranking order form, which was devised by the authors to reflect some of issues of clinical supervision to encourage students to participate in a group activity. This information was collated over two year period and included six different cohorts with an average number of 20 students in each cohort.

Table 6.1 Supervision statements: descriptive statistics showing the maximum/minimum scores including the mean and standard deviation for each ranked statement

Statement	Minimum	Maximum	Mean	Standard deviation	Rank order
Confidentiality is assured and agreed.	1.00	2.00	1.1667	0.4082	1
Members should provide support for each other.	2.00	7.00	3.5000	1.8708	2
The goals of supervision are explicitly formulated.	1.00	10.00	4.1667	3.5449	3
A written contract for supervision is completed.	3.00	9.00	4.8333	2.3166	4
Members' feelings should be considered during supervision.	3.00	10.00	5.5000	2.5884	5
Members should challenge each other's practice.	6.00	10.00	8.0000	1.2649	6
Time is allocated for each member by the supervisor.	5.00	13.00	8.0000	3.5214	7
The supervisor should direct the focus of the group.	5.00	15.00	8.0000	3.7947	8
Supervisees should be allowed to express negative feelings.	4.00	13.00	8.1667	3.1885	9
Supervision groups should be of closed membership.	2.00	13.00	8.3333	4.6762	10
Time should be allowed to facilitate personal issues if they emerge.	6.00	16.00	10.3333	3.3267	11
Each member should have the opportunity to facilitate supervision.	6.00	14.00	10.3333	3.3862	12
The supervisor should be an expert practitioner.	8.00	15.00	11.5000	2.2583	13
Supervisees should be of roughly equal experience and status.	10.00	16.00	13.3333	2.1602	14
Supervision notes should be maintained by the supervisor.	12.00	17.00	14.5000	2.0736	15
Supervisor and supervisees should share the same theoretical orientation.	14.00	16.00	14.8333	0.7528	16
The supervisor should be a manager.	16.00	17.00	16.8333	0.4082	17

Note
Statements are in rank order (1 = most agree, 17 = least agree).

The authors suggest that the data strongly reflects the concerns and issues, which have been discussed in previous literature on clinical supervision particularly in relation to:

- issues of confidentiality in clinical supervision;
- theoretical orientation of the supervisor and supervisee;
- the status of the supervisor in relation to the supervisee.

The following statements in Table 6.1 were drawn from the literature to act as a vehicle in which the students would be encouraged to participate in a group work exercise in relation to group supervision and group dynamics.

Table 6.1 contains the statements used in the group supervision exercise; the statements are originally in a different order and have now been included according to rank order of importance according to six different groups' results. The groups were not aware of previous groups' rankings.

Example of teaching and learning: group work exercise

The group work exercise involves half of the group sitting in a circle with the ranking form (see Table 6.1). The task is to consider the list of statements and come to a consensus of opinion. These are ranked accordingly, 1 being the most important and 17 the least important. They are encouraged to work as a total group and dissuaded from voting; the importance of total group consensus is reaffirmed. The other half of the group is briefed separately in relation to the task of the students who will be ranking the 'supervision statements'. This half of the group are also given a form (see Box 6.1), including description statements in relation to observable behaviour of individuals within groups.

Box 6.1 Some examples taken from the behavioural observation statements

Behaviour analysis sheet: examples of behaviour observation statements

Group task behaviours
- Initiating: Proposes aims, ideas action or procedures.
- Summarising: Pulls data together, so group may consider where it is.
- Clarifying: Illuminates or builds upon ideas or suggestions.

The observer group sits behind the students involved in the group ranking exercise in order to observe a student's behaviour on the other side of the circle.

The students on the outside of the circle are in effect 'fish-bowling' the students on the inner circle and making observations of an individual's behaviour using a behaviour analysis sheet as a guide.

Once the inner group has completed the task of ranking the statements in relation to group supervision, the observer joins the observed to feed back their observations of how that particular student performed in the group. The exercise works on several levels: it encourages discussion on the principles and practice of group supervision whilst participating in group processes and provides a workshop in which the students have the opportunity to observe group dynamics and provides feedback to colleagues.

Confidentiality

'Confidentiality is assured and agreed' ranked as the most important aspect of clinical supervision, perhaps reflecting the students' possible distrust of disclosing information to potential supervisors. Issues of confidentiality often arise in discussion with students and are of such concern that anecdotal reports of resistance to the uptake of supervision by potential supervisees may be attributed to the unclear boundaries of confidentiality and the accountability of each of the participants in the supervisory relationship. The rank order highlights this, as five of the six course intakes ranked this consistently as being the most important statement. Issues of confidentiality have been discussed by numerous authors (Hawkins and Shohet 1989), 'A contract of ground-rules should be negotiated at the start of any supervisory relationship to protect both the person giving and the person receiving supervision'. Cutcliffe *et al.* (1998) examined the need to develop agreed working principles in relation to ethics and the dilemmas of confidentiality. This has highlighted the complexities and ambiguities of the supervisory relationship incumbent with the accountability of the nurse's role in relation to the professional bodies and the law. It is clear that confidentiality is not only a concern to the supervisees but supervisors are equally uncertain when it comes to the rather murky boundaries of confidentiality.

The supervisory relationship must have a strong confidential ethic to encourage a trustworthy and safe environment in which nurses can discuss practice in an open and honest manner, which may include self-disclosure. Tschudin (1992) addresses the ethics of confidentiality by suggesting that we ask ourselves two questions:

1   What is meant by confidentiality?
2   What is confidential material?

By answering the first question, the answer to the second question will largely become apparent. Students are encouraged to discuss and engage in the initial stages of creating a contract for supervision as part of the clinical supervision practice groups. Kohner (1994) believes it is vital that the extent and limits of confidentiality are clarified and agreed with an understanding reached about what does and does not fall within the scope of clinical supervision. She further concludes that a contract of ground rules should be negotiated at the start of any supervisory relationship to protect both the person giving and receiving supervision.

Theoretical orientation and status of the supervisor and supervisee

Students ranked this statement consistently low, perhaps indicating that the supervisor and supervisee do not necessarily need to be from the same background. The theoretical background and orientation of the supervisor may be particularly important specifically in relation to the formative and normative function of clinical supervision. However the ability to choose an appropriate supervisor may not be an option for many nurses if supervision is structured and implemented by management. Whilst nurses undertaking the clinical supervision course are encouraged to be reflective and to promote reflection within their supervisees, many nurses report the urge and tendency to act as expert advisor and problem solver. This tendency seems to have a relationship to status and orientation: if the supervisor is of higher status or indeed also more experienced than the supervisee the 'expert advisor' pattern of interaction seems to emerge which has been characterised by Holloway and Poulin (1995) as the 'teacher–student' function. French and Raven (1960) refer to this process of advising as exerting expert and legitimate power where the supervisor provides information, opinions and suggestions based on professional knowledge and skill. Communication is largely controlled by the supervisor thus emphasising the hierarchy of the relationship; when the supervisory alliance is more equally matched in perceived expert power a decreased amount of advising may result.

Some of the supervisors have reported that the role of being an expert can get in the way of supervision. The tendency to encourage a more exploratory and reflective style of supervision is almost forced by the virtue of not having a similar orientation to that of the supervisee.

The supervisor may not be the expert 'knower' in relation to the supervisee's clinical speciality and to rely on the 'teaching of' rather than encouraging the 'reflection on' will continue to reinforce the status of the 'teacher–student' roles, thus reducing the supervisee's capacity for reflection and problem solving. This status position may continue to develop if nurses are unable to let go of the notion of clinical supervision being implemented in a hierarchical manner. Parallels from the supervision alliance may be drawn from the Japanese title 'Roshi' (Zen teacher or master) and 'Inka' the term given by the Zen master to a disciple who has completed his training and is now considered qualified to guide others. Zen stresses self-inquiry and independence of spirit: the teacher who, instead of liberating students, makes them dependent upon him has surely failed both his students and his Zen. These analogies are worthy of reminding us as teachers and students embarking on the journey of clinical supervision that clinical supervision is a developmental process whereby the confidence and competence to supervise others unfolds gently rather than being forced or thrust upon the unwilling.

The supervisor should be a manager

This statement was consistently ranked as the least important aspect of clinical supervision. Nurses undertaking the course frequently report that the development of their clinical supervision structures have been imposed from the top down rather than grown organically out of practice. Whether it is the framework in which supervision takes place, group, individual or peer, or it is hierarchically structured with higher grade nurses supervising lower grade nurses the discussions in many areas of clinical practice have been few or the options have not been considered. Many nurses have reported their suspicions to the authors that lip service is being paid to the implementation of clinical supervision and particularly the implementation of group supervision being based on economic principles rather than evidence of good practice. Nurses may resist entering into a supervisory relationship if they perceive it to be a management-led initiative and imposed upon them with little ownership of the way they may provide or receive clinical supervision. The course encourages a high degree of supervisee ownership of 'bringing your own agenda to supervision'. The King's Fund Centre (1994) stated 'Clinical supervision must not become yet another imposition from managers or academics'. Skoberne (1996) suggests the ideal supervisor is a person who possesses the necessary professional skills and knowledge to fulfil the role of enabling and supporting the supervisee to grow into an effective practitioner in ways that are unique and meaningful, also creating a relaxed and trustful atmosphere. As yet many managers still need to develop clinical supervisory skills and the evidence from course records would bear out that the uptake of clinical supervision training from those above, e.g. grade or ward manager level, is still minimal. There needs to be a clear recognition and delineation of competing agendas and roles for managers as supervisors.

Whilst we would not endorse managers as clinical supervisors based on the grounds of organisational structure alone, to exclude managers from developing supervisory responsibilities would be paramount to cutting out experienced staff undertaking a rewarding role which is to enhance quality care.

Supervision and training in the wider context

As providers of education in clinical supervision, we believe that training and education do make a difference and can influence practice; hopefully the implementation and take up of clinical supervision increases as a result of undertaking the course. Our personal hopes and visions are that clinical supervision becomes a cornerstone of practice, organised systematically with regular protected time that is valued by the participants and of value to patients. Overcoming resistance to the uptake of clinical supervision and converting the sceptical and non-believers perhaps sounds rather zealous, but the authors believe that the perceived benefits of clinical supervision are spreading. Those who are not involved are starting to ask themselves why not, it is becoming *wanted* rather than *needed*; the cultural acceptance of clinical supervision is creeping into practice – not yet the cultural norm but hopefully rooting itself permanently into quality care. We know of examples where previous students have been charged with the responsibility of implementing clinical supervision either in directorates or in some cases across the whole of a large trust as a condition of undertaking the course. There are numerous reasons why the uptake of clinical supervision is still patchy; as course providers we are considering ways forward for the course to be more influential in the uptake of clinical supervision in practice.

The possibility of a database including 'willing supervisor' profiles could offer choice and opportunity for those wishing to receive supervision. We can see that educational providers could have a role to play in this process and that the continuing development of supervisor competence could perhaps be monitored by the development of supervisor registers in conjunction with participating purchasers. This could encourage networking within directorates and trusts, and possibly across them. As clinical supervision becomes implemented more widely, some supervisors may have responsibility for the supervision of numerous staff. This raises the question of the supervisor not only receiving clinical supervision for their clinical practice but receiving supervision for their role as a supervisor. The educational needs of those 'supervising the supervisors' is possibly an as yet unmet demand, bearing in mind that there may be a future need for the possibility of requiring more than one supervisor for the complexity of the care provided.

Whilst the authors recognise that practising supervisors should meet a minimum prerequisite for supervising others we would argue that Wright's suggestion of a Master's degree level of education would presently preclude many potentially 'good enough' supervisors from undertaking this role.

There is much debate about clinical supervision training and education, mostly regarding when, how long and where it should take place, be it in pre-registration, post-registration, in-house; or whether it is offered at diploma, first degree or master's level. We would suggest that these issues are primarily a reflection of the developments and changes which are taking place both in practice and nurse education and will change again over time. Some may become proficient but it is our belief that this happens over a longer period of time with increased experience and responsibility for supervising others. It is a maturation process that cannot be taught within the confines of a curriculum, which sets out to meet the more immediate needs of preparing practitioners to embark on something for which they have little previous experience. Courses aimed at developing proficient supervisors may be required for some or it may be a future need as competent supervisors increasingly take on the role of supervising others. Many authors have commented on the need to be first an expert practitioner and, second, with a 'good enough' experience of clinical supervision oneself (Hawkins and Shohet 1989; Sharpe 1995; Carroll 1996). The need to be an expert practitioner prior to undertaking the role of supervising others is considered later when discussing theoretical orientation and status of the supervisor.

As providers of a course in clinical supervision the authors would suggest that the complexities of the supervisory relationship demands the need for designated training for supervisors and that previous experience of supervision itself is not sufficient to prepare for this role.

Conclusion

There is presently a need for courses on clinical supervision and to feature both within pre-registration and specialist post-registration curricula in a much more robust manner. This requires an investment of time and the skilled facilitation of learning which embraces experiential methods providing the opportunity to practise and not as isolated didactic lectures within an already crowded and competing timetable. The reflective practitioner has become synonymous with clinical supervision, Schön (1987) called for 'practice-led' curricula to enable a more reflective approach to practice. We would support the concept of learning by 'doing' and analysing that 'doing'. This approach to learning facilitates the development and improvement of the skills of supervision through observed critical feedback combined with self-evaluation.

This chapter has outlined the authors' learning and developmental model of training which has been built upon our visions generated from the classroom as well as our personal experiences of providing and receiving clinical supervision. The curriculum has matured and grown in tandem with consideration of the learners' perceptions, evaluation and feedback encompassing practice issues as they change and develop. We believe it is essential that supervisors use a developmental model to make reference to the process and stages of learning. We believe this also applies to ourselves as course facilitators, to map our personal skills, development and course curricula in an ongoing way.

References

Benner, P. (1984), *From Novice to Expert: Excellence and Power in Clinical Nursing Practice*, Reading, MA: Addison-Wesley.

Bond, M. and Holland, S. (1998), *Skills of Clinical Supervision For Nurses*, Buckingham: Open University Press.

Butterworth, T. and Faugier, J. (1992), *Clinical Supervision and Mentorship in Nursing*, London: Chapman & Hall.

Carroll, M. (1996), *Counselling Supervision: Theories Skills and Practice*, London: Cassell.

Cassedy, P. and Cutcliffe J.R. (1998), Empathy, students and the problems of genuineness, *Mental Health Practice*, 1(9): 28–33.

Connor, M. (1994), *Training the Counsellor*, London: Routledge.

Cutcliffe J.R. and Epling M. (1997), An exploration of the use of John Heron's confronting interventions in clinical supervision: case studies from practice, *Psychiatric Care*, 4(4): 174–180.

Cutcliffe J.R., Epling M., Cassedy P., McGregor J., Plant N. and Butterworth, T. (1998), Ethical dilemmas in clinical supervision 1: need for guidelines, *British Journal of Nursing*, 7(15): 920–923.

Dreyfus, S.E. and Dreyfus, H.L. (1980), A five-stage model of mental activities involved in directed skill acquisition, in P. Benner (ed.), *From Novice to Expert: Excellence and Power in Clinical Nursing Practice*, Menlo Park, CA: Addison-Wesley.

Faugier, J. (1992), The supervisory relationship, in T. Butterworth and J. Faugier (eds), *Clinical Supervision and Mentorship in Nursing*, London: Chapman & Hall.

French Jr., J.R.P. and Raven, B.H. (1960), The bases of social power, in D. Cartwright and A. Zander (eds), *Group Dynamics: Research and Theory*, 2nd edn, New York: Peterson, pp. 607–623.

Hawkins, P. and Shohet, R. (1989), *Supervision in the Helping Professions*, Milton Keynes: Open University Press.

Heron. J. (1990), *Helping the Client*, London: Sage.

Holloway, E.L. and Poulin, K. (1995), Discourse in supervision, in E. Holloway (ed.), *Clinical Supervision: A Systems Approach*, London: Sage.

Inskipp, F. and Proctor, B. (1993), *The Art, Craft and Tasks of Counselling Supervision, Part 1: Making the Most of Supervision*, Twickenham: Cascade Publications.

Inskipp, F. and Proctor, B. (1995), *The Art, Craft and Tasks of Counselling Supervision, Part 2: Becoming a Supervisor*, Twickenham: Cascade Publications.

Johns, C. (1994), Guided reflection, in A. Palmer *et al.* (eds), *Reflective Practice in Nursing*, Oxford: Blackwell Science.

King's Fund Centre (1994), *Clinical Supervision: An Executive Summary*, London: King's Fund Centre.

Kohner, N. (1994), *Clinical Supervision in Practice*. London: The King's Fund Centre.

Kolb, D.A. (1984), *Experiential Learning*, London: Prentice Hall.

Page, S. and Wosket, V. (1994), *Supervising the Counsellor*, London: Routledge.

Power, S. (1999), *Nursing Supervision: A Guide for Clinical Practice*, London: Sage.

Proctor, B. (1986), A Co-operative Exercise in Accountability, in M. Marken and M. Payne (eds), *Enabling and Ensuring: Supervision in Practice*, Leicester: National Youth Bureau and Council for Education and Training in Youth and Community Work.

Rogers, C.R. (1983), *Freedom to Learn in the 80's*, Colombus, OH: Charles Merrill.

Russell, R.K., Crimmings, A.M. and Lent, R.W. (1984), Counsellor training and supervision: theory and research, in S.D. Brown and R.W. Lent (eds), *Handbook of Counselling Psychology*, New York: Wiley & Sons.

Schön, D.A. (1987), *Educating the Reflective Practitioner*, San Francisco: Jossey Bass.

Sharpe, M. (1995), Training of supervisors, in M. Sharpe (ed.), *The Third Eye: Supervision of Analytic Groups*, London: Routledge.

Skoberne, M. (1996), Supervision in nursing: my experience and views, *Journal of Nursing Management*, 4(5): 289–295.

Tschudin, V. (1992), *Ethics in Nursing*, Oxford: Butterworth Heinemann.

Wright, S.G. (1992), Modelling excellence: the role of the consultant nurse, in T. Butterworth and J. Faugier (eds), *Clinical Supervision and Mentorship in Nursing*, London: Chapman & Hall.

7 Training requirements for clinical supervision in the United Kingdom

Graham Sloan and Mick Fleming

This chapter focuses on a challenging aspect in the substantive area of training/education in clinical supervision; that of deciding on what and how much of *what* to include in training/education programmes/courses designed to enable effective engagement in and effective use of clinical supervision. After reviewing the extant literature emanating from the United Kingdom and drawing on examples also from the UK, the chapters show how training in and for clinical supervision is far from homogenous. Nevertheless, the literature does indicate that there appears to be some common curricula content. The chapter concludes with recommendations for training for clinical supervision and advances an argument for establishing minimum competences for clinical supervision practice and accreditation criteria for clinical supervisors.

It is noteworthy that, even in the epoch of competency-driven education in many health-focused programmes, there is currently no consensus regarding minimum competences for the practice of clinical supervision and correspondingly, no common or core competencies to include in clinical supervision training curricula. Furthermore, examination of the extant literature indicates that the debate concerning core competencies is, as yet, unresolved. It seems to the editors that the creation of (or agreement on) clinical supervision competencies could quite easily still leave plenty of room for nuanced and/or particularised competencies and curricula that reflects the needs of specific, disciplinary groups, cultural idiosyncrasies etc. While the editors have some of their own views on what these minimum criteria might look like, we sincerely hope that a robust and open debate about these matters can occur soon.

Acknowledgment

The authors would like to express their gratitude to Allan Thompson, assistant psychologist for his assistance in undertaking a literature search in preparation of writing this chapter.

Introduction

According to Holyoake (2000), nurses often receive clinical supervision (CS) because they are expected to, usually by their managers, who in turn receive CS from their managers. Moreover, no formal qualifications or training are necessarily expected or required for nurses to be able to act as supervisors and provide CS. When describing CS in the psychotherapies, Milne and James (2002) noted that supervisors often draw on their skills as therapists and their past experiences as supervisees to guide their delivery of CS. There is evidence in the nursing literature of an assumption that skills can be transferred from a clinical context into CS (see for example, Driscoll 2000). There appears to be a wide scale consensus that many nurses may well possess some skills and attributes that can be transferred to and utilised in CS. Furthermore, it is imprudent to assume that nurses with these skills and attributes will automatically be effective supervisors. Despite the absence of mandated minimum qualifications/requirements, there is a strong degree of consensus within the extant literature that effective provision of CS requires additional skills and attributes that extend beyond those necessary for clinical practice.

As a result, this situation draws attention to the difficult task of deciding on what and how much of *what* to include in the training/education programmes/courses designed to enable effective engagement in and effective use of CS. Accordingly, this chapter focuses on the training/education requirements to facilitate the provision of effective CS. It begins with an overview of the nursing CS literature on training issues in the United Kingdom (UK). It draws on two examples of training from Scotland to illustrate key aspects that require inclusion in training programmes for CS. It describes the CS training provision which has been established for several years in one National Health Service (NHS) Board. Following this, a further initiative is described: a collaborative project between NHS Ayrshire and Arran and the University of the West of Scotland which developed a Master of Science (MSc) module on CS. The chapter concludes with recommendations for training for CS and includes the argument for establishing minimum CS competences and accreditation criteria for clinical supervisors.

Overview of the literature in UK: training for clinical supervision

The following databases were explored for the purpose of this review: CINAHL, Medline and British Nursing Index, using the key words: clinical supervision, supervisors, training and/or supervisees. Published material from 1995–2009 was reviewed. One finding of the review is that there remains a great deal of variation regarding the curricula content and educational 'delivery' methods in training/education for CS in nursing. There has been an absence of agreement on the content of training/education for CS from any of the nursing specialisms. Such an absence of agreement is echoed in the recent reviews of mental health nursing (Scottish Executive 2006; Department of Health 2006): for example, they offer little in the way of recommendations for best practice relevant to CS generally and specifically its training requirements. Perhaps not surprisingly, the published material on CS training/education in the UK varies considerably in its mode of delivery and duration. The duration of training ranges from two hours (Jones 1998) to five days on a part-time basis (Bulmer 1997) through to university provision of a 13-week module/course (Sloan 2006). The two-hour seminar (Jones 1998) aimed to introduce CS to nurses in such a way as to model the skills and competences required for developing productive working relationships, a considerable expectation for a two-hour training session. Interestingly, the issue of adequate preparation was highlighted in the UKCC's commissioned review of CS literature. Gilmore (2001 p. 130) cited Cutcliffe's (1997) assertion that if a nurse receives insufficient or inadequate training, then the quality of their CS would likely be incapable of producing change in the supervisee. The review undertaken for this chapter perhaps further highlights that the issue of receiving inadequate training/education in CS and high quality outcomes from participating in CS has yet to be reconciled.

A strong argument for education/training in CS as a prerequisite to the implementation process throughout the UK was proposed by Cutcliffe and Proctor (1998a, 1998b) and acknowledged/advanced by McKeown and Thompson (2001) and Clifton (2002). According to Bartle (2000), successful implementation will be significantly influenced by participants' understanding of CS. In a collaborative approach between a Primary Care Trust and a school of nursing, aimed at implementing CS (Spence *et al.* 2002), two-day training for supervisors was provided. In addition to providing two training days for supervisors, McKeown and Thompson (2001) offered four two-hour coaching sessions for supervisors. As part of a strategy for the implementation of supervision across a Trust, Clifton (2002) described three-day training for CS. Cutcliffe and McFeely (2001) reported on the lived experiences of 17 practice nurses, each of whom had attended and participated in a four-day training programme for CS. Bulmer (1997) describes a slightly longer period of training/education and an additional support system used during the implementation of CS. The education/training was delivered over five days: an initial three days, followed by a period of practice which lasted several weeks, then a further two days to reflect on experiences. Importantly, Bulmer identified that the training programme was insufficient and so created a supervisors' support group, which met for half a day each month during the first year of implementation. Cassedy *et al.* (2001) described how two mental health nurses provided group CS over the six month duration of a pilot project to registered general nurses who were about to take on their new role of clinical supervisor.

Sloan's previously mentioned CS module is a level 3 (undergraduate degree level), 20-credits module consisting of 12 hours of lectures and 12 hours of seminars, and attended on a part-time basis over 13 weeks (Sloan 2006). During this, students were encouraged to engage in three formats of CS: group supervision facilitated by the module leader, individual peer supervision with a colleague from the student's workplace and individual supervision with their line manager. The aim of the module was not necessarily to prepare practitioners for the role of clinical supervisor; rather students were introduced to, and prepared for the experience of CS.

Common curricula content

Supervisor training in the UK usually incorporates:

- defining CS (Jones 1998; McKeown and Thompson 2001; Clifton 2002);
- benefits of clinical supervision (McKeown and Thompson 2001);
- skills of supervising (McKeown and Thompson 2001; Clifton 2002; Spence *et al.* 2002);
- use of models and frameworks in CS (Jones 1998; McKeown and Thompson 2001; Clifton 2002; Spence *et al.* 2002);
- formats of CS (McKeown and Thompson 2001);
- contracts/contracting (Jones 1998; McKeown and Thompson 2001; Clifton 2002; Spence *et al.* 2002);
- introducing CS (McKeown and Thompson 2001); and
- examining/challenging performance (Clifton 2002).

It would appear that after some initial introductory training, clinical supervisors in many settings throughout the UK are left to get on with the task of delivering CS with limited opportunities for ongoing support and continued training. Significant exceptions to this include the initiative described by Bulmer (1997) which, in addition to the supervisors' support group, provides a further four development days each year. Spence *et al.* (2002) have also reported the provision of one day each month for additional training. Nonetheless, while acknowledging notable exceptions (e.g. see Cutcliffe and Proctor 1998a, 1998b), the published work indicates that there appears to be an emphasis on training for potential clinical supervisors with limited training opportunities for supervisees.

There are some who argue that the success of CS is greatly dependent on the clinical supervisor (Bishop 1998; Gilmore 2001); others hold an alternative viewpoint which has received empirical support in recent research findings. It has been suggested that training/education for supervisees is also warranted (Cutcliffe and Proctor 1998a, 1998b; Tate 1998). A one-day training course for supervisees was described by Tate (1998) which had to be attended by anyone engaging in CS. The study day was devised to ensure supervisees engaged in supervision with realistic expectations, appropriate knowledge and skills, and confidence in taking control of their supervision. Cutcliffe and Proctor (1998a, 1998b) introduce a more radical idea when they suggested incorporating CS training into pre-registration nurse education. The student nurse would be trained to be a supervisee rather than a clinical supervisor.

The supervisees' contribution to their CS emerged in a qualitative investigation illuminating the reciprocal interactions between clinical supervisor and supervisee (Sloan 2006). Findings from this study highlighted that supervisees (registered mental health nurses) endeavoured to prepare for their CS; had their own agenda items and attempted to introduce these into the discussion; and demonstrated knowledge of the issues discussed. The findings underscored how CS was not something that was done to the supervisee; rather it is a process to which both clinical supervisor and supervisee can and should contribute.

Clinical supervision training initiatives in Scotland

In NHS Ayrshire and Arran, one of the 14 NHS Boards in Scotland, education/ training for both clinical supervisors and supervisees has been established for several years. These programmes have developed in accordance with the publication of CS research, best practice guidelines, expert consensus, collaboration between key stakeholders and evaluation/feedback from course participants. Gaps in the CS practices of experienced nurses (Scanlon and Weir 1997; Duncan-Grant 2000; O'Riordan 2002) have been identified. This work suggests that educational/training requirements of those participating in CS extend beyond its underpinning theory and related skills. It would appear that inclusion of interpersonal relations, research awareness and evidence-based practice is also required. *While there are some transferable clinical skills and attributes that nurses can use in their CS practice, the goals are very different from those of clinical nursing and require reflection to enable the careful and effective provision of CS.* Education/training in clinical supervision should highlight the ways in which supervision and the clinical practice of nursing are similar and different. But training in clinical supervision has more important priorities and should focus on those approaches which facilitate learning, take cognisance of the interpersonal context of helping relationships and delineate clear boundaries of the supervisory relationship.

At the time of writing this chapter, a half-day training programme for supervisees and a six-half-days training programme for clinical supervisors is available (see Box 7.1: half-day training for supervisees; and Box 7.2: training programme for clinical supervisors). Regarding the education/training session for supervisees, 'Getting the most from clinical supervision', participants are introduced to the educational material using a variety of teaching aids, taking cognisance of learning styles and adult experiential learning principles. The session is highly interactive, facilitating discussion, engagement in experiential exercises and creating thinking space for participants to reflect on their CS experiences prior to training and forward planning for subsequent engagement in CS. A considerable number of practitioners have received this preparatory training; they often leave the session with new ideas on how to get more from their CS. Course evaluations are favourable; many participants, following the development of their skills as a supervisee, go on to receive clinical supervisor education/training with subsequent experience in providing CS. Approximately 200 practitioners, mostly from the mental health directorate, particularly community services, have participated in training for supervisees.

Box 7. 1 Half-day training for supervisees

- Introductions.
- Identifying aims for session.
- Defining and clarifying the purposes of clinical supervision.
- Key drivers for clinical supervision in nursing.
- Presenting potential benefits from clinical supervision.
- Getting the most from clinical supervision.
- Supervisee contribution.

For several years, an education/training programme for clinical supervisors, 'Giving your best to clinical supervision', has been available for practitioners working in NHS Ayrshire and Arran. At the time of writing this chapter this programme consists of six half-day sessions and a half-day follow-up session, usually organised six months following the initial education/training. Sessions are arranged at two-weekly intervals; this is thought to provide participants with time to incorporate learning, reflect on content of training, follow-up with discussions with colleagues, supervisees and other course participants. As illustrated in Box 7.2, homework or follow-up tasks are agreed at the end of each session and reviewed at the beginning of subsequent session. Again this education/training programme was developed in accordance with findings emanating from empirical research (supervision literature pertaining to nursing, psychotherapy, counselling and clinical psychology), best practice guidelines, expert consensus, collaboration between key stakeholders and evaluation/ feedback from course participants. Certain principles are introduced, discussed and reflected on:

- A collaboratively negotiated CS agreement serves as a solid foundation for the establishment of an effective supervisory relationship, which should be reviewed frequently (Sloan 2005).
- We all have different preferences as to how we learn which should be discussed and clarified between clinical supervisor and supervisee.
- *CS provides a forum for the celebration of good practices as well as reflecting on and reso-lution of clinical problems.*
- *Reciprocity of learning: in addition to CS providing an opportunity for supervisee learn-ing, it serves as an educational resource for the clinical supervisor; clinical supervisors have much to learn from their supervisees.*
- *Reciprocity of evaluation: too much emphasis has been given to the evaluative function of the clinical supervisor. Supervisees should be encouraged to contribute to the frequent evaluation of their supervision and enabled to provide feedback on the processes central to, and outcomes arising from, CS.*
- *Supervisees are encouraged to follow-through by putting into practice those changes emerg-ing from discussions during CS.*

Again, the educational material is presented using a variety of teaching mediums, including DVD footage, role plays and reflective exercises taking cognisance of dif-fering learning styles and adult experiential learning principles. The sessions are highly interactive, facilitating discussion, engagement in experiential exercises and enable thinking space for participants to reflect on their CS experiences prior to training and their forward planning for subsequent provision of CS. Box 7.2 presents an outline of the content of the six half-day sessions.

Participants are encouraged to provide CS incorporating their learning from the education/training programme. The final session provides time to contemplate indi-vidual action/learning plans. A follow-up session is negotiated for participants, usually six months following the initial training. Furthermore, clinical supervisors' provision of CS is nurtured with opportunities for CS of the CS they themselves provide in addi-tion to supervisor's support groups. Approximately 250 practitioners, including mental health nurses, occupational therapists, clinical psychologists and psychothera-pists have participated in this training programme, which is positively evaluated.

The supervisory relationship is regarded as the cornerstone to effective clinical supervision (Bond and Holland 1998; Chambers and Cutcliffe 2001). It has been recognised that achieving and maintaining an effective supervisory relationship is demanding and requires a considerable level of theoretical understanding and skills competence (Sloan 2006). Consequently, the supervisory relationship and related issues take centre stage in the training programme, concentrating on healthy begin-nings and the productive working phase of the CS trajectory. The establishment of a collaboratively negotiated supervision agreement is viewed as a solid foundation for such a relationship (Howard 1997; Beinhart 2004; Jones 2006). See Box 7.3 for Session 2 of the training programme for clinical supervisors.

MSc in psychosocial interventions: the Level 11 supervision module

Psychological approaches such as Cognitive Behaviour Therapy, Family Interven-tions, Early Interventions and Motivational Interventions delivered to individuals or

Box 7.2 Overview of training programme for clinical supervisors

Session 1: Getting the most from clinical supervision

- Introductions
- Establishing aims for the sessions
- Clarifying and defining clinical supervision
- Highlighting key drivers for the introduction of clinical supervision into nursing
- Getting the most from CS: the supervisee's contribution
- Homework.

Session 2: Giving your best: providing effective clinical supervision

- The clinical supervision agreement
- Establishing agreement on the purpose of clinical supervision
- Supervisory relationship – getting to know each other
- Practical arrangements
- Identifying learning objectives/goals for clinical supervision
- Models and methods
- Evaluation of processes and outcomes
- Confidentiality
- Accountability, responsibility and ethical practices
- Documentation and clinical supervision records
- Dual relationships
- Problem resolution
- Homework.

Session 3: Providing effective supervision

- Clinical supervision models and methods
- Clinical supervision frameworks
- Clinical supervision frameworks guided by psychotherapy models
- Models of reflection
- Learning theory
- Discussion of clinical supervision related issues
- Homework.

Session 4: Providing effective supervision

- Clinical supervision models and methods
- Clinical supervision frameworks
- Clinical supervision frameworks guided by psychotherapy models
- Models of reflection
- Learning theory
- Discussion of clinical supervision related issues
- Homework.

Session 5: Providing effective supervision

- The empirical literature: 'good enough' clinical supervision
- Discussion of clinical supervision related issues
- Homework.

Session 6: Pulling it together and moving forward

- Discussion of clinical supervision related issues
- Action plans to move forward with clinical supervision.

Box 7.3 Session 2 of training programme for clinical supervisors

Session 2: Giving your best: providing effective clinical supervision

- Welcome participants to Session 2
- Collaboratively establish agenda for session:
  - Review Session 1
  - Feedback and questions
  - Feedback and discussion on homework (which might include participants reading Chapter 3 from Driscoll (2007) *Practising Clinical Supervision: A Reflective Approach for Healthcare Professionals*, which presents and discusses boundaries and responsibilities in clinical supervision; reflections on participants contribution to their receipt of clinical supervision).

- Celebrating skills and attributes as a practitioner using 'Gallery of my Assets' experiential exercise
- Discussion on which skills and attributes can be transferred from clinical context into supervision
- Before moving onto agreements, participants are encouraged to reflect and discuss their experiences of supervision agreements.
- The clinical supervision agreement:
  - Establishing agreement on the purpose of clinical supervision (reflect on discussion from Session 1).
  - Supervisory relationship – getting to know each other (DVD example and discussion).
  - Practical arrangements (best practice recommendations incorporated into discussion).
  - Identifying learning objectives/goals for supervision (DVD example and discussion).
  - Models and methods (participants are given the opportunity to decide which frameworks are covered during training).
  - Evaluation of processes and outcomes (DVD example and discussion).
  - Confidentiality.
  - Accountability, responsibility and ethical practices.
  - Documentation and supervision records.
  - Dual relationships (empirical research incorporated into discussion).
  - Problem resolution.
  - Experiential exercise (role play) practicing discussing a supervision agreement with a supervisee.

- Questions from session
- Review session
- Collaboratively establish homework assignment (which may include participants reading educational material on clinical supervision frameworks and methods; discussing agreements with supervisees and supervisors; reflecting on what guides their current provision of supervision)
- Feedback on session
- Thank participants for their contribution

through groups, have come to prominence through their effectiveness with people, and their carers, who experience serious and complex mental health problems (Velleman *et al.* 2006). Additional research suggests these approaches can be successfully utilised with clients who have long-term physical health conditions such as diabetes, cardiac disease and cancer (Steed *et al.* 2005; Linden *et al.* 2007). In keeping with such findings and approaches, a new MSc in Psychosocial Interventions programme promotes understanding of the influence that psychosocial factors have, and how skills development in practitioners can benefit health outcomes for these groups of people. The Postgraduate Diploma/MSc in Psychosocial Interventions at the University of the West of Scotland has been designed with this purpose in mind. Health practitioners are educated to utilise a range of psychosocial skills, validated through research and which have been demonstrated to be effective in addressing the needs of people who suffer from long-term conditions. It is based on the principle that the research evidence base has a significant influence on clinical work and its delivery.

The programme is a 120 credit Postgraduate Diploma/180 credit M.Sc course (See Figure 7.1: Postgraduate Diploma/MSc programme structure). There are ten modules within the programme. Practitioners complete three core modules: 'Core Values', 'Cognitive Behavioural Therapy' and 'Research Methods in Health Care'. Practitioners can then choose three further option modules from a possible six available: 'Family Intervention', 'Motivational Enhancement Skills', 'Forensic Mental Health Skills', 'Early Intervention', 'Group Facilitation Skills' and 'Clinical

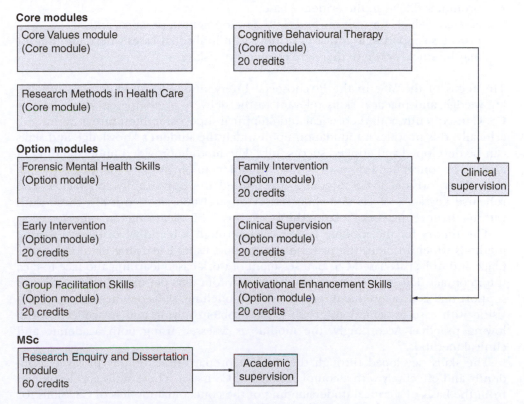

Figure 7.1 Postgraduate Diploma/MSc programme structure.

Supervision'. At the Masters level, students are expected to utilise a full range of academic and research skills in order to undertake a piece of empirical research, which needs to be related to their service/clinical area and their area of interest. CS is provided throughout each of the clinical modules in both the workplace (clinical environment) and in a group format at the university. CS not only provides the expertise and support for clinical skills development but ensures practitioners are exposed to the effective delivery of CS so that they can develop these competences.

The Matrix: A Guide to Delivering Evidence-Based Psychological Therapies in Scotland was commissioned by National Health Service Education for Scotland (NES) and the Scottish Government (NES and Scottish Government 2008). Within this document, it is recommended that staff delivering psychological therapies/psychosocial interventions should receive frequent, competently delivered CS (in accordance with guidelines for the particular therapeutic modality and relevant accreditation standards). Accordingly, the guidance contained within *The Matrix* had a significant influence on the curriculum design for the CS component of the MSc in psychosocial interventions.

It is acknowledged that CS has a key role in supporting the effective delivery of evidence-based psychological therapies and psychosocial interventions. In this context, it is argued (NES and Scottish Government 2008: 11) that CS:

- ensures that the supervisee practices in a manner which conforms to ethical and professional standards;
- ensures adherence to the therapeutic model;
- promotes fidelity to the evidence base;
- acts as a vehicle for training and skills development in practice; and
- provides support and advice in dealing with individual cases where the therapy may be stuck, or where there are elements of risk.

The focus of the MSc in the Psychosocial Interventions CS module is to develop knowledge and practical skills relevant to the delivery of competent and effective CS. Consequently both theoretical and empirical supervision literature is appraised, critically; this provides a foundation upon which the student's knowledge and skills can be developed and applied successfully. The module provided understanding of a range of conceptual frameworks, formats and technologies and the means to evaluate the provision of CS. Students are offered the opportunity to practice and rehearse key skills of CS and then reflect on and appraise, critically, these skills within current supervisory relationships (see Box 7.4 for learning outcomes).

The theory for the module is delivered through a blend of distance learning methods which includes the provision of support using e-learning materials; workplace and university-based CS, an assessment of work-based learning and face-to-face tutor contact. The skills element is supported by four days per module direct contact support that is structured and includes skills modelling, skills practice, group supervision with case presentation, group work, problem solving and self-reflection following practice. Accordingly, the module is assessed using both academic and clinical methods.

The skills developed through the module prepare practitioners to work confidently and effectively with a complex range of CS issues. These skills are developed from the basis of a critical understanding of the conceptual models of CS. Skills for the facilitation of effective CS in a variety of formats, offered by a range of practi-

---

Box 7.4 Learning outcomes for clinical supervision module

At the end of the clinical supervision module the student will be able to:

L1 Critically appraise the literature regarding a variety of conceptual models of clinical supervision.

L2 Apply knowledge and skills of clinical supervision in varying formats of clinical supervision: individual, triads and small groups.

L3 Demonstrate both practical and theoretical knowledge of case formulation relevant to a broad range of psychosocial problems.

L4 Demonstrate leadership and creativity in the implementation of the knowledge and skills of clinical supervision.

L5 Evaluate both the processes integral to and the outcomes resulting from the provision of effective clinical supervision using a range of valid and reliable measures.

---

tioners from different disciplines are explored. These are a sophisticated array of skills which promote the integration of knowledge and skills for independent and autonomous practice; they are congruent with the Scottish Credit and Qualifications Framework (SCQF) level 11 descriptors for knowledge and skills (SCQF 2002) (i.e. descriptors for postgraduate and master's level study). These skills are assessed academically through the submission of a 2,500 word essay which needs to provide evidence of a critical review of the literature pertinent to CS and a critical reflection on the preparation, delivery and evaluation of a format of CS for health practitioners in the student's clinical area.

The module has three clinical learning outcomes which assess the student's ability to apply theory to their CS practice. In order to achieve these clinical outcomes, the students are required to provide evidence that demonstrates the use of a range of enhanced CS skills. The first outcome relates to negotiating a CS agreement for individual, triad or small group CS. The recommended evidence is a completed and signed supervision agreement, which would include coverage of those issues regarded as central to this process (Sloan 2005). The students include excerpts from an audio recording of one of their CS sessions as evidence of the collaboratively negotiated agreement. The second outcome relates to the implementation of the knowledge and skills of CS. Students are required to demonstrate leadership and creativity in the integration of the knowledge and skills of CS. The recommended evidence is an audio recording of a CS session of at least 60 minutes' duration and a completed and signed CS record. The third outcome is related to evaluating the processes and outcomes from CS. The recommended evidence is excerpts from an audio recording which includes an evaluation of CS. Further evidence should include a completed formal measure of evaluation and a completed and signed CS record. The evidence for each of the clinical outcomes is accompanied be a reflective report of 500–700 words which critically reviews the evidence that students have provided and the skills utilised within their evidence portfolio. Workplace clinical supervisors and university academic staff will advise about the amount and quality of the evidence that can be submitted in support of their achievement of the clinical learning outcomes.

Conclusion

This chapter has presented two training programmes emanating from Scotland, one that has been established for several years, the second a more recent initiative involving the collaboration of university and health care staff. Both programmes are underpinned by recognition that education/training opportunities for the participants of CS should focus on those theories and related approaches that facilitate learning, take cognisance of the interpersonal context of helping relationships and delineate clear boundaries of the supervisory relationship. During these programmes, particular ideas are introduced, discussed and reflected on and these include:

- A collaboratively negotiated CS agreement serves as a solid foundation for the establishment of an effective supervisory relationship, which should be reviewed frequently.
- People have different preferences as to how they learn: these need to be discussed and clarified between clinical supervisor and supervisee.
- CS provides a forum for the celebration of good practices as well as reflecting on and the resolution of clinical problems.
- Reciprocity of learning: in addition to clinical supervision providing an opportunity for supervisee learning, it serves as an educational resource for the clinical supervisor; clinical supervisors have much to learn from their supervisees.
- Reciprocity of evaluation: too much emphasis has been given to the evaluative function of the clinical supervisor. Supervisees should be encouraged to contribute to the frequent evaluation of their supervision and enabled to provide feedback on the processes central to, and outcomes arising from, supervision.
- Supervisees are encouraged to follow through by putting into practice those changes emerging from discussions during CS.

It is noteworthy that nursing has been remiss in establishing competences for the practice of CS. Some might argue that there is insufficient evidence derived from empirical work in nursing to formulate such competences. *Nonetheless, it is proposed that the development of supervision competences for CS practices in nursing, which can incorporate evidence from related fields, will contribute to the creation of sound training opportunities for the future.* Following on from this, nursing may be able to establish accreditation criteria for clinical supervisors. We remain hopeful.

References

Bartle, J. (2000), Clinical supervision: its place within the quality agenda, *Nursing Management*, 7(5): 30–33.

Beinart, H. (2003), Models of supervision and the supervisory relationship and their evidence base, in I. Fleming and L. Steen (eds), *Supervision and Clinical Psychology: Theory, Practice and Perspectives*, New York: Brunner-Routledge.

Bishop, V. (1998), *Clinical Supervision in Practice: Some Questions, Answers and Guidelines*, Basingstoke: Macmillan/NTResearch.

Bond, M. and Holland, S. (1998), *Skills of Clinical Supervision: A Practical Guide for Supervisees, Clinical Supervisors and Managers*, Buckingham: Open University Press.

Bulmer, C. (1997), Supervision: how it works, *Nursing Times*, 93(48): 53–54.

Cassedy, P., Epling, M., Williamson, L. and Harvey, G. (2001), Providing cross discipline group supervision to new supervisees: challenging some common apprehensions and myths, in J.R. Cutcliffe, T. Butterworth and B. Proctor (eds), *Fundamental Themes of Clinical Supervision*, London: Routledge.

Chambers, M. and Cutcliffe, J. (2001), The dynamics and processes of 'ending' in clinical supervision, *British Journal of Nursing*, 10(21): 1403–1411.

Clifton, E. (2002), Implementing clinical supervision, *Nursing Times*, 98(9): 36–37.

Cutcliffe, J.R. (1997) Evaluating the success of clinical supervision, *British Journal of Nursing*, 6(13): 725.

Cutcliffe, J.R. and McFeely, S. (2001), Practice nurses and their 'lived experience' of clinical supervision, *British Journal of Nursing*, 10(5): 312–323.

Cutcliffe, J.R. and Proctor, B. (1998a), An alternative training approach in clinical supervision: part one, *British Journal of Nursing*, 7(5): 280–285.

Cutcliffe, J.R. and Proctor, B. (1998b), An alternative training approach in clinical supervision: part two, *British Journal of Nursing*, 7(6): 344–350.

Department of Health (2006), *From Values to Action: The Chief Nursing Officer's Review of Mental Health Nursing*, London: Department of Health.

Driscoll, J. (2000), *Practising Clinical Supervision: A Reflective Approach*, London: Bailliere Tindall.

Driscoll, J. (2007), *Practising Clinical Supervision: A Reflective Approach for Healthcare Professionals*, 2nd edn, London: Bailliere Tindall, pp. 35–49.

Duncan-Grant, A. (2000), Clinical supervision and organisational power: a qualitative study, *Mental Health Care*, 3(12): 398–401.

Gilmore, A. (2001), Clinical supervision in nursing and health visiting: a review of the UK literature, in J.R. Cutcliffe, T. Butterworth, and B. Proctor (eds) *Fundamental Themes of Clinical Supervision*, London: Routledge.

Holyoake, D.D. (2000), Using transactional analysis to understand the supervisory process, *Nursing Standard*, 14(33): 37–41.

Howard, F.M. (1997), Supervision, in H. Love and W. Whittaker (eds) *Practice Issues for Clinical and Applied Psychologists in New Zealand*, Wellington: The New Zealand Psychological Society.

Jones, A. (1998), Getting together with clinical supervision: an introductory seminar, *Journal of Advanced Nursing*, 27(3): 560–566.

Jones, A. (2006), Clinical supervision: what do we know and what do we need to know? *Journal of Nursing Management*, 14(8): 577–585.

Linden W., Phillips, M.J. and Leclerc, J. (2007), Psychological treatment of cardiac patients: a meta-analysis, *European Heart Journal*, 28(24): 2972–2984.

McKeown, C. and Thompson, J. (2001), Implementing clinical supervision, *Nursing Management*, 8(6): 10–13.

Milne, D. and James, I. (2002), The observed impact of training on competence in clinical supervision, *The British Journal of Clinical Psychology*, 41(1): 55–72.

NES and Scottish Government (2008), *The Matrix: A Guide to Delivering Evidence-Based Psychological Therapies in Scotland*, Edinburgh: NES and The Scottish Government.

O'Riordan, B. (2002), Why nurses choose not to undertake clinical supervision: the findings from one ICU, *Nursing in Critical Care*, 7(2): 59–66.

Scanlon, C. and Weir, W.S. (1997), Learning from practice: mental health nurses' perception and experiences of clinical supervision, *Journal of Advanced Nursing*, 26(3): 295–303.

Scottish Executive (2006), *Rights, Relationships and Recovery: The report of the National Review of Mental Health Nursing in Scotland*, Edinburgh: The Scottish Executive.

SCQF (Scottish Credit and Qualifications Framework) (2002), *Handbook Volume 1: Scottish Subjects Benchmarks*, Edinburgh: The Scottish Executive.

Sloan, G. (2005), Clinical supervision: beginning the supervisory relationship, *British Journal of Nursing*, 14(17): 918–923.

Sloan, G. (2006), *Clinical Supervision in Mental Health Nursing*, London: Wiley & Sons.

Spence, C., Cantrell, J., Christie, I. and Samet, W. (2002), A collaborative approach to the implementation of clinical supervision, *Journal of Nursing Management*, 10(2): 65–74.

Steed L., Cooke, D. and Newman, S. (2005), A systematic review of psychosocial outcomes following education, self-management and psychological interventions in diabetes mellitus, *Centre for Reviews and Dissemination*, York: University of York.

Tate, S. (1998), Helping supervisees to get the most out of their supervisory experience, *Nursing Times Learning Curve*, 2(2): 10–11.

Velleman R., Davis, E., Smith, G. and Drage, M. (2006), *Changing Outcomes in Psychosis*, London: Blackwell Publishing.

8 Postmodernising clinical supervision in nursing

Chris Stevenson

This chapter adopts an approach that has infrequently been used to frame the discourse around clinical supervision; it attempts to reconstruct clinical supervision from a postmodern perspective. After providing a useful and succinct overview of (one view of) postmodernism in nursing, Chris then used a postmodern critique to enable a revisioning of clinical supervision using some of her earlier published work (Stevenson and Jackson 2000) in which clinical supervision is reconstructed as 'egalitarian consultation meetings'. Case study extracts of group clinical supervision with 'G' grade community psychiatric nurses are then used to illustrate how the supervisors divested themselves of the role of 'expert' by inducting the attendees into the postmodern approach.

The chapter draws the editors' attention to an important issue: should we as an academe (and/or collection of health-focused clinicians, educators, researchers and managers) strive for one best approach to operationalising clinical supervision, or should we embrace multiple approaches? Clearly this issue is inextricably tied to that of common or core competencies for clinical supervision and perhaps as a result of such an association, parallels might be drawn. Drawing on Barney Glaser's (2001) work, it seems to the editors that 'shared' psychosocial processes exist within the (social) world of clinical supervision and that these transcend individual substantive areas. Notwithstanding the possible existence of a formal level theory of an approach to clinical supervision, this would still clearly allow room for substantive level particularised approaches (and interventions) that are idiosyncratic to various substantive areas of psychiatric and mental health nursing care.

Introduction

High profile individuals/organisations have identified that clinical supervision (CS) is not a homogeneous practice (Cutcliffe *et al.* 2001; Department of Health 1994; Fowler 1996; Paunonen 1991) or located in a single 'correct' model. Indeed, there has been a proliferation of models that claim to be tailored to the needs of specific nursing groups (for example Hawkins and Shohet 1989; Johns 1998; Page and Wosket 1994; Proctor 1986). Despite this, much CS has been organised around five core principles, implying that there is a reality of what constitutes good clinical supervision practice. These principles are themselves grounded in modernist assumptions, such as:

- there are real mental health problems (otherwise described as diagnoses, signs, imbalances, illnesses, etc.) that are lodged within people and/or their social networks;

- the problems can be treated (by bio/psycho/social approaches) by professionals;
- it is possible for an external, expert supervisor to spot the problem, even if it has been missed by the involved practitioner, and identify treatment solutions when the practitioner cannot;
- that the ability to practice and supervise grows with grade, so that it is only appropriate to have a hierarchy of supervision, where senior nurses (referred to as 'I' grades in the United Kingdom) accordingly supervise less senior nurses (referred to 'H' grades in the United Kingdom) and so on down the 'command chain', implicitly (if not explicitly) a management function. This applies across different supervision structures, for example individual, triadic or group; and
- that there is a 'form' of supervision based on Proctor's triad of functions – normative, formative and restorative (see Butterworth 1994, 1996; Kipping 1998; Sloan and Watson 2002) – that shapes the supervisee through promoting self-awareness (Cutcliffe and Epling 1997) or reflection, but without being psychotherapeutic (Faugier 1998; Severinsson 1995). This implies that there is linear progress towards the practically perfect practitioner.

There is an abundance of existing literature that supports, picks over, or is based in the principles, and some references is made to it below. However, this chapter does not seek to review comprehensively but to reconstruct CS from a postmodern perspective.

Postmodernism in nursing

Stevenson and Beech (2001), drawing on Lyotard (1984), take postmodernism as a rejection of 'grand' theories in relation to how we make sense of our worlds. Rather, we tend to know from 'being in' situations. Knowledge is inseparable from the context in which it comes into existence. Taking a social constructionist stance within postmodernism, language is the means by which we construct our world. We create 'stories' together, which we treat as realities and which we base our practices on. Of course, this means that there are multiple realities rather than a single truth.

Turning to CS, we can re-evaluate the principles outlined above. Firstly, we have to question the idea that there are real mental health problems that are anchored in some kind of biological or psychological or social pathology that can be remedied by clever professionals. While we are, undoubtedly, biologically based beings, how we talk about our bio-psycho-social functioning seems to be critical in getting on, or not getting on, with our lives. For example, in working with families, I have been struck by how often there is a family story about what is wrong with a member. The story serves to organise the family in relation to every aspect of their lives – who has to be at home, what level of achievement is possible at work, and so on. By using a process that invites dialogue (Seikkula *et al.* 1995) or trialogue (Amerling *et al.* 2002) it is possible to loosen the dominant family story and open up possibilities to construct other stories and allow the family members more scope to function. Seikkula *et al.* (1995) present convincing case summaries that describe less reliance on medication, less hospitalisation, and less re-presentation of psychotic symptoms when a different, shared vision is available.

Once we surrender the idea of broken machines that need fixing, the function of the expert clinical supervisor, reaching conclusions that other professionals cannot reach, becomes extinct. If knowledge is joined into the situation, then the person who is expert is the person most closely connected to that situation. In relation to CS, the practitioner who is working with the person in distress must be more knowledgeable than the detached supervisor. The practitioner and person in mental health difficulties co-create a narrative about the problem situation. Thus, by definition, it will be the practitioner most intimately involved with the person-in-context who will be the co-constructor and relayer of stories. Any 'stuckness' may be attributed to the practitioner (and person) becoming organised by their dominant story rather than that the practitioner has failed to detect the real problem. The new description of stuckness as an unhelpful story means that the supervisor only needs to help create different stories, a point I return to below. Finally, the whole hierarchy of supervision, and its assumed form, comes tumbling down when we admit that we are all creators and tellers of stories; that each of us is steeped in the expertise of living and can contribute to an ecology of stories or narratives in a clinical setting.

The above critique may be a welcome alternative to some authors who have begun to challenge the processes of CS from *without* the postmodern turn. For example Van Ooijen (1994) sees CS as punitive for some nurses and Jones (1995) notes that it can involve criticism and discipline. Yegdich (1998) suggests that the supervisor can cruelly exploit a supervisee's 'blind spots' towards supposedly increasing self-awareness. Clouder and Sellars (2004) question whether the reflection-on-action, often explicit within CS, actually improves learning and practice. Bulmer (1997) in a study of 136 'F' grade nurses (junior charge nurses/ward sisters) who were receiving regular supervision found that the supervisees did not think that their supervisors necessarily needed more knowledge or higher clinical grade. In the same vein, Chambers (1995) and Bowles and Young (1998) want to dismantle hierarchical CS, although they continue to make a distinction between the educated and practiced supervisor and the supervisee who is seen as gaining insight through the CS process away from her/his novice state. Thus, there is a critique without the postmodern turn, but it lacks the radical edge that this chapter provides.

So what does the new clinical supervision look like?

Drawing on the postmodern critique outlined above, I offer a re-visioning of CS using and developing earlier work (Stevenson and Jackson 2000: 493) which reconstructed CS as 'egalitarian consultation meetings'.

Egalitarian consultation meetings (ECMs)

ECMs were an approach to CS that grew out of the desire of Stevenson and Jackson (2000) to take the 'super' out of supervision. As researchers and practitioners, they favoured a postmodern stance that provided the underpinning philosophy for the ECMs (adapted from Stevenson and Jackson 2000):

- Imposed structure/content is problematic. It creates an illusion of CS as a homogeneous process and practice, with right and wrong approaches to care (the 'reality' of diagnosis and treatment). For example, much CS begins with a description of 'the case', structured around categorical information – gender, age, class, occupation, diagnosis, number of treatment sessions and kinds of interventions. The personal narrative, the person's story, is less prominent. The task is to dig into the information in order that the CS can discover a) the real problem; b) the weaknesses in the supervisee's approach to date; and c) the correct intervention. This may limit the creativity needed to promote excellent care and, instead, be a conservatising force. For example, the quality of CS may be dependent on the degree to which the individual supervisor can step outside existing understandings rather than recycling them to fit the new case (Ekstein and Wallerstein 1972).

- Clinical supervision should be separate from line management. When there is a hierarchical structure, innocent questions asked by the supervisor, e.g., 'How is the case going?' can be interpreted as surveillance and imbued with coercive connotations to induce a 'confession' (Clouder and Sellars 2004). This leads to a cycle of power and resistance in which supervisees moderate what they take to supervision (op. cit.) in order to avoid close scrutiny, but supervisors only become more intrusive wondering whether they are being consulted only on cases that are not particularly stuck. Alternatively, the expert supervisor/manager creates dependency in supervisees.

- CS should be democratic. The all-seeing, all knowing, all-powerful, ever-present clinical supervisor is mythical (Farrington 1995). Indeed, Bobele *et al.* (1997) note that practiced expertise can close down the possibility for new meanings to arise in CS. One implication might be convergence on a limited number of interventions, or even on the best evidence-based treatment. Yet, evidence-based practice is notoriously difficult to enact (McSherry *et al.* 2002). It frequently does not take account of the specific context – the person, her/his existing illness narratives. For those who embrace postmodernism, the construction of an intervention is a conjoint dialogical process. Without a shared narrative, it is likely that the evidence-based approach will not be a difference that makes a difference. In a democratic system, there are multiple knowledges (plural rather than singular), as there are multiple sources of expertise. Such ecology can help both the supervisor and supervisee to 'move beyond their present knowledge states' (Hawes 1993: 4). More importantly, the multiple versions can be processed by the expert practitioner in relation to what s/he understands might be a story of interest for the person experiencing mental health difficulties.

Participants' constructs of 'real' group supervision based in the ECM approach

Chris Stevenson and Barry Jackson (BJ) (2000) were also interested in how 'real' group supervision based in the above philosophy might be constructed by participants. Accordingly, they engaged a group of 'G' grade community psychiatric nurses (CPNs) for a series of six ECMs within which they divested themselves of the role of 'expert'[1] by inducting the attendees into the postmodern approach. So that, in Session 1, Lesley[2] stated:

> I came in here this morning with the old view, and I've had a realisation since I came in about supervision, and I've done all these classic things where I think BJ's the expert. If I have a problem I will take it to BJ to help sort it out.
>
> (Stevenson and Jackson 2000: 495)

The group constructed a meaning of egalitarian consultation as liberating. They found benefit in having a space created by the reworking of the 'rules' of supervision (which they could further recreate at will). Losing the omnipotent supervisor appealed to Claire:

> I don't mind taking away people's ideas, but I don't like people saying you must do this when you're your own person … That whole feeling of being an expert is taken away from us because everybody has their own little idea of what we should be working from. What they think you should do with that person.
>
> (Stevenson and Jackson 2000: 497)

While Jean was aware that being seen as an expert was validating in relation to putting ideas into practice:

> I think that some of the paranoia (amongst staff) comes from the word supervision. I have certainly found in my previous job that supervision has a punitive feel to it. We're all individuals and we all work as different personalities, and we interpret whatever we learn in different ways and use it differently with each client. I think it's just validations and accepting that.
>
> (Stevenson and Jackson 2000: 497)

The group members were pleased to move away from existing patterns of case presentation in favour of relaying people's narratives, elaborating cases rather than reducing them. As Lesley described it:

> I can't remember information from the top of my head like dates of birth, etc. I can remember the things to his life story, and that's the things that interest me.
>
> (Stevenson and Jackson 2000: 497)

When a multiplicity of truths about the world is allowed, stories breed stories. Storytelling often concerned the interpersonal relationship between the person defined as in psychiatric distress and the professional. The stories rarely concerned personal characteristics of the CPN and how s/he needed to use self-awareness to adapt her/himself to be a better practitioner. Deborah's version stated:

> I think there was an incredible benefit in bringing it [a case] here. I took a lot of the things I discussed here back to M when I was talking to her. I was doing a lot of thinking about what we'd been talking about here when I was talking to her…
>
> (Stevenson and Jackson 2000: 497)

The group had a sense of cohesion that does not necessarily occur in more hierarchical arrangements for the reasons outlined above. As Tom described it:

> If there's some cohesion and some value amongst us … and we're actually talking openly about the professional roles we have, then maybe … we're almost in a separate world to our colleagues…
>
> (Stevenson and Jackson 2000: 498)

This led to more radical thought that questioned practice of colleagues. For example, Keith responded to the idea of blacklisting a General Practitioner (GP, physician) who had put a CPN at risk:

> I would find that quite a difficult thing if I'd gone through doing that myself ... I would rather appreciate that would come as a collective thing because that could be more powerful.

(Stevenson and Jackson 2000: 499)

However, the group members were still cautious in relation to the potential for surveillance from without the group, or from self-surveillance. Talking about a group that was organised in a way similar to the ECMs, Lesley said:

> We have these very formal staff meetings once a fortnight and the alternating weeks we have seminars. We invite speakers down. It's all very formal. Everybody has their supervision through the hierarchical structure. So, what we [Community Psychiatric Nursing Group] thought that we would have a group meeting once a month where nobody took minutes. There was no agenda written down anywhere and that we would literally just meet. If people just sit and they don't say anything that's fair enough. We've had one of these meetings so far and everybody talked non-stop. There were no awkward silences or anything and we are more relaxed. I suppose it's similar to this ... but we all felt really, really guilty as if we were skiving doing this. After the first one everyone went away feeling positive ... it was really good ... but the interesting thing is that we felt that we couldn't broadcast it to the outside world, because there was no agenda there, there was no name for it.

(Stevenson and Jackson 2000: 500)

Whilst Tom and Jean were aware of how they retreated from a political agenda:

> Tom: We always feel safer talking about patients.

> Jean: ... by saying that [we] talk about patients we're getting paid for that, you know dealing with patients and making yourself feel a bit more comfortable if you discuss cases.

(Stevenson and Jackson 2000: 500)

Discussion

Modernist, hierarchical supervision has a stranglehold on CS practice, yet, it can hardly be said to be unproblematic; it is heavily critiqued from both outside and within the post-modern turn. Although CS is apparently sustaining for practitioners (Butterworth *et al.* 1997), it is well known that CS is often a casualty in busy clinical environments. Given the experience of some in relation to the critical, punitive and deskilling aspects of CS, it is unsurprising that it is shunted to the bottom of the clinical agenda. Reconstructing CS from a postmodern position might well address some of the existing problems. ECMs are one example. In the case of ECMs, when the assumptions of traditional supervisory practice are set aside, practitioners have the opportunity to construct their own meanings in relation to CS. Having a negoti-ated meaning is experienced as liberation, as hoped for by Chambers (1995).

The supervision group members preferred thinking of themselves as experts by experience in relation to the people they were working with. From a postmodern stance, the actions that a practitioner reports cannot be judged out of context. The alternative of being scrutinised, criticised and corrected is, understandably, unat-tractive. In a situation where the supervisee feels the need to be defensive, it is unlikely that supervision will be a site where complex challenging practice issues are viewed as opportunities as Cutcliffe and Proctor (1998) propose.

The postmodern ambience facilitated the production of an ecology of stories. These stories were a response to the story relayed by the practitioner as the expert on the person in context. Stories were offered spontaneously. This contradicts work that suggests that CS proceeds best when there is a clear contract in respect of content and process (Oxley 1995; Porter 1997). In traditional dyadic supervision there is the potential for non-connecting monologues. The supervisee tells the case history, following an accepted format. S/he may have the information elicited by a challenging or confronting interventions model like Heron's (1990) approach. The supervisor responds by offering an expert monologue consisting in a formulation of the person's diagnosis or illness or problem and the preferred intervention. Con-versely, in ECMs, stories were rich, personal and meaningful. They were presented as tentative suggestions, rather than exemplars. They invited dialogue, which, in turn, aided new narratives to emerge. The external dialogue created the opportun-ity for internal dialogue as the supervisee explored the relevance of the supervision stories for the person 'in view'.

Hawes (1993: 4) has provided an excellent summary of the above points:

> Collaboration in the supervisory process can be understood to include at least three defining characteristics: bidirectionality, non centrality of expertise, and circularity in modelling practices. These characteristics speak to the reciprocity of interpersonal obligations, the absences of rigidly enacted hierarchy in a working relationship, and an outcome or object that is a shared construction of every participant.

ECMs were a place where radical talk could occur in relation to how practice might be better organised. The group members drew strength from being together physi-cally and emotionally in relation to the macho practice environment. As Cutcliffe and Proctor (1998) note, comradeship and cohesion between peers can protect against a culture of divide and rule. However, the participants were nervous about the extent to which they could share and create stories about the organisation which paid them, and which promoted hierarchical supervision. Narrow definitions of what constitutes work weighed heavily on the group members.

Conclusion

The chapter has sought to challenge existing ideas about CS and to construct an alternative approach. In the postmodern spirit, there is no 'truth claim' about the effectiveness of ECMs. Rather, practitioner narratives have been presented as descriptors and testimonials to the experience of ECMs. However, one reading is that ECMs were a site where practitioners began to feel 'powered up' in relation to casework and the system. Being part of a polyvocal community, that is a group where different narratives were valued and people are valued beyond a diagnostic label, appeared to be important. However, no approach is without a political dimension and the group was not immune to the broader, modernist culture. Thus, change in CS practices needs to be at multiple levels of the system.

Notes

1 As far as it is ever possible to do so.
2 Pseudonyms are used to protect confidentiality.

References

Amerling, M., Hofer, H. and Rath, I. (2002), The 'first Vienna Trialogue' – experiences with a new form of communication between users, relatives and mental health professionals, in H.P. Lefley and D.L. Johnson (eds), *Family Interventions in Mental Illness: International Perspectives*, London: Praeger.

Bobele, M., Gardner, G. and Biener, J. (1995), Supervision as social construction, *Journal of Systemic Therapies*, 14(2): 14–25.

Bowles, N. and Young, C. (1998), Partnerships for sound practice, *Nursing Times Learning Curve*, 2(2): 7–8.

Bulmer, C. (1997), Supervision: how it works, *Nursing Times*, 93(48): 53–54.

Butterworth, T. (1994), *A Delphi Study of Optimal Practice in Nursing*, Manchester: University of Manchester.

Butterworth, T. (1996), Primary attempts at research-based evaluation of clinical supervision, *Nursing Times Research*, 1(2): 96–101.

Butterworth, T., Carson, J., White, E., Jeacock, J., Clements, A. and Bishop, V. (1997), *It Is Good to Talk: An Evaluation Study in England and Scotland*, Manchester: University of Manchester.

Chambers, M. (1995), Supportive clinical supervision: a crucible for personal and professional change, *Journal of Psychiatric and Mental Health Nursing*, 2(5): 311–316.

Clouder, L. and Sellars, J. (2004), Reflective practice and clinical supervision: an interprofessional perspective, *Journal of Advanced Nursing*, 46(3): 262–269.

Cutcliffe, J.R. and Epling, M. (1997), An exploration of the use of John Heron's confronting interventions in clinical supervision: case studies for practice, *Psychiatric Care*, 4(4): 174–180.

Cutcliffe, J.R. and Proctor, B. (1998), An alternative training approach to clinical supervision 2, *British Journal of Nursing*, 7(6): 344–350.

Cutcliffe, J.R., Butterworth, T. and Proctor, B. (2001), Introduction, in J.R. Cutcliffe, T. Butterworth and B. Proctor (eds), *Fundamental Themes in Clinical Supervision*, London: Routledge, pp.1–5.

Department of Health (1994), *Clinical Supervision for the Nursing and Health Visiting Professionals*, CNO Letter 94(5), London: Department of Health.

Ekstein, R. and Wallerstein, R.S. (1972), *The Teaching and Learning of Psychotherapy*, New York: New York International Universities Press.

Farrington, A. (1995), Defining and setting the parameters of clinical supervision, *British Journal of Nursing*, 4(15): 874–875.

Faugier, J. (1998), The supervisory relationship, in T. Butterworth, J. Faugier and P. Burnard (eds), *Clinical Supervision and Mentorship in Nursing*, 2nd edn, Cheltenham: Stanley Thornes.

Fowler, J. (1996), The organisation of clinical supervision within the professions: a review of the literature, *Journal of Advanced Nursing,* 23(3): 471–478.

Glaser, B.G. (2001), *The Grounded Theory Perspective II: Description's Remodeling of Grounded Theory,* Mill Valley, CA: Sociology Press.

Hawes, S. (1993), *Reflexivity and Collaboration in the Supervisory Process: A Role for Feminist Post-structuralist Theories in the Training of Professional Psychologists,* chapter presented to the National Council of Schools and Programs in Professional Psychology, winter meeting, La Jolla, CA.

Hawkins, P. and Shohet, R. (1989), Approaches to the supervision of counsellors: the supervisory relationship, in W. Dryden and B. Thorne (eds), *Training and Supervision for Counselling in Action,* London: Sage.

Heron, J. (1990), *Helping the Client: A Creative, Practical Guide,* London: Sage.

Johns, C. (1998), Opening the doors of perception, in C. Johns and D. Freshwater (eds), *Transforming Nursing Through Reflective Practice,* Oxford: Blackwell Science.

Jones, A. (2006), Clinical supervision: what do we know and what do we need to know? A review and commentary, *Journal of Nursing Management,* 14(8): 577–585.

Kipping, C. (1998), Learning from the experiences of mental health nurses, *Nursing Times Learning Curve,* 2(3): 6–8.

Lyotard, J.F. (1984), *The Postmodern Condition: A Report on Knowledge,* G. Bennington and B. Massumi (trans.), Minneapolis: University of Minnesota Press.

McSherry, R., Simmons, M. and Abbott, P. (2002), *Evidence Informed Nursing: A Guide for Clinical Nurses,* London: Routledge.

Oxley, P. (1995), Clinical supervision in community psychiatric nursing, *Mental Health Nursing,* 15(6): 15–17.

Page, S. and Wosket, V. (1994), *Supervising the Counsellor,* London: Routledge.

Paunonen, M. (1991), Promoting nursing quality through supervision, *Journal of Nursing Staff Development,* 7(5): 229–233.

Porter, N. (1997), Clinical supervision: the art of being supervised, *Nursing Standard,* 11(45): 44–45.

Proctor, B. (1986), Supervision: a co-operative exercise in accountability, in M. Marken and M. Payne (eds), *Enabling and Ensuring,* Leicester: National Youth Bureau and Council for Education and Training in Youth and Community Work.

Seikkula, J., Aaltonen, J., Alakare, B., Haarakangas, K., Keränen, J. and Sutela, M. (1995), Treating psychosis by means of open dialogue, in S. Friedman (ed.), *The Reflecting Team in Action,* New York: Guilford.

Severinsson, E.I. (1995), The phenomenon of clinical supervision in psychiatric health care, *Journal of Psychiatric and Mental Health Nursing,* 2(5): 301–309.

Sloan, G. and Watson, H. (2002), Clinical supervision models for nursing: structure, research and limitations, *Nursing Standard,* 17(4): 41–46.

Stevenson, C. and Beech, I. (2001), Paradigms lost, paradigms regained: defending nursing against a single reading of postmodernism, *Nursing Philosophy,* 2(2): 143–150.

Stevenson, C. and Jackson, B. (2000), Egalitarian consultation meetings: an alternative to received wisdom about clinical supervision in psychiatric nursing practice, in *Journal of Psychiatric and Mental Health Nursing,* 7(6): 491–504.

Van Ooijen, E. (1994), Supervision: whipping up a storm, *Nursing Standard,* 9(8): 48.

Yegdich, T. (1998), How not to do clinical supervision in nursing, *Journal of Advanced Nursing,* 28(1): 193–202.

9 Solution-focused clinical supervision

Using solution-focused techniques within clinical supervision

John Fowler

This chapter explores how the principles and techniques used in solution-focused therapy can be transferred to the clinical supervision relationship. Clinical supervision should never be confused with therapy, but some of the techniques used by therapists such as listening skills, helping people to focus and clarifying points are transferable skills to any sort of relationship. Similarly the author argues that there are a number of key techniques that have been developed by the solution-focused therapists that transfer to the clinical supervision relationship. Even the core principle of being positive and looking for solutions can transform a clinical supervision meeting.

We believe that the relationship between the supervisor and the supervisee is key in the process and outcome of clinical supervision. Each relationship will be different and it would restrict the natural growth and development of that relationship if each supervisor conformed to a prescribed approach. However if supervisors are aware of different skills and techniques that they can use to build upon their natural way of working, then they can develop and grow as supervisors. In the words of solution-focused philosophy (O'Connell 2005): 'if it isn't broken don't fix it' (p. 29) but 'if it's working keep doing it' (p. 32).

Introduction

'How do you prevent clinical supervision from becoming a moaning session?' This must be one of the most frequent questions I am ever asked, when working with staff involved in clinical supervision. The second most frequent question is usually, 'How should I structure a clinical supervision session?' and the third most commonly asked question which usually comes from the managers, is 'What are the measurable outcomes of clinical supervision?' These are all good, valid questions. The last thing anyone wants from clinical supervision is for it to degenerate into an unstructured session in which staff complain about their workload, do nothing about it and leave the session feeling worse than when they went in. Sadly, however, in any objective evaluation of clinical supervision, this negative scenario often typifies those sessions in which clinical supervision fails. Philosophically these failing groups and individuals adopt a problem-focused approach. They identify the problems and then wallow in them. For many this is a passive response, one of least resistance, a consequence of feeling a small cog in a big wheel. For others there is almost an intentional propagation of the negative, in which they seem to receive some perverse pleasure in other people's misery. I am sure you recognise these stereotypes; the latter are some of the most perniciously destructive people to have in any group or team.

One of the most effective ways I have found of helping people in these sorts of situations, both the positive and the negative scenarios, is by the application of some of the techniques and ideas developed in solution-focused therapy. Solution-focused therapy is becoming increasingly popular as a therapeutic model in social work, and other counselling-type professions (Kim 2007; O'Connell 2005). The aim is not to turn clinical supervision into some sort of therapy session, but to use and apply some of the ideas and techniques that have become identified with this solution-focused model.

Solution-focused clinical supervision offers a simple, yet quite profound philosophy and structure for the clinical supervision relationship. It has a positive focus and offers a relatively simple structure. The aim of incorporating solution-focused techniques into clinical supervision is to enhance the supervisor's range of options with which to assist the supervisees to move forward positively. Its use can give structure, focus and direction when at times the way forward seems unclear.

As the name suggests 'solution focus' is about looking for solutions rather than dwelling on problems (Iveson 2002; O'Connell 2005). At the heart of solution-focused work is what Waskett (2006) calls 'spacious simplicity' a simplicity that comes from a basic attitude of mutual respect; combined with the intention of moving forward positively (Fowler 2005). In the traditional setting of therapy, solution-focused techniques are used to help the person to live in the present; to identify small achievable steps to moving forward; and to build on inner resources in a positive way.

> I asked for some help because I felt decisions at work were getting on top of me, I was taking work home with me, dwelling on problems with staff at home, which was beginning to put a strain on my marriage. I knew my staff were not happy with me as well, but I didn't know what to do. My manager arranged for some one-to-one clinical supervision with one of the lecturers from the local university. We met up for one hour, once a month and for me that session was like a lifesaver. It was a time to collect thoughts and reflect. I'm sure that I would never do a reflection if I didn't have clinical supervision. I was not given advice or told how to do things, rather I was encouraged to look at myself and draw upon my own resources. The only thing I was asked to do was to write a short account of one situation at work, what it was about and what I did. I then discussed that in the supervision session. The solutions came from me. If I was feeling cross or aggressive I had to see how I could use that energy in a positive way, rather than letting it weigh me down. I've stopped taking unnecessary work home and changed my way of thinking. I feel far more in control of my work and have regained my enjoyment of work.
>
> (Senior Nurse Manager)

From a professional perspective, the NMC updated (NMC 2006) the original (UKCC 1995) guidance which identifies the aims of clinical supervision within the UK as:

- identify solutions to problems;
- increase understanding of professional issues;
- improve standards of patient care;
- further develop their skills and knowledge;
- enhance their understanding of their own practice.

A generally accepted umbrella definition of clinical supervision is that given by Butterworth and Faugier: *'An exchange between practising professionals to enable the development of professional skills'* (Butterworth *et al.* 1998: 12). However, many employers have developed clinical supervision to meet their specific circumstances and often refocus clinical supervision with a specific aim. As an example, in one place I was employed this was identified as: *To enable staff to meet together in a regular and structured way to reflect upon issues that arise from their own professional work and move forward positively* (Fowler 2005). Note the emphasis on 'moving forward positively'.

In the early 1990s, a number of accounts appeared in the literature describing how clinical supervision could work, or was working, in a variety of clinical settings. Different models of clinical supervision began to emerge. At the more humanistic end of the spectrum, Faugier (1992) described a growth and support model of the supervisory relationship, the prime focus being the relationship between the individuals. Then, using the interactions within the relationship, it focuses on the role of the supervisor to facilitate both educational and personal growth for the supervisee. At the same time, the relationship must be one that provides support for the developing clinical autonomy of the supervisee.

From a more behaviourist perspective, Nicklin (1995) argued that clinical supervision would become rhetoric, promoting the illusion of innovation without producing change. While supporting the developmental elements, he felt that tangible outcomes are required. He proposed that clinical supervision be used to analyse issues and problems, clarify goals and identify 'strategies for goal attainment and establish an appropriate plan of action'. Nicklin (1997) developed these ideas into a six-stage process of supervision. Focusing on practice, it starts with practice analysis, problem identification, objective-setting, planning, implementation action and evaluation.

'Solution-focused clinical supervision' identifies with both the humanistic and behavioural models in that it values the enriching humanistic relationship that enhances growth and development, whilst at the same time using that relationship to help the supervisee to move forward in a positive step by step, 'measurable' way. In practice, very few supervision relationships would reflect a 'pure' humanistic or pure behaviourist model of working. Human relationships are far too complex (Byrne 1998) to encapsulate them into narrow boxes. What can be seen in practice is that some people work more predominantly towards one end of a spectrum than others. *What solution-based clinical supervision is suggesting however, is these two models are not mutually exclusive and that the combination of a warm, genuine trusting relationship which is used to help a person focus on achievable, positive outcomes, is an extremely powerful way to help people move forward.*

Solution-focused brief therapy: a summary

Solution-focused brief therapy falls within the 'talking therapies' and was developed as a therapeutic technique in the early 1980s, by Steve de Shazer and colleagues (de Shazer 1985). The underpinning principles are, as the name suggests, the two fold aspects of focusing on solutions, rather than problems and, second, it being time limited or brief, as opposed to the months and years associated with psychotherapeutic therapies. Koss and Butcher (1986) summarised a lot of the early research into brief therapy as:

- there is a focus on the here and now;
- the therapist is openly active and influential;

- the therapist takes on a confident, positive and competent stance;
- specific and achievable goals are identified.

As a therapy it acknowledges that for the majority of time, the majority of people, live successful lives using their own inner resources to cope with and manage their lives. On occasions when part of their lives becomes problematic, or they enter a new situation which is causing them difficulties the 'problems' can begin to dominate. A downward spiral can begin in which the person begins to feel out of control of their life, at the mercy of outside forces. Solution-focused therapy helps the person to identify a preferred or future goal, and then to identify manageable steps that lead in that direction. It helps the person to remember or discover what inner resources they have that have solved similar problems in the past, and to re-engage those resources for the present situation.

Barrett-Kruse (1994) summarises the main features of brief therapy as:

- viewing yourself and others as essentially able;
- accepting the client's definition of the problem;
- focusing objectively on the client's behaviour rather than their personality;
- creating a therapeutic alliance;
- crediting the client with success.

As a 'talking therapy', a solution-focused approach can be an effective intervention for a range of problem presentations in a variety of contexts (Iveson 2002), not just therapy sessions. A meta-analysis of 22 studies (50 per cent experimental and 50 per cent quasi-experimental designs) showed a cautious acknowledgment of the effectiveness of solution-focused therapy (Kim 2007). Kim's analysis suggests that it appears to be more effective with internalised behaviour problems such as anxiety, self-concept and self-esteem, but not so effective with externalised problems such as aggression, hyperactivity and behaviour problems. This is particularly interesting when we take its application into clinical supervision, for it is often the self-esteem, confidence and self-concept issues that underpin a number of topics presented by the supervisee at supervision.

Solution-focused therapy contains a number of techniques to assist a person in identifying existing skills, strengths, resources and goals. It is these techniques that can be transferred so effectively to clinical supervision. They include the use of scales, the miracle question, searching for exceptions, constructive feedback and follow-up tasks (George *et al.* 1999). *The solution-focused techniques can be used equally effectively in both one-to-one and the various forms of group clinical supervision.* Use of these techniques assists the clinical supervisor to engage collaboratively with supervisees and focus on solutions. It gives the sessions an underpinning philosophy which translates into a tangible structure. It encourages a focus on the supervisee drawing upon their own inner resources, rather than seeing the supervisor as one with all the answers. Both the solution-focused session and the clinical supervision session encourage a relationship which is based on mutual respect and equality. This encourages openness and honesty and an opportunity to reflect on work related issues in a safe and non-judgemental environment.

Although focused-based clinical supervision uses some core techniques, it is not just a collection of these techniques that are used in a routine, dehumanised way.

They are tools that should be used within this mutually respectful relationship. It is the genuine respect for the person combined with the reinforcement of their own ability to positively move forward. The role of the supervisor is to help them realise their strengths and existing ways of coping and then to help the person build upon these existing strengths. A number of the techniques will now be explored.

Application of solution-focused techniques to clinical supervision

The curious inquirer

When identifying the supervisee's skills, strengths and resources, the supervisor adopts the stance of a curious inquirer. For example, being interested about how they managed a particular situation, despite the difficulties they faced, enables the supervisee to acknowledge their ability to identify the skills they used in order to have discovered that particular solution.

> Supervisor: 'So this was the first time that you were in charge of the ward. When bereaved relatives came back onto the ward, how did you go about organising it? What did you do?'

Positive self-affirming questions

The following questions encourage a positive way forward at the same time as helping the supervisee(s) to identify their own inner resources:

- So what did it take to do that?
- What helped you to achieve that?
- How did you do that?
- How did you get through that time/experience/deal with that difficulty?
- What did you learn about yourself managing to do that?
- What do you think that that might have taught others about you?

> Supervisor: 'What did you have to do to organise it in that way?'.... 'What did you learn about yourself in how you handle that sort of situation?'

Scaling

One of the techniques is the zero-to-ten scale. This can be used in a number of ways in a clinical supervision session. First, it can be used to identify the ultimate goal, where ten represents the absolute best achievement of the person's goals and zero is the worst case scenario. The person then uses the scale to assess their current position. Their satisfaction with this position can be determined and they are also able to identify their preferred position.

> *Staff Nurse Anita was concerned that the health care assistants on her ward did not seem to respect her authority when she was in charge of the shift. In supervision she was asked to rate this on a scale of zero to ten, 'zero' being a total disregard for everything she says*

and *'ten' being treated with great respect. She rated herself as five.* To reinforce the positive aspects of her current actions she was asked if there was ever a time when she would have rated that as less than five. She gave details of the previous year when things seemed worse, and she would have rated herself as a three. She was then asked what had caused the improvement from three to five. The reason she gave was: *One of the existing HCAs left and a new one started, I was responsible for her induction and supervision.* She was then asked if there was anything she could learn from that positive experience that she could use in the next week or two with the other HCAs. She identified that *'spending one-to-one time with her and being interested and supportive had worked well with the new HCA'.* Between them they agreed that she would: 1. Spend some one-to-one time with each of the HCAs; 2. Show interest in them; and 3. Try to be supportive. This was a positive, measurable and achievable set of actions that she would monitor and report back on at the next clinical supervision meeting. At the next meeting they would use the zero-to-ten scale to re-evaluate her position.

Thus positioning oneself on such a scale can help put into perspective one's position in relation to the worst scenario, it can help focus on achievable targets, it can reinforce success and monitor progress.

The miracle question

In addition to scales, use of the 'miracle question' can determine preferred futures or goals. If during supervision a problem is posed then the supervisor can ask the following question, *'if a miracle occurred what would be the first thing you would notice?'* Asking *'what else'* several times elicits the finer detail of the supervisee's preferred future. The supervisee is then encouraged to consider, *'are there times when some of the preferred future already happens?'* This can help them to realise that there are times when a problem does not occur and identify what is different at those times. Those 'differences' can then be the key to developing actions and behaviours for future action.

> During a group clinical supervision session a number of staff identify that they do not feel valued or appreciated by the doctors, the senior staff, the patients, relatives and generally everyone, they felt that they were viewed as an *'anonymous pair of hands'.* The supervisor asked the question, *'If you came to work tomorrow and a miracle had occurred and people appreciated you, what would be the first thing you would notice?'* Some of the comments were: *'to be greeted by name as we come on shift, to be thanked by the ward sister, not to have to tidy up after the doctors, for relatives to say thank you, to be told what your duties are for the shift...'* The supervisor then asked if there were times when the ward sister had thanked anyone and most of the group could actually cite at least one occasion. The same was done with the other examples. The supervisor then began to explore with the group when and why these 'preferred solutions' occurred and if they could be 'prompted' to reoccur.

Identifying exceptions

This is a development of the miracle question in which the supervisee is encouraged to consider if there are times when some of the miracle is already happening, 'the exceptions' which enables the preferred future to be identified. This can help them to realise that there are times when a problem does not occur and identify what is different at those times and what is already working. Those differences or exceptions can be the key in identifying actions and behaviours that are currently within the supervisee's mode of action that could be a positive way forward. It reinforces that the supervisee has the skills and abilities currently within them.

Positive communication

Subsequent clinical sessions should focus on solutions rather than dwelling on old problems. Asking *'What is better'* at the beginning of a session, as opposed to *'How are things'* encourages the supervisee to focus on positive aspects of their practice. At the end of each supervision session, the supervisor provides a summary of the supervisee's strengths, skills and resources. It is the supervisor's role to provide this feedback based upon what they have heard. The importance of adopting good communication cannot be over-emphasised. The following are important:

- acknowledgement of the issue or difficulty being discussed, but at the same time looking for positive outcomes within these difficulties;
- listening with a constructive ear for evidence of resources e.g. skills, strengths, supportive relationships;
- encouraging self-belief – treating the other person/people within the supervisee relationship with equity and a genuine belief that they have the ability and skills to move forward positively;
- reinforcing the positive – this involves feeding back the skills, strengths and abilities that are evident in the supervisee that have emerged during the session.

Positive questions

Appropriate use of questions can aid communication and exploration enabling the supervisees to be specific:

- Questions which are likely to draw out resourceful answers.
- Questions that lead to exploration.
- Questions of who, where, what, when, how.
- Questions that focus on one point at a time.
- Questions that help imagination of new behaviour, new self image.

(George *et al.* 1999)

Jean was a reasonably experienced community nurse but her manager felt that she was not fulfilling her full responsibilities and always seemed to be presenting them with problems. Her sick record was poor, with a number of odd days taken periodically. Following her annual 'individual performance review' her managers asked if she would like to meet with someone from outside of the employing authority for individual clinical supervision. She agreed to this.

I phoned Jean and we agreed a time to meet up. For the first meeting she turned up appearing flustered. We had a cup of tea together and I emphasised the voluntary nature of the clinical supervision and the general principle that it was her time, to focus on what she felt important and that it was completely confidential. She quickly relaxed with me and told me of her work and life, all of which seemed to be full of difficulties and problems. I reinforced to her that this was not a counselling session and explained the principles of focusing and reflecting on aspects of clinical practice. We talked for some time about the nature of her work (the curious inquirer) and identifying the positive qualities that she possessed (self-affirming question). I asked her to scale her current job satisfaction and then explored via the 'miracle question' how she would recognise an improvement. I then left her with 'homework' of writing down if any of these 'improvements' occurred over the forthcoming month and we were to discuss them at the next clinical supervision meeting. Over the next few meetings we began building on the exceptions and moving forward positively. The supervisee began to recognise in herself her own abilities to look for and build upon the positive.

Solution-focused clinical supervision provides a structured framework that can be used by a range of practitioners to assist colleagues to reflect upon their practice and enhance their existing skills, moving forward in a positive way. Although presented here as a series of techniques, it is better to see it as a philosophy of practice in which the supervisee looks for the positive and encourages positive self-belief in the supervisee. In one-to-one clinical supervision, the application is obvious and straightforward. Also with a 'facilitator led' group clinical supervision, the application is again fairly straightforward. However for 'peer group' clinical supervision the application is not so simple. In peer group clinical supervision, facilitation rather than leadership summarises the group dynamics and part of the structure of solution-focused work is positive and confident 'leadership'. However even in peer groups, if the members have a little coaching into the philosophy of solution-focused clinical supervision and are encouraged to use affirming questions, positive communication, looking for exceptions and any of the other techniques, then the peer group can use solution-focused techniques equally effectively.

Supervisor training

The final point just to touch on in this chapter is to ask what degree of training the supervisor requires to use solution-focused techniques. There is no standard answer to this question. If supervisors and group facilitators already have supervision skills and a general knowledge of counselling-type techniques, then they can begin incorporating this way of working quite naturally into their own working model. Bill O'Connell's short book on *Solution Focused Therapy* (O'Connell 2005) would make good preparatory reading. Other staff, who have not had training and little prior knowledge, would be advised to undertake some formal supervision/solution-focused course, which hopefully encompasses its own supervision. *Unlike some other 'therapeutic' skills, a little knowledge of solution-focused skills is not a dangerous thing.* The worst outcome of a little knowledge poorly applied and executed, is that the supervisor may be perceived as somewhat patronising. So in the words of solution-focused techniques (O'Connell 2005), 'if it isn't broken don't fix it' (p. 29) and 'if it works, keep doing it' (p. 32), but be honest in your reflections.

References

Barrett-Kruse, C. (1994), Brief counselling: a user's guide for traditionally trained counsellors, *International Journal for the Advancement of Counselling*, 17(2): 109–115.

Butterworth, T., Faugier, J. and Burnard, P. (1998), *Clinical Supervision and Mentorship in Nursing*, 2nd edn, Cheltenham: Stanley Thornes.

Byrne, D. (1998), *Complexity Theory and the Social Sciences*, London: Routledge.

de Shazer, S. (1985), *Keys to Solution in Brief Therapy*, New York: W.W. Norton.

Faugier, J. (1992), The supervisory relationship, in T. Butterworth and J. Faugier (eds), *Clinical Supervision and Mentorship in Nursing*, London: Chapman & Hall.

Fowler, J. (2005), *Clinical Supervision: Making a Space for Reflection*, Vision Statement, Leicester: Leicester City West PCT Information Leaflet.

George, E., Iveson, C. and Harvey, R. (1999), *Problem to Solution*, 2nd edn, London: BT Press.

Iveson, C. (2002), Solution-focused brief therapy, *Advances in Psychiatric Treatment*, 8(2): 149–157.

Kim, J. (2007), Examining the effectiveness of solution focused brief therapy: a meta-analysis, *Research on Social Work Practice*, 18(2): 107–116.

Koss, M. and Butcher, J. (1986), Research on brief psychotherapy, in S. Garfield and A. Begin (eds), *Handbook on Psychotherapy and Behaviour Change*, 3rd edn, New Yorks: Wiley & Sons.

Nicklin, P. (1995), Super supervision, *Nursing Management*, 2(5): 24–25.

Nicklin, P. (1997), A practice centred model of clinical supervision, *Nursing Times*, 93(46): 52–54.

NMC (2006), *Advice Sheet – Clinical Supervision*, London: Nursing and Midwifery Council.

O'Connell, B. (2005), *Solution-Focused Therapy*, 2nd edn, London: Sage Publications.

UKCC (1995), *Position Statement on Clinical Supervision for Nursing and Health Visiting*, Registrar's Letter 4/1995 Annexe 1, London: UKCC.

Waskett, C. (2006), Solution focused supervision, *Healthcare Counselling and Psychotherapy*, 6(1): 9–11, also online, available at: www.northwestsolutions. co.uk/ sf-supervision-res.php.

Part II

Introducing, implementing and developing clinical supervision

10 Clinical supervision and clinical governance

Veronica Bishop

This chapter examines the relationship between clinical supervision and clinical governance. Both terms are somewhat imprecise and the variety of definitions that surround both terms only adds to the confusion that is experienced by clinicians and managers alike. The author carefully examines both concepts and draws them together with a convergence model. Veronica is unique among the authorities on clinical supervision. She held one of the highest strategic positions in nursing and was a key figure in the implementation of clinical supervision within the UK. Since then she has continued to research, write and be actively involved in clinical supervision at all levels of the nursing profession. Within this chapter she manages to draw together the clinical supervision practice of the individual nurse and the implications of developing clinical supervision at strategic level.

We believe that clinical supervision should not be seen as a substitute for poor staffing levels, or lack of clinical leadership. As this chapter demonstrates, clinical supervision is part of a companion of structural and strategic systems that contribute to effective and efficient patient care.

Introduction

Clinical supervision (CS) has the potential to place nursing firmly at the forefront of policymaking, reflecting clinical needs. So why has it not been grasped more fully? Taking part in CS is taking a journey. Any journey needs a map, and the link between effective and quality care (and the two are not synonymous) has only recently been forged, through clinical governance, thus providing the ideal route. To signpost the way to effective CS, I begin by considering why there is a need for it, before going into more depth on the issues essential to get CS on the mainstream health agenda. Central to any initiative with resource implications, which CS has, is the need for evidence. In this chapter I offer examples that provide the opportunity to adopt/adapt evidence from both the United States and the United Kingdom. Other chapters in this book will emphasise the need for reflection, self-knowledge and constructive peer review; this chapter seeks to lead the reader, through their personal involvement with CS, to the core of their employing organisation. How to achieve this is illustrated through the convergence model of clinical supervision which includes audit, necessary for clinical governance, and lends itself well to initiatives such as the widely acclaimed Magnet hospitals in the US and subsequent work in the UK. In highlighting how clinical supervision can

impact effectively on clinical governance, the touchstone of organisational standard setting, and professional competence, the text provides an essential map to
make CS a journey worth taking.

What is clinical supervision? Why do we need it?

As a key player in the UK in the introduction of clinical supervision (CS) in the
early 1990s I have discussed the policy drivers for the introduction of CS elsewhere
(Bishop 2007), and they are rehearsed in other chapters in this book. The interest
that CS engendered is significant as it reflects a sustained interest amongst practitioners to develop approaches to care that enhance quality as well as developing
their personal motivations, a point well described by McCormack and Henderson
(2007). The subsequent implementation of CS across the UK, Scandinavia, Australia, New Zealand and the United States is further proof of a need, but I would
suggest that its potential to support good care is undervalued, despite studies, some
of which are discussed later in this text, that have clearly identified some outcomes.
Initially there was no overt link between CS and employing organisations' management strategies that connected safety, quality and professional development with
practitioners. The demand for evidence-based practice, driven by policy initiatives
that strive to contain healthcare within finite resources, has led to considerable conflict. Conflict, not only between users of health care services and their providers, but
also between employing organisations and their staff, on both sides of the Atlantic.
While clinical supervision has to be aligned with the evidence-based practice movement – indeed I argue that it should be leading the way in issues that impact on the
quality of direct patient care – it has lacked the mechanism to bridge professional
and managerial requirements. It took the introduction of clinical governance in
1998 (Scally and Donaldson 1998) to provide a great opportunity for all clinical
practitioners to hold sway at the board table, despite the fact that it was a medically
driven initiative to elicit quantitative data in evidence-based treatments. To make
the connection between clinical supervision and clinical governance it is necessary
first to define clinical supervision and then to highlight how it can underpin good
clinical governance. Several useful definitions will have been aired in other chapters
in this book, but the one that I favour, as it was developed with a variety of clinical
staff, explains where the important focus of clinical supervision has to be – in the
safe and supported delivery of quality care.

> Clinical supervision is a designated interaction between two or more practition-
> ers within a safe and supportive environment, that enables a continuum of
> reflective critical analysis of care to ensure quality patient services, and the well
> being of the practitioner.
>
> (Bishop 2007)

As other chapters in this volume indicate, policy and educational approaches to CS
have varied over the past decade, with equally varying degrees of success. Why is
this? Many managers appear to have been too preoccupied with government targets
and have given minimal thought to overstretched nurses and vulnerable patients. A
combination of staff shortages, overburdened staff and lack of funds and/or facilities provide compelling reasons to implement clinical supervision and thus protect

staff from failing in their duty of care; a situation that too often prevails, as media coverage regularly demonstrates. There is also the underestimated problem of staff who do not see the importance of investing in themselves. That age-old enemy of progress – apathy! The mind set of 'I can't change anything' which generally means that if you don't expect anything – that's what you'll get! There is a leadership issue here – staff who are not inspired to invest in themselves and to contribute more to their employing organisation are not only disempowered, their negativity will block progress within their team. Somehow the link between clinical governance and the individual practitioner has not yet been grasped, yet this is where the authority lies for an accountable professional, and where the impact that professional has on patient care can be maximised.

Berwick (2004) acknowledged the tremendous power of nursing, set against the fragility of the relationship with an individual patient. For nursing to realise that power, and to use it in a therapeutic way, must be what being a professional provider of health care it about. But how to achieve this? What framework will consistently support each individual nurse or healthcare worker in balancing their workload, in feeling empathy with their patients and clients despite a fast turnover, and in driving forward standards of care without burning out? How important is it to anyone dealing with people in often fraught circumstances to mirror what they are doing, to 'play back' and reflect on current practices, to self-critique and to grow both personally and professionally? Very important – indeed crucial for any thinking practitioner – and this reflection is most effective if done with peers, a person, or people who have some understanding of what you need to achieve and how to succeed in those goals (Freshwater 2007). Despite the lack of nationwide clarity, the cynicism and the resistance to the professional development offered through CS, the concept has been, and is still, promoted from our more visionary and possibly more stubborn colleagues. They have identified it as, at worst, a mechanism to safeguard minimum clinical standards and public safety, and at best to sustain and develop excellence in practice. However, it must be realised that:

> while clinical supervision will help nurses to achieve the best level of care possible, it cannot compensate for inadequate facilities, poor management or unmotivated staff. However it will create a culture within which nurses can flourish if they are willing to embrace it, and if management is supportive.
>
> (Bishop 1994: 36)

Accountability, peer review and empowerment

Today, in the UK, all healthcare professional regulators are subject to the terms of the United Kingdom Council of Healthcare Regulators. This Council aims to ensure that each regulatory body works according to principles of public protection. Health care regulators are also active in *defining* the individual professions within health care, controlling entry to them, setting standards of conduct and imposing sanctions on individual professionals whose practice falls below these standards. Each practitioner is accountable to their own regulatory body for their standard of professional practice and to the employer for working within mutually agreed parameters.

Nursing does not have a culture of peer review. Learning to critique and value other people's work in a constructive way is not easy, and requires a great deal of tact and honesty. However learning to give and to receive comments on one's work is the professional fertiliser for growth and confidence. Butterworth (1992: 12) pointed a finger at nurses for not 'indulging' in critical debate as a matter of routine. Team working is central to health care services, and that means that each team member has an inherent responsibility to both give and receive feedback on their effectiveness within that team – everyone has something to learn and to share.

> The results of a Delphi study in the UK on what facilitated good practice indicated that practitioners rated CS very highly as an empowering and stress-reducing mechanism.
>
> (Butterworth and Bishop 1995)

What perhaps is most important with regard to the semantics of CS is the use of the word 'clinical' – the focus is on clinical practice, the heart of what nursing is about. I have always held the view (Bishop 1998) that the terminology must focus on clinical practice and support the best possible standards of care. Power (1999: 29) took this view further by categorically stating that if CS is to work it should not be allowed to become linked with management issues, perhaps unwittingly introducing a schism between organisational and professional needs. It is undoubtedly this lack of differentiation between management and CS that has hindered many in taking it forward. A similar lack of differentiation – that of distinction between leadership and management – has seriously impeded any real UK strategy for the future of nursing to date (Bishop 2009; Stanley 2009).

What is clinical governance and where is the link with CS?

The UK government document *A First Class Service – quality in the New NHS* (Department of Health 1998) stated that one of the key strategies for achieving quality was the introduction of clinical governance which was intended to herald a new approach to quality. Scott (2001: 38) noted that

> considering the focus in healthcare in recent years has been on the financial agenda and managerial framework, we are presented with a challenge that demands a radical change in thinking, which will in essence require a fundamental change in culture.

This culture change is still to occur, and the opportunities integral to clinical governance are not being realised in the current narrowness of its interpretation.

Clinical governance is primarily concerned with standards and with the dissemination of best evidence. The term 'governance' aims to ensure accountability and excellence in the corporate and financial management of an organisation. Clinical governance is an extension of financial governance into clinical practices, and the need for health care providers to provide effective, quality health care has been the subject of a number of policy and strategy documents in the United Kingdom within both the National Health Service (NHS) and the independent sector. Several national and international initiatives have been developed to facilitate clinical governance, which focus on implementation of evidence-based practice, including the establishment in the United Kingdom of the National Institute for Clinical Effective-

---

Box 10.1 Donabedian's (1990) seven pillars of quality

- Efficacy
- Effectiveness
- Efficiency
- Optimality
- Acceptability
- Legitimacy
- Equity.

---

ness (NICE), though this is not without its critics. The most important principle of clinical governance is a commitment to high quality, safe, patient-centred services in clinical practice. The guru of quality since the 1960s, Donabedian described the seven pillars of quality.

While Donabedian himself acknowledged the equal importance of *processes* as well as outcomes, this understanding has not been embedded in the drive within health care in the UK to provide evidence-based care, meet targets, and reduce staff costs. However, recently, in the UK, government policy has shifted from target setting to issues of safety and quality practice (*Journal of Research in Nursing* 2009) and a wider view of what clinical governance should embrace is being considered.

Models used in clinical governance tend to work well for care interventions that are clearly defined and measurable, but are less sensitive to many of the interventions and interactions carried out by nurses. To address this, in the UK, health care is now to be measured through the twin indicators of finance and quality (quality includes safety, clinical effectiveness and patient satisfaction). The newly formed Care Quality Commission will base its measures on recommendations within *A High Quality Care for All* (Department of Health 2008) focusing care into discrete clinical networks, reflecting earlier recommendations from health policy leaders. While these initiatives are to be welcomed we still have a long way to go. Integral to clinical governance is patient satisfaction, which is an area which nursing can and should influence.

Clinical governance is something that nursing in the United Kingdom as a whole appears to embrace, but there is little evidence that the profession really understands its role within this framework, and most importantly, how to maximise the effectiveness of nursing. Currently there is no overt link between the individual and clinical governance that explicitly expresses the power of the individual practitioner to influence the employing authority. But there is! CS, carefully applied, can make that philosophical lead from reflection to hard evidence.

Bridging the gap: a model for clinical and organisational guidance

The most commonly cited model of CS was devised by Proctor (1988) who identified formative (developmental and educational), normative (professional standard setting) and restorative (de-stressing, recharging) components as essential for effective CS. It has provided a solid base from which to build a more accountable structure. If you add to this the work of Sarafino (2002) it contributes greatly, the focus being quite specifically on support and professional development, raising the potential to nurture the individual practitioner. However, in the current culture of clinical governance, there is still lacking a structure that explicitly expresses the power of the practitioner to influence standards, and indeed, sit at the high table of the employing organisation. Working with clinical staff from general hospitals, the community and prisons has led me to develop the model identified in Figure 10.1. This illustrates how, by building on earlier models, we can marry or converge the concepts described by Proctor and widened by Sarafino, 'stitching in' the need for standard setting and audit to feed into clinical governance, but quite separate from any individual appraisal system.

Taking a pyramid as the main structure through which to develop CS you will see that the following essential components of quality care are stacked in three blocks placing the patients/client at the pinnacle. The three components, normative, restorative and formative, are demonstrated by the overlapping circles within the pyramid.

- *Block 1.* Restorative and supportive needs of staff and the importance of reflective practice are highlighted. The buffer mechanism that through CS may prevent staff from 'crashing' e.g. burning out or taking detrimental short cuts in practice is in place, creating an environment that is empathetic and facilitates constructive critique.

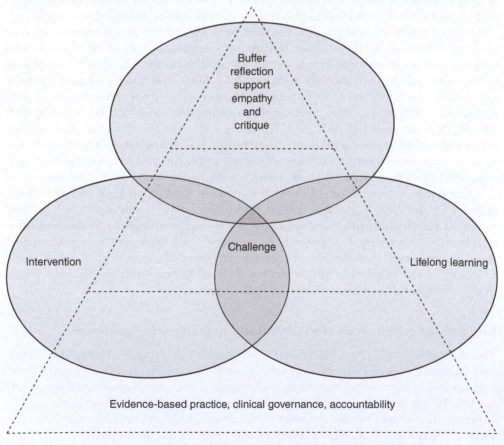

Figure 10.1 Convergence model of clinical supervision (source: Bishop 2007: 45).

- *Block 2.* The importance of formative and normative interactions that affect clinical interventions – those of lifelong learning, being up to date on your work, using research and challenging out-of-date practices are firmly in place, being integral to good CS.
- *Block 3.* All of which feed into and from personal professional development, underpinned with evidence-based practice that informs clinical governance. Each individual must find their connection with standard setting within their organisation, be it through their line manager or through staff within their clinical speciality. *Clinical governance is not solely for the board room – it is a matter of personal professional accountability and while it is incumbent on the employing organisation to facilitate CS, its effectiveness is dependent on staff involvement with standards of care.*

This convergence of theories and concepts places the practitioner firmly in the centre of the organisation, while maintaining their personal cycle of professional development, and points to quality patient care. However, remember 'models' in themselves are no value unless they are used to guide a philosophy or plan of action!

Convergence model of clinical supervision: clinical excellence

- *Normative, formative and restorative functions.*
- *Support, buffer mechanisms, empathy.*
- *Reflection, feedback, critique, advice.*
- *Challenge and intervention.*
- *Clinical governance, standard setting, evidence-based practice, accountability.*

This model offers a framework that integrates staff development, peer review and clinical effectiveness and embraces clinical governance in its totality. It would sit well within the Magnet accreditation system developed in 1991 in the United States by the American Nurses Credentialing Centre (ANCC).

Magnet hospitals

The publication of the first 'Magnet hospital' report in 1983 (McClune *et al.* 1983) had a marked effect, coming at a time of severe nursing shortages in the US. As Buchan noted (1999: 102), *'the characteristics identified in the study were not in themselves new but what the report did was emphasize the need to plan for, and integrate, these characteristics within a strategic framework.'* It also provided some research-based confirmation that the identified characteristics were related to organisational success in recruiting and retaining nursing staff. A later series of further comparative studies (Kramer and Schmalenberg 1991; Kramer 1990) identified that nurse turnover and vacancy rates in the Magnet hospitals were significantly lower, and reported nurse job satisfaction higher, than in 'control' hospitals. Later research on Magnet hospitals examined the links between the organisational characteristics of hospitals and outcomes of care, reflecting new priorities in the management of nursing resources in the US. Research in the area had suggested links between lower mortality rates and the organisation and delivery of nursing care, amongst other relevant variables. In a detailed study that attempted to assess the possible link between mortality rates as an indicator, Magnet hospitals were found to have a lower mortality rate for

Medicare patients than the control hospitals (Aiken *et al.* 1994). As Buchan (1999) noted, the significance of this study was that it pushed the policy research agenda on Magnet hospitals into new territory; that of quality of care and organisational efficiency. Since the publication of the work by Aiken *et al.* (1994) the focus on Magnet hospitals has been further increased and taken up by the ANCC who control their sought after accreditation. A nice example of nursing setting the criteria!

More recently, bringing the issue of quality of care and organisational efficiency into the spotlight for nursing again, Rafferty *et al.* (2001) undertook a postal survey of over 1,000 staff nurses in 32 hospitals in England to explore the relationship between interdisciplinary teamwork, nurse autonomy on patient and nurse outcomes, and nurse assessed quality of care. The key variables of nursing autonomy, control over resources, relationships with doctors, emotional exhaustion and decision making were found to correlate with one another as well as having a relationship with nurse-assessed quality of care and nurse satisfaction. Nursing autonomy was positively correlated with better perceptions of the quality of care delivered and higher levels of job satisfaction. Nurses with higher teamwork scores were significantly more likely to be satisfied with their jobs, planned to stay in them, and had lower burnout scores. Higher teamwork scores were associated with higher levels of nurse assessed quality of care, and perceived quality improvement over the last year. A strong association was found between teamwork and autonomy, this interaction suggesting synergy rather than conflict. The results of a study on nurses' support and work performance among 365 nurses in Jordanian hospitals indicated a positive effect on their work when properly supported (Amarneh *et al.* 2010). These are all issues that properly implemented CS should pick up and feed into the clinical governance agenda.

Clinical governance and leadership: a way forward

Ownership of health care is now very diverse with the traditional authority of medical colleagues restrained and with the blurring of many professional boundaries leaving many nurses feeling powerless. While no patient wants a powerless professional taking care of them, nurses who generally have the majority of patient contact tend not to own any significant level of power in policymaking terms. Nursing has been caught in a web of strong threads which stem from such sources as gender stereotyping, medical dominance and inadequate professional leadership (Bishop 2002). With current global changes all health professionals should be playing a central role in making changes that improve their health care system, however Marinker (1994) noted that nursing is not recognised for its leaders and that the ability to guide, direct or lead is a quality often lacking in the nursing profession. Johns (2003) contends that clinical leadership is the cornerstone for innovation and development, and who would dispute him? However, clinical leadership requires courage and support, it will not happen in isolation. Leadership is not a one person act – it is a play for everyone with the energy and inspiration to change for the better what they do where they are, and clinical supervision is the gateway to make this happen! *(For further reading on leadership in health care see Bishop 2009.)* For the purposes of this chapter and to make the essential link between clinical supervision and clinical leadership the following key points are helpful:

- Leadership is essential to the effective functioning of groups and societies.
- Effective leadership involves having a vision, and the passion and intellect to sell it to your peers.
- Leadership, to be successful, must have a power base e.g. knowledge, funding, authority.

(Bishop 2009: 29)

The overt link here is the final point – knowledge. Formal knowledge, tacit knowledge, organisational knowledge, knowledge of oneself – these are the key personal movers and shakers, the essential personal attributes for successful CS. As Cottrell (2001) noted there are conceptual and methodological difficulties that make it very difficult to attribute any change in a client's health status to the actions of an individual practitioner's CS. However, evaluation of CS by a range of researchers and practitioners have found that CS has had a positive effect on their practice and their professional growth (eg. Kemppainen 2000; McCormack and Henderson 2007). Basing her work on the questionnaire developed for a multi-site Department of Health funded study in the 1990s (Butterworth *et al.* 1996), Winstanley (2000) further developed the Manchester Clinical Supervision Scale which now arguably has the largest database available on CS. This is currently being used by White and Winstanley in a randomised controlled trial (RCT) in Australia involving nurses receiving CS in mental health settings (2009). Although the notion that a happy nurse equals a happy patient may be true, it is unlikely to be sufficient basis upon which to construct a compelling argument to introduce, maintain or increase financial resources for clinical supervision. Confidence to do so requires unequivocal evidence of a causal relationship between CS and improved patient outcomes. To this end the RCT will focus not only on outcomes for individual nurses but will also examine the quality of care that they provide, and the effects of both on patient outcomes. Such data will add significantly to the studies previously mentioned. All this may sound a bit academic to those less interested in research but remember it is your ammunition – knowledge!

Moving from theory to practice: how?

This is not rocket science! But it does require real commitment, a shared vision and a lot of reflection and honesty. It is not a 'tick box' activity if it is to be effective, and if it is not effective it is a waste of resources and a lost opportunity to provide better care. Clinical supervision is a mechanism to empower practitioners and requires time and investment. It is not, when properly carried out, a cheap option, but the benefits must be set against the advantages of safe, confident, motivated practitioners. High staff turnover and heavy litigation costs must be a penalty no organisation wants or can afford; consider here the Magnet principles discussed earlier. As has been stated previously (Bishop 1994) clinical supervision is not a substitute for poor management or a back door means of staff appraisal. To be effective it needs strong management commitment and funding for supervisees' time and, at least for supervisory training. If an organisation is not proactive in any initiative the staff are unlikely to perceive it as a useful road to travel. Butterworth *et al.* (1996) in the multi-site study of clinical supervision identified organisational requirements that are essential for the successful implementation of clinical supervision. See Box 10.2.

Box 10.2 Organisational requirements that are essential for the successful implementation of clinical supervision

- Management commitment at every level
- Protected resources in terms of budget, time, manpower and training
- Supervision for supervisors
- Establishment of evaluation techniques
- Application of evaluation data to service management.

Many practitioners are developing the skills of giving an account of practice, through the processes of reflective practice and through attending or taking part in research conferences at local, national and international level. Many nurses to whom I have spoken across the UK who have taken part in clinical supervision say that they have developed an unexpected confidence – a bonus, if you like, over and above the expected support and professional exchange. They attribute this to taking time to examine their work and reflect with another experienced person; the sharing of knowledge and participation in agreed standards of care. The value of this interaction should not be underestimated, but neither should the courage it takes to enter into a challenging yet trusting relationship. Many practitioners have found that after participating in clinical supervision for a while they are far more active in the health care team in which they work and more likely to speak up rather than leave a meeting wishing that they had spoken their view if it did not coincide with more senior staff. The acceptance of one's own accountability is part and parcel of being a professional, as is audit of one's work. The framework of clinical supervision gives nurses the opportunity to reflect on their practice, identify short-comings and build on strengths, and with the confidence gained, to promote the quality of care in their clinical areas and impact on policy decisions.

Conclusion

We have journeyed through the 'whys' and some of the 'hows' of CS, collecting evidence on the way with which to persuade others to travel this route. The advantages to clinical staff are stressed, with the concomitant benefits to patients and clients. Most importantly, here, is the recognition of the value of clinical governance and the connection that can be forged between it and CS. Current work on staff perceptions of their work and patient outcomes serve only to strengthen the argument for the implementation of CS. The convergent model illustrated offers an inclusive format that encompasses the personal as well as the organisational, broadening earlier formats but maintaining their integrity. The importance of leadership in clinical areas as well as in the board room has been stressed. A journey of self-discovery may be considered a luxury that the health care services cannot afford, and indeed were that the case this would be fair comment! But a journey that extends the boundaries of personal knowledge, that impacts positively on the employing organisation and – most importantly – on patients and clients, has to be worthwhile. Travel well...

References

Aiken L., Smith H. and Lake E. (1994), Lower Medicare mortality among a set of hospitals known for good nursing care, *Medical Care*, 32(8): 771–787.

Amarneh, B.H., Abu Al-Rub, R.F. and Al-Rub, N.F. (2010), Co-workers' support and job performance among nurses in Jordanian hospitals, *Journal of Research in Nursing* (in press).

Berwick, D.M. (2004), *NHS Live Masterclass*, online, available at: www.doh.gov.uk.

Bishop, V. (1994), Clinical supervision for an accountable profession, *Nursing Times*, 90(39): 35–37.

Bishop, V. (1998), Clinical supervision: what is it? in V. Bishop (ed.), *Clinical Supervision in Practice: Some Questions, Answers and Guidelines*, Basingstoke: Macmillan/NTResearch.

Bishop, V. (2002), Editorial, *Journal of Research in Nursing* (formerly *Nursing Times Research*), 7(4): 240.

Bishop, V. (2007) *Clinical Supervision in Practice: Some Questions, Answers and Guidelines for Professionals in Health and Social Care*, 2nd edn, Basingstoke: Palgrave Macmillan.

Bishop, V. (2009), What is leadership? in V. Bishop (ed.), *Leadership for the Nursing and Allied Health Care Professions*, Maidenhead: McGraw Hill.

Buchan, J. (1999), Still attractive after all these years? Magnet hospitals in a changing health care environment, *Journal of Advanced Nursing*, 30(1): 100–108.

Butterworth, C.A., Carson, J., White, E., Jeacock, J., Clements, A. and Bishop, V. (1996), *It is Good to Talk. The 23 Site Evaluation Project of Clinical Supervision in England and Scotland*, Manchester: Manchester University.

Butterworth, T. (1992), Clinical supervision as an emerging idea in nursing, in T. Butterworth and J. Faugier (eds), *Clinical Supervision and Mentorship in Nursing*, London: Chapman & Hall.

Butterworth, T. and Bishop, V. (1995), Identifying the characteristics of optimum practice: findings from a survey of practice experts in nursing, midwifery and health visiting, *Journal of Advanced Nursing*, 22(1): 24–32.

Cottrell, S. (2001), Occupational stress and job satisfaction in mental health nursing, *Journal of Psychiatric and Mental Health Nursing*, 8(2): 157–164.

Department of Health (1998), *A First Class Service: Quality in the New NHS*, London: Department of Health.

Department of Health (2008), *High Quality Care for All: NHS Next Stage Review*, Darzi Final Report, London: Department of Health.

Donabedian, A. (1990), The seven pillars of quality, *Archives of Pathology and Laboratory Medicine*, 114(11): 1115–1118.

Freshwater, D. (2007), Reflective practice and clinical supervision, in V. Bishop (ed.), *Clinical Supervision in Practice: Some Questions, Answers and Guidelines for Professionals in Health and Social Care*.

Johns, C. (2003), Clinical supervision as a model for clinical leadership, *Journal of Nursing Management*, 11(1): 25–35.

Journal of Research in Nursing (2009), *Special Issue: Safety, Quality and Effectiveness*. 14(4), London: Sage Publications.

Kemppainen, J. (2002), The critical incident technique and nursing care quality research, *Journal of Advanced Nursing*, 32(5): 1264–1271.

Kramer, M. (1990), The Magnet hospitals: excellence revisited, *Journal of Nursing Administration*, 20(9) 35–44.

Kramer, M. and Schmalenberg, C. (1991), Job satisfaction and retention: insights for the 1990s, *Nursing*, 21(3): 50–54.

Marinker, M. (1994), *Controversies in Health Care Policies: Challenges to Practice*, London: BMJ Publishing Group.

McClure, M., Poulin, M., Sovie, M. and Wandelt, M. (1983), *Magnet Hospitals: Attraction, Retention of Professional Nurses*, Kansas City, MO: American Academy of Nursing.

McCormack, B. and Henderson, L. (2007), Critical reflection and clinical supervision: facilitating transformation, in V. Bishop (ed.), *Clinical Supervision in Practice: Some Questions, Answers and Guidelines for Professionals in Health and Social Care.*

Power, S. (1999), *Nursing Supervision: A Guide for Clinical Practice*, London: Sage.

Proctor, B. (1988), *Supervision: a cooperative exercise in accountability*, in M. Marken and M. Payne (eds), *Enabling and Ensuring*, Leicester: Leicester National Youth Bureau and Council for Education and Training in Youth and Community Work, pp. 21–34.

Rafferty, A.M., Ball, J. and Aitken, L.H. (2001), Are teamwork and professional autonomy compatible, and do they result in improved hospital care? *Quality in Health Care*, 10(Supplement II): ii32–ii37, online, available at: www.ncbi.nlm. nih.gov/pmc/articles/PMC1765758/pdf/v010p0ii32.pd.

Sarafino, E.P. (2002), *Health Psychology: Biopsychosocial Interactions*, 4th edn, New York: Wiley & Sons.

Scally, G. and Donaldson, L.J. (1998), Clinical governance and the drive for quality improvement in the new NHS in England, *British Medical Journal*, 317 (7150): 61–65.

Scott, I. (2001), Clinical governance: a framework and models for practice, in V. Bishop and I. Scott (eds), *Challenges in Clinical Practice*, Basingstoke: Palgrave Macmillan.

Stanley, D. (2009), Leadership and management: a new mutiny? in V. Bishop (ed.), *Leadership for the Nursing and Health Care Professionals*, Maidenhead: McGraw Hill.

White, E. and Winstanley, J. (2009), Clinical supervision for nurses working in mental health settings in Queensland, Australia: a randomised controlled trial in progress and emergent challenges, *Journal of Research in Nursing*, 14(3): 263–276.

Winstanley, J. (2000), Manchester supervision scale, *Nursing Standard*, 14(19): 31–32.

11 Implementing clinical supervision in a National Health Service Community Trust
Sharing the vision

Jenny Bennett, Bob Gardener and Fiona James

This chapter outlines how a group of practitioners (lead professionals) facilitated the widespread implementation and development of clinical supervision within a NHS Community Trust. Drawing on the experiences of health visitors, general nurses and community psychiatric nurses, the authors describe the phases or stages of this implementation process. Furthermore, they describe their particular roles involved in the implementation and use case examples of the introduction of clinical supervision into each practice discipline. The chapter concludes with reflections on the implementation process and identifies some of the barriers to introducing clinical supervision.

The widespread introduction of clinical supervision within the NHS is not a development that can be introduced using a 'quick fix' technique. We believe that in order to bring about the widespread introduction, a shift in culture throughout the NHS may be required, a shift towards a culture that welcomes and encourages the examination of one's practice, the ventilation of any feelings, openness and transparency within practitioners, and views such endeavours as supportive, necessary and enabling.

Introduction

This chapter describes how a group of three lead professionals underwent the task of facilitating the implementation and development of clinical supervision (CS) within our Community Health Care Trust. Our organisation is a Community Trust including several community hospitals which serves a wide geographical area with both rural and urban locations with a population of 370,000. Our roles as lead professionals were new within our organisation and were part of the Quality and Professional Development Directorate, which took the lead on the clinical governance agenda. We had specific responsibility for the facilitation of professional and practice development within our nursing disciplines of community hospital nursing, mental health nursing and health visiting.

A central aspect of the role of lead professional for the first two years of the post was the promotion, implementation and development of CS. We were to focus on our own nursing disciplines but also to forward recommendations for the long-term strategic implementation of CS throughout the organisation. Our implementation plans were guided by:

- *The national United Kingdom picture* – responding to national policy documents on the health service and the development of nursing which highlighted the need for lifelong learning and the role of CS in providing a quality service (UKCC 1996; Department of Health 1997, 1998).

- *Local picture* – within our organisation a comprehensive nursing review had recently been conducted, guided by the document *A Vision for the Future* (Department of Health and NHS Management Executive 1993). All of the nursing disciplines involved in our Community Trust identified a role for CS in supporting clinical practice and a major recommendation was to plan for its introduction.

Throughout this chapter we therefore describe how we worked in our own nursing disciplines to facilitate the implementation of CS. This involved working with community mental health teams, health visitors working within primary health care teams and the wards/departments of community hospitals.

Planning

Following our appointment as lead professionals we allocated time to enable all three of us to have a full discussion and debate on CS. This was guided by our experience of CS, our own beliefs about its value and limitations, discussions with other colleagues and the extant literature on CS. As a group we had a shared belief in the value of CS to be able to provide a pathway to improving the quality of services provided by clinicians. We debated the role, purpose and function of CS and adopted the three interactive elements of educative, supportive and personal management and monitoring, as the primary functions of CS depicted in Proctor's model (1991; see also Chapter 3 in this book). We found that this common understanding and agreement on the function of CS was essential in enabling us to share a vision of how we could facilitate the implementation and development of CS and communicate this to others.

We used the knowledge and understanding we had gained during our discussion to produce a project plan. The stages of the rational planning process, described in Box 11.1, guided the production of our project plan:

Box 11.1 Identified stages of the planning process

- What are we trying to do?
- What is the best way of doing it?
- What are we going to have to do?
- In what order?
- What resources will we need?
- Let's review it: is it going to work?
- Who is going to do what and when?

Through this planning process we were able to identify the practical tasks we would need to undertake and the personal, professional and organisational issues we would need to address. We set ourselves clear objectives with timescales for review. *A central tenet supporting the project plan was for us to openly express our enthusiasm for and belief in CS, inspiring others to be involved in developing a true shared vision of the potential of CS in enhancing the quality of clinical practice.* A shared vision has been shown to be an important element in achieving successful organisational change (Kouzes and Posner 1995; Poole *et al.* 2000). We would be seeking to develop relationships that encouraged others to become actively involved and inspired to participate in the change process. Bass and Avolio (1994) and Guastello (1995) describe how this approach can transform work areas to become more productive and more responsive to change.

In her discussion on introducing CS, Kohner (1994) highlighted the need for all staff (clinician, managers and administrators) to be involved in the local process of planning for its introduction. We wanted to engender an approach to change that encouraged commitment and used the strengths and creative ideas of practitioners. Therefore our approach to the implementation and development of CS was to encourage its introduction from the practitioner level in the first instance and was underpinned by the following principles:

1   To build on the good practice that was already taking place within the organisation with respect to CS.
2   To provide information, advice and support to practitioners that would facilitate individual areas to make informed decisions as regard to the implementation and development of CS.
3   To respond enthusiastically to the positive requests from individual areas within our organisation with regard to their desire to implement/develop CS.
4   Where available, to work alongside clinical leaders in individual areas to develop their knowledge base and experience, promoting local ownership and their role and strengths as change agents.
5   To use a flexible approach that was responsive and sensitive to practitioners' level of knowledge, experience and professional confidence.

Using these as our guiding principles we reflected on what our roles as leaders and facilitators in the implementation process should involve. We identified the following key elements:

1   *Change agent*
    To act as key change agents with a formal responsibility for advising on the implementation and development of CS. Our leadership style would promote ownership and commitment by individuals in local areas, building on their strengths and talents.
2   *Partner*
    To work alongside practitioners and managers to meet shared objectives.
3   *Educator*
    To organise and deliver informal and formal training on the role, function and benefits of clinical supervision.
4   *Advisor and supporter*
    To develop a resource library on CS and respond to managers' and practitioners' requests for information and support.
5   *Communicator*
    To ensure managers and practitioners are informed of the local and organisational developments regarding CS.

6   *Networker and co-ordinator*
   To promote the sharing of good practice across the organisation and the
   sharing of strategies to overcome difficulties.

Establishing a baseline

One of our first tasks on the project plan was to establish what CS was already taking
place within our individual nursing disciplines and what practitioners' knowledge,
thoughts and attitudes were regarding CS. We devised a comprehensive questionnaire, based on the issues identified in a review of the relevant theoretical and
empirical literature, in conjunction with the clinical audit and research team and
sent this to all practitioners in our disciplines. In total 377 questionnaires were distributed and there was an overall response rate of 55 per cent. This was an encouraging response and perhaps reflected a positive attitude towards CS which was
evident in the qualitative sections of the questionnaire. The questionnaire covered
areas such as: baseline provision, practitioners' level of knowledge and understanding and their views as to how CS should be developed further. The results highlighted an overall lack of knowledge and experience with regard to CS and
therefore a high level of training needs. However, within community mental health
teams, CS was established though its purpose and content was in need of review.
Guided by the results we devised a flexible introductory training package on CS and
decided to meet with all areas to give individuals within these the opportunity to be
informed about CS and take part in its implementation.

Sharing the vision

We therefore visited individual areas and were enthusiastic to inspire others in our
belief that CS had a valuable contribution to make in improving the quality of
service we provide. We initially targeted receptive clinical leaders or teams that we
had identified through meetings during our induction as lead professionals or by
direct interest that we had received. *Working with individuals that had a positive interest
enabled us to initiate a change process and these individuals were able to act as motivators
and role models for others.* While we had a desire to share our enthusiasm it was important that during our initial meetings with individuals we actively listened to their
beliefs and opinions about the functions of CS, the implementation process and
their expectations of us. This proved essential to the development of shared and
realistic implementation plans. Time was spent discussing and clarifying all aspects
of CS that we had uncovered in our review of the literature/personal discussions. It
was important that there was a shared understanding of the aims and functions of
CS and its potential impact upon clinicians' practice and development. Our
approach in supporting the development of local implementation plans was to
empower clinicians/managers/administrators to reflect on their current situation
and be enthusiastic about what could be achieved. Their central role in the implementation process was reinforced and we informed them that we were available to
provide them with help, advice and formal training. When discussing the implementation process there was open and honest communication regarding the difficulties
that could be encountered.

Case study examples

Below are three examples that illustrate the implementation process in action in each of our respective disciplines. As discussed previously, to support this work we provided awareness-raising sessions across the organisation. These sessions were organised around individual areas' work patterns so that they were accessible to as many practitioners as possible. We also provided more in-depth supervisee and supervisor training as requested. The provision of a formal clinical supervisor's course for practitioners from all nursing disciplines was then purchased from a local university and following on from the success of this, a contract was agreed for them to provide further courses.

Example one: health visiting

The results of the baseline questionnaire highlighted that the majority of health visitors within the organisation did not, at the time of the data collection, give or receive CS. Of those that did report being involved in the process of CS, the results of the questionnaire suggested that there were different interpretations of the term amongst health visitors including confusion with 'mentorship' and 'child protection supervision'. It was identified that there was a need to clarify and clearly define what is meant by the term CS and, in addition, its aims and objectives, with 62 per cent of health visitors reporting that they had only an average knowledge of CS and 20 per cent reporting having a poor knowledge base. Overall, however, health visitors were positive about the concept of CS and welcomed its introduction into practice.

Within the organisation, health visitors worked in widespread geographical areas and many were based within individual Primary Health Care Teams. Initial discussions with health visitors across the district raised several key issues and concerns. These included how CS could be organised and resourced within each geographical area, in addition to who would co-ordinate this, as for many areas there was no designated team leader or health visitor with a practice development role. There was also a debate as to which health visitors would become clinical supervisors of others and whether one-to-one, group or peer supervision would be the most appropriate format for health visitors. There was also the issue that no one was trained as a supervisor. Reflection on these discussions highlighted that there was a diversity of opinions amongst health visitors as to a strategic way forward in health visiting and that there was no easy solution to these questions.

Returning to the principles that we had set in our initial discussions as lead professionals and a certain level of pragmatism proved to be the way forward. As lead professional, I wrote to all health visitors offering them the opportunity to become a 'pilot site' for CS with support and access to individual training. One group of health visitors who worked together in a clinic setting came forward requesting to undertake peer group CS. Within this group, one health visitor did have some previous experience of CS and a further health visitor had previously received some training. Two morning (half-day) workshops were spent exploring the concept of CS, models of reflection, contracting and documentation and how to conduct a group session. The health visitors were keen to proceed and began meeting on a monthly basis with regular review. Their continued interest and motivation was essential to the success of this pilot.

Simultaneously, four health visitors from different geographical locations were invited to attend the external clinical supervisor's course. Nominations were requested from individuals who would be prepared to undertake this role after completion of the course and act as champions for CS in their area. These health visitors formed a supportive group and it was arranged for them to receive group CS from an external supervisor for six months following the course. This gave the health visitors valuable experience in receiving CS and proved to be very successful in building up their confidence, particularly in CS. During these six months, I organised supervisee training workshops in each of the geographical locations and conducted these alongside the four 'champion' health visitors. The aim of these sessions was to support them in facilitating their colleagues' knowledge of and interest in CS and to encourage other health visitors to either receive CS or to attend supervisor training. The result of this was very positive as health visitors wanting to receive CS approached the four 'champion' clinical supervisors and they have set up both one-to-one and group CS, depending on what was requested, with a small number of health visitors in their area. In addition, the 'champion' supervisors continued to meet for peer group CS.

Through individual health visitors beginning to set up CS arrangements on either a one-to-one or group basis, more health visitors were becoming aware of the purpose and benefits of CS and were either requesting their own CS or attending clinical supervisor training. The implementation was therefore an incremental process and it evolved, flexibly, with input and participation from health visitors and in response to local needs.

Example two: community hospitals

This section describes three examples of how ward nurses introduced CS. They illustrate that a diverse approach to the implementation of CS was taken within community hospitals.

It is important to note that prior to implementing CS in the community hospitals, a selection of nurses from such facilities attended a leadership course. This acted as a catalyst for discussion on CS. These nurses identified that they would need to experience CS for themselves before being able to develop CS in/on their ward and day hospital areas. Monthly, one-to-one external CS was subsequently purchased by the organisation for a fixed period of six months. Several of the nurses who had experienced the external CS put forward formal plans to implement CS into their wards and day hospitals. They adopted different approaches, according to their view of local needs as shown by the following examples.

One ward manager decided to supervise all the qualified nurses on their ward for a fixed period of time and then review the whole process. As the lead professional for this clinical area, I made the ward manager aware of the constraints of hierarchical supervision: the ward manager put forward a logical reason for this approach. The ward manager felt it was a starting point, as initially there were no CS available and it would be a good way to demonstrate to ward nurses that dedicated time was available for them to reflect on their practice. The longer-term aim was to train nurses from the ward to become supervisors, then ultimately removing the hierarchical structure.

The second example involves a manager from another community hospital who allocated supervisors to all nurses. The rationale for this approach was, in the manager's words, 'to get CS started in our hospital'. As the lead professional for this clinical area, I discussed and challenged this approach making the manager aware that it was important that nurses should be actively involved and own the implementation process. However, the manager continued with this approach and I advised him that they should consider reviewing progress at an early date.

In the third example, a ward manager encouraged and supported two nurses from the ward to receive CS from the lead professionals. In time, one of the practitioners went on to facilitate group supervision for four ward colleagues. This approach to implementation has proved successful and it continues to meet.

Example three: mental health – community team

The lead professional for mental health nursing met with all the Community Mental Health Teams (CMHT) within our organisation. The following is a brief outline of the discussions with one specific team, which highlights the issues facing the majority of the teams. The key discussion points were guided by the results of the questionnaire, and the discussions occurred within meetings with the lead nurse within the CMHT and with all the CMHT nurses.

On a positive note, the majority of nurses reported that they were receiving CS on an individual basis, at monthly intervals. While there were nurses who reported they were not receiving CS on a monthly basis, this was the frequency they were aiming for. There was a history of CS taking place within the CMHT and it was valued and seen as 'much needed'. However, there were issues raised by the lead nurse and the nurses within the CMHT as to the way CS was organised and carried out.

The lead nurse within the CMHT, who had designated management responsibility for all the nurses, provided clinical and management supervision within one session, dividing the time between both areas. This structure of provision had developed in an unplanned way and was a response to a rapid increase in the number of nurses working within the CMHT, who needed both types of supervision. Interestingly, the nurses expressed (anecdotally) a positive view of the CS they received from the lead nurse. *However there was confusion between clinical and management supervision and concern that the sessions were dominated by management issues.*

Other issues that arose out of the discussions were that prior to commencement of CS there had been no contract drawn up between the clinical supervisor and supervisee, and that in the subsequent session, little or no documentation was used. It was also apparent that there was no choice of clinical supervisor. The lead nurse within the CMHT was motivated to further explore the issues raised by the discussions and the results from the questionnaires. I therefore continued to meet with the lead nurse, providing written information and offering guidance about the issues that had been raised. The lead nurse, after discussion with the nurses from the CMHT, decided to implement the following changes:

1 CS would be held separately from management supervision.
2 Management supervision would be termed caseload management.
3 The lead nurse within the CMHT would continue to be clinical supervisor for all the nurses but it had been openly acknowledged that there could be potential conflict in a line manager providing CS.

4   The supervisee would be responsible for setting the agenda within the CS sessions. The lead nurse had provided all nurses with a booklet in which to document the sessions. This was their property and they were encouraged to use it in support of their professional portfolio.
5   A contract would be drawn up based around the discussions that had taken place as to the aim and function of CS; sample contracts were available to the team.

While it should not be regarded as a formal evaluation, numerous positive verbal comments from the lead nurse and by some of the nurses from the CMHT were forthcoming, especially indicating that the changes allowed them to focus and reflect on their issues with regard to clinical practice.

In implementing these changes, the lead nurse within the CMHT has been able to promote clarity as to the function of CS and caseload management and as to how both processes can be used to support the nurses in their demanding role. The lead nurse dealt positively with the change process and educated his manager as to the need for and benefit of the changes made.

Finally two other points raised are worthy of mention. First, while most nurses had some experience of CS, very few had received any formal education/training. Second, some nurses identified a need for 'specialist' clinical supervision to enable them to practice a specific therapeutic approach i.e. Cognitive Behavioral Therapy.

Reflections on the implementation process

There are relatively few studies that specifically discuss the local implementation of CS (Fowler 1996). Authors have generally highlighted specific areas that need considering and/or potential problems that need to be overcome (Devine and Baxter 1995). Below are our reflections on the process of facilitating the local implementation of CS. Our aim during the first year of the implementation process within our organisation was to develop a culture that supported and valued CS. To add clarity to this, we have divided our discussion into the separate areas of: ownership; developing an organisational approach; and barriers to change.

Ownership

The importance we gave to the need for practitioners to own the implementation process, to value and want CS has proved to be successful. In areas where there are identified clinical leaders motivated to promote CS, the process of implementation moved forward. We have positive examples of areas where CS is now happening on a regular basis and is valued by practitioners. We have since built upon this success, in part by sharing the good practice and positive experiences of CS to other clinical and geographical areas. At an organisational level we are considering how we identify and develop future clinical leaders to progress the implementation of CS in areas where minimal supervision is taking place. The need to maintain local ownership will remain important as will the need to work in partnership with the managers of the service.

Developing an organisational approach

As discussed in our reflections on ownership, in the first instance we were keen to promote individual practitioners' understanding of CS and their role in developing supervision locally. We became acutely aware that this needed to be supported by an organisational approach to CS. Practitioners have an important role in developing CS but they also need the support of managers and the organisation to do this. As we worked with practitioners they raised this issue. For example, practitioners were keen to know that they were entitled to CS and questioned whether there was an organisational policy to support this. They were also requesting standard guidelines for issues such as setting up contracts between the supervisor and supervisee and the documentation of CS sessions.

Throughout the first stages of the implementation process we worked with practitioners' line managers on an individual basis but we also led a formal session for managers on their role in supporting CS and the difference between CS and management supervision. The implementation of CS was seen to need a 'partnership approach' to be successful: both managers and nurses would need to see its value and be committed to its development. In order to promote an organisational strategy for CS, including the provision of resources to ensure that the implementation moved forward, we produced an interim report after 12 months in post. The report detailed current progress with the implementation process and put forward recommendations for a future organisational approach to implementation including resource and training implications. Together with the director and assistant director of nursing we presented the report to the senior management board and the senior nursing and professional advisory groups.

As a result of this process and significant background work, we have made progress in promoting practitioner involvement and local implementation supported by an organisational approach. We now have a written validated CS policy in addition to guidelines on the aims and function of CS; the role and responsibilities of supervisors and supervisees; and the use of documentation. Importantly we have agreement on the need to draw up contracts prior to commencing CS that cover the issues of confidentiality and information that needs to be disclosed/shared and the need for regular review. We have also set up a CS steering group that includes senior management and practitioner representation to strategically take forward the implementation of CS. We formulated a five-year implementation plan and monitored the status and progress of the plan via the CS steering group. This has produced evidence to indicate that local geographical areas have developed implementation plans and as they report on their progress, this evidence has been used to both underscore the benefits of engaging in CS and has also informed (and help revise) our continued implementation process.

Barriers to change

Implementing CS has involved a change process. As with any change process, as lead professionals we were aware that we might encounter barriers to change and resistance. Our leadership approach within our disciplines has aimed to minimise barriers and resistance, and has promoted a positive approach. Our approach of sharing a vision of the potential of CS for nursing practice and promoting

---

Box 11.2 Examples of barriers to change

- Resources: e.g. lack of clinical supervisors
- Individual resistance: e.g. some practitioners expressed that they did not need CS
- Workload factors: e.g. high caseloads, shortage of qualified nurses
- Concurrent change: e.g. other practice developments taking place
- Lack of knowledge: e.g. high level of training needs.

---

practitioner involvement, enabled practitioners to be committed to receive CS and finding realistic ways of achieving its implementation. It would be unrealistic to suggest that we have not encountered barriers. Examples of barriers to change that lead professionals and practitioners have identified are summarised in Box 11.2. These have ranged from individual factors to wider organisational issues.

We have openly recognised these barriers to change and through our ongoing discussions and support within the lead professional team we have developed the following strategies for addressing them:

1   developing supportive relationships with practitioners which encouraged them to identify potential problematic areas and develop creative approaches to deal with them;
2   the use of informal and formal training sessions in an environment that allowed practitioners to openly express their beliefs and concerns regarding CS;
3   developing implementation plans with individuals and their areas that were realistic, achievable and encouraged an incremental approach;
4   building on success and empowering practitioners to motivate their colleagues;
5   our use of self to provide ongoing positive support and encouragement through time of resistance and change.

Conclusion

As a result of our experiences, we would assert that the implementation of CS should not simply be seen as a task that staff need to be trained/educated and then to do; CS should be seen as part of an overall (overarching) framework that enables nurses and others to provide a quality health care service to clients and families. It needs to be introduced into the culture of the organisation, one that promotes individuals to maximise their strength, promotes autonomy and encourages reflection. In order to achieve this culture, managers and practitioners need to work in partnership and the organisation needs to be committed to being a learning organisation that aims to facilitate lifelong learning (Haire 1997). Planning for the implementation of CS therefore needs to include a long-term goal of aiming for it to be become a routine and valued practice.

References

Bass, B.M. and Avolio, B. (1994), *Improving Organisational Effectiveness through Transformational Leadership*, London: Sage.

Department of Health and NHS Management Executive (1993), *Vision for the Future: The Nursing, Midwifery and Health Visiting Contribution to Health and Health Care,* London: HMSO.

Department of Health (1997), *Modern and Dependable,* London: HMSO.

Department of Health (1998), *A First Class Service: Quality in the New NHS,* London: HMSO.

Devine, A. and Baxter, T.D. (1995), Introducing clinical supervision: a guide, *Nursing Standard,* 9(40): 32–34.

Fowler, J. (1996), The organization of clinical supervision within the nursing profession: a review of the literature, *Journal of Advanced Nursing,* 23(3): 471–478.

Haire, C. (1997), Life-long learning, *Nursing Management,* 3(9): 24–25.

Kohner, N. (1994), *Clinical Supervision in Practice,* London: King's Fund Centre.

Guastello, S. (1995), Facilitative style, individual innovation and emergent leadership in problem solving groups, *Journal of Creative Behaviour,* 29(4): 225–239.

Kouzes, J.M. and Posner, B.Z. (1995), *The Leadership Challenge: How to Keep Getting Extraordinary Things Done in Organizations,* San Francisco: Jossey-Bass.

Poole, M.S., Van de Ven, A.H., Dooley, K. and Holmes, M.E. (2000), *Organizational Change and Innovation Processes: Theory and Methods for Research,* Oxford: Oxford University Press.

Proctor, B. (1991), On being a trainer, in W. Dryden and B. Thorne (eds), *Training and Supervision for Counselling in Action,* London: Sage, pp. 49–73.

UKCC (1996), *Position Statement of Clinical Supervision for Nursing and Health Visiting,* London: UKCC.

12 Clinical supervision in the United Kingdom – ten years on

A review of the United Kingdom clinical supervision literature

Graham Sloan

In *Fundamental Themes in Clinical Supervision*, Gilmore (2001) presented a summary of her comprehensive United Kingdom Central Council (UKCC)-commissioned literature review of clinical supervision for nurses and health visitors in the UK. As a logical follow up, this chapter presents a review of the nursing literature relating to clinical supervision which has been published between 1999 and 2009. After reminding readers of the UKCC's (now the Nursing Midwifery Council's) endorsement of clinical supervision, the chapter includes a critical appraisal of both the empirical and conceptual literature, including anecdotal accounts, expert opinion and position papers which have pervaded the nursing literature during the past decade. The chapter concludes with some recommendations on how clinical supervision can be further embedded into nursing practice.

Graham's chapter reminds the editors that while the consensus of the academe is that engaging in high quality clinical supervision brings about significant benefits for supervisees, supervisors, receivers of health care (e.g. clients/patients) and the health care organisations, there remains a high degree of resistance to operationalising clinical supervision in some organisations. This resistance can be underpinned by: economic concerns; inappropriate approaches to operationalising clinical supervision (e.g. top down, hierarchical, cascading models of supervision); a lack of understanding of the purpose and function of clinical supervision; and/or individual practitioner resistance. Clearly, a more developed evidence base is needed to help address some of these problems, as is more open mindedness on the part of some. While the editors are mindful of the economic climate in which health care operates, organisations (and the key individuals within them) might consider the long-term economic benefits of having a healthy and happy health care workforce; something which clinical supervision appears to be able to help bring about.

Acknowledgment

The author would like to express his gratitude to Allan Thompson, assistant psychologist, for his assistance in undertaking a literature search in preparation of writing this chapter.

Introduction

When consideration is given to the multitude of publications describing where and how clinical supervision (CS) has been implemented across the United Kingdom (UK) and the knowledge and experiences from further afield presented throughout some of the chapters of this text, there can be little doubt that familiarity with CS within the discipline of nursing has expanded. In *Fundamental Themes of Clinical Supervision* (Cutcliffe *et al.* 2001), Gilmore (2001) presented a summary of her comprehensive United Kingdom Central Council (UKCC)-commissioned literature review of clinical supervision for nurses and health visitors in the UK. Given that this book is development from *Fundamental Themes in Clinical Supervision*, it is logical to follow Gilmore's original review with a review of the more recently published work, in the hope that this will help identify and enhance our understanding of how the knowledge base of CS has advanced during the intervening years. Accordingly, this chapter presents a review of the nursing literature relating to CS which has been published between 1999 and 2009. An important aim of the review was to develop an appreciation of the recently published literature and the associated knowledge of CS in nursing in the UK. In particular, this chapter focuses on a critical appraisal of both the empirical and conceptual literature, including anecdotal accounts, expert opinion and position papers which have pervaded the nursing literature during the past decade. The chapter will conclude with some recommendations on how CS can be further embedded into nursing practice. First, the UKCC (now the Nursing Midwifery Council's) endorsement of CS will be reiterated.

United Kingdom Central Council's position on clinical supervision

The UKCC (1996) delivered its much-anticipated position statement on CS, clarified the context within which it works and the principles which underpin its implementation. The Council argued that the potential impact on care and professional development for practitioners was enough to warrant investment. *Nonetheless, the UKCC also suggested that possible benefits are not limited to patients, clients or practitioners: 'A more skilled, aware and articulate profession should contribute effectively to organisational objectives' (UKCC 1996: 2).* The six key principles offered by the UKCC (Box 12.1) emphasised CS. Consequently, this fuelled the expectations of academics, managers and practitioners. Not surprisingly, CS has been implemented into a broad range of clinical settings in the UK.

Box 12.1 The UKCC's six key statements (UKCC 1996)

1   Clinical supervision supports practice, enabling practitioners to maintain and promote standards of care.
2   Clinical supervision is a practice-focused professional relationship involving a practitioner reflecting on practice guided by a skilled supervisor.
3   The process of clinical supervision should be developed by practitioners and managers according to local circumstances. Ground rules should be agreed so that practitioners and supervisors approach clinical supervision openly, confidently and are aware of what is involved.
4   Every practitioner should have access to clinical supervision. Each supervisor should supervise a realistic number of practitioners.
5   Preparation of supervisors can be effected using 'in house' or external education programmes. The principles and relevance of clinical supervision should be included in pre- and post-registration education programmes.
6   Evaluation of clinical supervision is needed to assess how it influences care, practice standards and the service. Evaluation systems should be determined locally.

Literature review strategy

A comprehensive search of the literature on CS published during the past decade was conducted. Literature was reviewed from a variety of sources. Keywords to locate literature on computerised databases – CINAHL, Medline, Psychlit and the British Nursing Index included 'supervision', 'clinical supervision', 'support', 'stress', 'relationship', 'evaluation', and 'benefits'. This provided the foundation for the literature search. Reference lists in the literature sourced were also scrutinised for any potentially unlisted or inaccessible sources. A manual scrutiny of more recent journals was conducted to ensure that potential sources not yet listed in the computerised databases had not been overlooked. This search strategy was supplemented by networking via email with researchers and educators from the international community. The Internet was also used to obtain useful resources related to the field of interest.

Clinical supervision: growing popularity in nursing

The increasing popularity of CS in nursing has been evidenced by the plethora of articles featured in the leading nursing journals and the publication of related texts and policy statements. Some of this work has attempted to demystify the concept (Lyth 2000). While its implementation appears to be widespread (Clough 2001; Spence *et al.* 2002), sizeable proportions of nurses claim never to have received CS (Davey *et al.* 2006). There have been descriptions of specific CS models (Sloan *et al.* 2000; Proctor 2001). While some have challenged the way in which CS is represented in nursing in the UK (Yegdich 1999), others suggest a multitude of alleged benefits.

Formats and frameworks

Reports of how CS has been introduced to district nursing, health visiting, mental health nursing, older adult mental health services, intensive care nursing, a day-surgery unit, a haematology nursing development unit, theatre nursing, occupational health nursing and practice nursing have been published (see, for example, Styles and Gibson 1999; Ashmore and Carver 2000; Clough 2001; Spence *et al.* 2002). Descriptions of its implementation into these nursing contexts reveal that CS can be delivered in a variety of formats.

CS delivered in a one-to-one format is probably the most common mode of delivery in nursing in the UK (Edwards *et al.* 2005; Sloan 2006; Ho 2007; Sines and McNally 2007). In this context, and in keeping with UKCC (1996) recommendations, the clinical supervisor is often a nurse. More often than not, the supervisor is also the supervisee's line-manager (Duncan-Grant 2003; Sines and McNally 2007; Sloan 2006; Rouse 2007), something according to Bishop (2006) that is contrary to initial policy spirit and professional ideals. Though less common, descriptions of group and triad formats have been published (Price and Chalker 2000; Sloan *et al.* 2000) as have examples of when the supervisor has been provided by another health care professional (Sloan *et al.* 2000).

Results from a validation study of the Manchester Clinical Supervision Scale support the view that supervision sessions should be of significant length to be effective, recommending that clinical supervision should be either monthly or bi-monthly in frequency and, at the least, last for an hour (Winstanley and White 2003). For community staff there may be some benefit from extending supervision sessions to last longer than one hour. Similarly Edwards *et al.* (2005) highlighted that when sessions lasted longer than an hour and were provided monthly, clinical supervision was evaluated as being more effective. Achieving this goal, according to Edwards *et al.* (2005), will involve both organisational and cultural change. *Moreover, it will require significant investment and creativity in developing an adequate resource to enable the provision of effective clinical supervision. While it is encouraging to have such recommendations, when agreements between supervisee and clinical supervisor are established, consideration of the supervisee's work context, developmental level, complexity of clients, learning needs and the supervisor's availability should also be taken into account when establishing the duration and frequency of clinical supervision.*

Conceptual frameworks

Consideration has been given to the frameworks guiding the delivery of CS. There are few theoretical frameworks that specifically explain the processes of CS as adopted in nursing. However, some nurse scholars have suggested frameworks used by other professional groups to conceptualise the purposes and processes of CS. Proctor's model (1987) is probably the most frequently cited CS model in the UK nursing press (see for example, Davey *et al.* 2006; Buus and Gonge 2009). Using this model, supervisors can focus on all or any one of three areas at any time. In nursing's adoption of this model, the *formative* function is concerned with skills development and increasing the supervisee's knowledge; the *normative* function concentrates on managerial issues including the maintenance of professional standards and the *restorative* function is focused on providing support in an attempt to alleviate the stress evoked by doing nursing work. The original description of the three-function interactive model (Proctor 1987) did not provide any guidance on how a clinical supervisor might operate when working within any of its three functions. However, the supervision alliance model (Proctor 2001) clarifies how supervisors might provide helpful responses when guided by this framework.

Advancing earlier work (see, for example, Fowler 1996; Cutcliffe and Epling 1997), Driscoll (2000) described a model based on Heron's (1989) six-category intervention analysis. This model, as a CS framework, has been subjected to at least one study in the UK. Devitt (1998) explored the nature of the supervisory relationship and the labour of supervision through the eyes of the supervisor, using a grounded theory approach. Analysis of data from a focus group, self-reported reflective diaries and in-depth interviews highlighted that prescriptive and informative interventions (authoritative interventions) were used most frequently. This was inconsistent with an initial agreement that the use of Heron's framework should be limited to the use of four of the six categories, confronting, cathartic, catalytic and supportive (mainly facilitative interventions).

Another CS framework, taken from psychotherapy and adapted for nursing, is the cognitive therapy supervision model (Todd and Freshwater 1999; Sloan *et al.* 2000; Sloan 2006). While Todd and Freshwater (1999) illustrated the similarities between reflective practice and guided discovery, Sloan *et al.* (2000) clarified that while the approach was devised to help develop the therapeutic competence of cognitive therapists, its use in nursing contexts merits consideration.

This model differentiates between modes and foci (Padesky 1996). A supervision mode is the means by which supervisee learning and discovery occurs, for example, case discussion (nursing care), reviewing audio recordings of therapy sessions (nurse-patient interactions) or the provision of relevant educational material. The focus can include the mastering of new therapeutic skills (nursing interventions), conceptualising a client's problems (care plan), progressing the therapist's under-standing of the client–therapist relationship (nurse–patient relationship) and working through the therapist's (nurse's) emotional reactions to their clinical work. These modes and foci appear relevant for the practice of CS in nursing where clini-cal practice has a therapeutic intention and it is recognised that knowledge and skills may develop as a result of practitioners reflecting on their interpersonal rela-tions with clients. It has been argued that cognitive therapy CS, by addressing both the processes and content of CS, highlights its essential purpose: the development of the supervisee's therapeutic competence (Sloan *et al.* 2000).

There has been a gradual increase in the number of conceptual models described in the nursing press (Spence *et al.* 2002), but research investigating their utility and effectiveness is scarce. To date, nursing research has focused almost exclusively on Proctor's framework; future investigations should consider exploration and evalu-ation of alternative frameworks. Nonetheless, regardless of which framework has been adopted, and irrespective of an absence of research supporting its efficacy, CS is considered to have far-reaching benefits and potential outcomes. A great deal has been written about the expectations for CS and a plethora of anecdotal accounts are depicted in the literature.

Great expectations or a heavy burden?

By introducing formalised CS, anecdotal accounts and expert opinion suggest that nursing staff will develop their clinical competence and knowledge base (Ashmore and Carver 2000), experience less stress, burnout and sickness absence (Winstanley 1999). There has also been speculation that patient care will be improved (Jones 2006; Alleyne and Jumaa 2007) and that it provides opportunity for nurses to reflect on practice (Ashmore and Carver 2000; Jones 2006). Additional potential benefits of clinical supervision are its use as a risk management tool (Herron 2000) and the promotion of the clinical governance agenda (McSherry *et al.* 2002).

There is a dearth of published research evidence to support many of these claims (Gallinagh and Campbell 1999; Buus and Gonge 2009). In the UK, CS is considered an effective means of reducing nurses' experience of stress and burnout and that it facilitates knowledge development and skills acquisition (Butterworth *et al.* 1997). Since previous reviews have summarised these works (see, for example, Sloan 2006) this review concentrates on some of the contextual and process-focused investiga-tions that have been conducted in the past ten years. Some studies have attempted to clarify factors that contribute to the effectiveness of CS.

Effectiveness literature

Using the Manchester Clinical Supervision scale, Edwards *et al.* (2005) reported from a sample of 260 (32 per cent) community mental health nurses that CS was more positively evaluated where sessions lasted for over one hour and took place on at least a once-monthly basis. *Perceived quality of CS was also higher for those nurses who had chosen their clinical supervisor and where sessions took place away from the workplace. Time, space and choice emerge as important factors influencing the effective provision of CS.*

Following a survey of current CS practice with stakeholders in Northern Ireland, including all twelve mental health trust directors and all heads of education, Rice *et al.* (2007) formulated a number of best practice guidelines. All participants reported experiencing problems implementing the guidelines. A lack of information on the development and introduction of the guidelines contributed to fear and apprehension of engaging in CS among mental health nurses. However, respondents felt that implementing the following recommendations would be useful:

- A definition of CS should be agreed.
- Managers should ensure that practitioners are facilitated to participate in CS.
- Managers should ensure that robust operational policies are put in place in their organisations.
- Operational policies should include contracting arrangements between supervisor and supervisee.
- Organisations should provide appropriate time within the working day for CS.
- Supervisors must have sound clinical skills, a strong knowledge base and be a practicing clinical nurse.
- Supervisors should demonstrate clear commitment to the role of clinical supervisor.
- Supervisors should have the capacity to inspire supervisees to reflect on and evaluate their clinical and therapeutic work.
- Supervisors should complete recognised training.
- Trusts should evaluate and monitor impact of CS.
- Supervisors and supervisees should agree a mechanism for collecting data and information that would inform the evaluation.
- Though a difficult task, obtaining and including patient/client feedback may be worth considering.

Contextual and process-focused investigations

Aspects of the health care environment and its influence on how nurses receive CS have been generally overlooked. Nevertheless, there is a growing body of literature that has uncovered a number of organisational dynamics (barriers) affecting the successful implementation of effective CS.

Barriers to the implementation of clinical supervision

In the UK it is common for supervisory arrangements to be hierarchical (Cutcliffe 2000; Sloan 1999, 2006; Duncan-Grant 2000; Kelly *et al.* 2001; Bishop 2006; Davey *et al.* 2006; Rice *et al.* 2007; Sines and McNally 2007). While there is some support for a management-led model for the delivery of CS (Darley 2001), there are many others who suggest managerial supervision should exist parallel to, not concomitant with, clinical supervision (Yegdich 1999; Cutcliffe 2000; Cutcliffe and Hyrkäs 2006). It has been identified that management agendas pervade discussions during clinical supervision (Sloan 1999, 2006; Duncan-Grant 2000; Kelly *et al.* 2001). Moreover, the hierarchical provision of CS appears to have had some negative influence on how nurses experience engaging in CS. According to O'Riordan (2002) staff withdrew from CS as a result of the supervisor being an insider to the unit and because it was hierarchical. Furthermore, CS was viewed negatively as it involved feeding back to management, was associated with a sense of being watched, and did not appear to be regarded by management as important (Rouse 2007). Sloan's (2006) investigation found that CS discussions were filled with talk about performance appraisals, professional development planning, annual leave and off duty and staff relations. Managerial agendas overshadowed clinical issues. *Such hierarchical provision is predetermined and therefore contrary to the notion that the supervisee should have some choice regarding a clinical supervisor.*

Duncan-Grant (2000) argued that hierarchy within the organisation in particular appears to poison the spirit and operation of CS for mental health nurses. It is suggested that this leads to an absence of ownership at all levels, tension between managers and staff and resistance among staff to a process that should, according to the literature, be to their benefit. More recently, Duncan-Grant (2003) proposed that problematic organisational dynamics will continue to undermine and threaten the successful implementation of CS.

As a result of the lack of acknowledgement having been given to the broader organisational and cultural context within which CS takes place, there has been a failure to appreciate how this may shape CS practice. Within the hierarchical cascading forms of CS, supervisees manage the supervision agenda by focusing on 'safe talk' (Duncan-Grant 2003). Consequently, discussions related to direct client care are overshadowed by other agendas (Sloan 2006). Ultimately this threatens any possibility of reflection on client care.

Following a systematic literature review of CS in psychiatric nursing, which included some of the empirical studies conducted in UK, Buus and Gonge (2009) argued that the lack of consensus on a definition of CS is the most serious obstacle for developing the field. *Perhaps the lack of an agreed definition delineating its core essence is the most significant barrier affecting the successful implementation of effective CS. It is suggested that absence of such clarity has and will continue to influence how CS is applied, the frameworks guiding its delivery, expectations on what it can achieve and ultimately the training programmes for its participants.*

Training practitioners for their engagement in clinical supervision

As described in Chapter 7 the content and methods of delivering sufficient or adequate training for CS in nursing in the UK remain elusive. There has been an absence of guidance on the content of training for CS; the published material varies considerably in its mode of delivery and duration. It is argued that developing the opportunities of CS training will contribute to increasing the availability of adequately trained clinical supervisors, its effective delivery, support a counter-challenge to the unhelpful dynamics that serve as a significant barrier to, and therefore the realisation of, useful practice-focused outcomes.

There are some who argue that the success of CS is greatly dependent on the clinical supervisor (Gilmore 2001). Consequently, training opportunities are often confined to clinical supervisors. It is noteworthy that CS is not something done to the supervisee; rather it is a process to which both supervisor and supervisee can contribute. Interestingly, the supervisees' contribution to their CS, by endeavouring to prepare for it, having their own agenda items and attempting to introduce these into the discussion and, demonstrating knowledge of the issues discussed, was highlighted in a qualitative investigation (Sloan 2006). It is suggested that training opportunities should be made available to both supervisors and supervisees. Unsurprisingly, the supervisee–supervisor dyad has, to some extent, been overlooked.

The supervisory relationship

In nursing, the supervisory relationship is regarded as an important aspect of CS (Chambers and Cutcliffe 2001). There was little evidence in the empirical literature from the UK of any attention afforded to this specific aspect of CS in nursing. Nonetheless, a small quantity of work attempted to clarify helpful characteristics of the clinical supervisor.

Characteristics of a good supervisor

Unlike the research conducted in North America (Pesut and Williams 1990) and the Scandinavian countries (Severinsson and Hallberg 1996) which focused on the perceptions of the supervisor, research in the UK investigating the desirable characteristics of the clinical supervisor focused on the supervisee's perspective. Guided by Fowler's earlier (1995) study, Sloan (1999) conducted a descriptive investigation of the characteristics of a good clinical supervisor with staff nurses working in a mental health setting. The ability to form supportive relationships, having relevant knowledge and clinical skills, expressing a commitment to providing CS, and having good listening skills were perceived as important characteristics. Supervisees viewed their supervisor as a role model, someone whom they felt inspired them, whom they looked up to and had a high regard for their clinical practice and knowledge base. These perceptions are consistent with Fowler's 1995 findings.

Interpersonal interactions during clinical supervision

Sloan (2006), in turning attention to processes integral to CS, investigated the interpersonal interactions between supervisor and supervisee. It emerged that the work context within which CS was provided had a significant influence on how it was experienced. Aspects of the instructional system, particularly an NHS Trust document and description of a clinical supervision module, were unable to penetrate the rigid and inflexible routine hierarchical provision of CS. It emerged that when supervisors also assumed a line-management function, because of dual role incompatibilities, covert tensions impinged on the experiences of both supervisors and supervisees (Sloan 2006). These tensions were illuminated as the reciprocal interpersonal interactions between the supervisor and supervisee were brought into focus. Not surprisingly, unhelpful exchanges were apparent; discussion of client-related issues was infrequent and mental health nurses' emotional responses to their work were rarely discussed during CS. Similarly, participants in Ho's (2007) small scale study informed that while one-to-one CS was commonly experienced, very little attention was paid to dealing with the emotions arising from mental health nurses' work with patients. Instead, participants coped with their emotional responses to their work through alternative means, mostly away from work, for example, going to church, talking to a loved one or playing sports.

Conclusion

This chapter presents a selective review of the CS literature pertaining to nursing in the UK. In closing the chapter, returning to the UKCC's (now the Nursing and Midwifery Council) position on CS is warranted and from which reflections and implications from the literature reviewed are presented (Box 12.2).

The increasing popularity of CS is obvious; nevertheless, there is considerable evidence informing that too few nurses are able to access it. While there is a plethora of guiding frameworks, there is too little research supporting their utility. The lack of an agreed definition, contributes to the burdensome expectations which perhaps detract from its core value. Clinical

---

Box 12.2 Revisiting the UKCC's six statements

1   Clinical supervision supports practice, enabling practitioners to maintain and promote standards of care.
    The Nursing and Midwifery Council (NMC) should emphasise the significant purpose of clinical supervision for all nurses by making it a statutory requirement for registration.
2   Clinical supervision is a practice-focused professional relationship involving a practitioner reflecting on practice guided by a skilled supervisor.
    Clarity from the NMC on the precise purpose of, and agreement of a definition for, clinical supervision for nursing is required.
3   The process of clinical supervision should be developed by practitioners and managers according to local circumstances. Ground rules should be agreed so that practitioners and supervisors approach clinical supervision openly, confidently and are aware of what is involved.
    Guidance from the NMC, based on current empirical evidence, is required, which should facilitate the implementation of effective clinical supervision to local circumstances.
4   Every practitioner should have access to clinical supervision. Each supervisor should supervise a realistic number of practitioners.
    The NMC should make it a statutory requirement that every nurse embraces clinical supervision.
5   Preparation of supervisors can be effected using 'in house' or external education programmes. The principles and relevance of clinical supervision should be included in pre- and post-registration education programmes.
    Having clinical supervision as a requirement for the registration for nurses could contribute to the establishment of supervision competencies which in turn could provide guidance for supervision training programmes.
6   Evaluation of clinical supervision is needed to assess how it influences care, practice standards and the service. Evaluation systems should be determined locally.
    Useful evaluation of the outcomes derived from clinical supervision will only become meaningful if supervision competencies are developed so that effective supervision provision can be evidenced and measured.

supervision is a gift, a golden opportunity. When embraced without apprehension and provided effectively it has the potential to enable high quality nursing care. It requires considerable investment and commitment: all stakeholders, supervisees, supervisors, management, educators and regulatory bodies can contribute.

References

Alleyne, J. and Jumaa, M.O. (2007), Building the capacity for evidence-based clinical nursing leadership: the role of executive co-coaching and group clinical supervision for quality patient services, *Journal of Nursing Management*, 15(2): 230–243.

Ashmore, R. and Carver, N. (2000), Clinical supervision in mental health nursing courses, *British Journal of Nursing*, 9(3): 171–176.

Bishop, V. (2006), The policy-practice divide, *Journal of Research in Nursing*, 11(3): 249–251.

Butterworth, T., Carson, J., White, E., Jeacock, J., Clements, A. and Bishop, V. (1997), *It Is Good To Talk: An Evaluation Study in England and Scotland*, Manchester: University of Manchester.

Buus, N. and Gonge, H. (2009), Empirical studies of clinical supervision in psychiatric nursing: a systematic literature review and methodological critique, *International Journal of Mental Health Nursing*, 18(4): 250–264.

Chambers, M. and Cutcliffe, J. (2001), The dynamics and processes of 'ending' in clinical supervision, *British Journal of Nursing*, 10(21): 1403–1411.

Clough, A. (2001), Clinical leadership: turning thought into action, *Primary Health Care*, 11(4): 39–41.

Cutcliffe, J.R. (2000), Should line managers be supervisors? *British Journal of Nursing*, 9(22): 2268.

Cutcliffe, J.R. and Epling, M. (1997), An exploration of the use of John Heron's confronting interventions in clinical supervision: case studies from practice, *Psychiatric Care*, 4(4): 174–180.

Cutcliffe, J.R. and Hyrkäs, K. (2006), Multidisciplinary attitudinal positions regarding clinical supervision: a cross sectional study, *Journal of Nursing Management*, 14(8): 617–627.

Cutcliffe, J.R., Butterworth, T. and Proctor, B. (eds) (2001), *Fundamental Themes of Clinical Supervision*, London: Routledge.

Darley, G. (2001), Demystifying supervision, *Nursing Management*, 7(10): 18–21.

Davey, B., Desousa, C., Robinson, S. and Murrells, T. (2006), The policy-practice divide: who has clinical supervision in nursing? *Journal of Research in Nursing*, 11(3): 237–248.

Devitt, P. (1998), A grounded theory investigation into the nature of the supervisory relationship and the labour of supervision through the eyes of the supervisor, *Department of Nursing*, Manchester: University of Manchester.

Driscoll, J. (2000), Clinical supervision: a radical approach, *Mental Health Practice*, 3(8): 8–10.

Duncan-Grant, A. (2000), Clinical supervision and organisational power: a qualitative study, *Mental Health Care*, 3(12): 398–401.

Duncan-Grant, A. (2003), Is clinical supervision in mental health nursing a triumph of hope over experience? *Mental Health Practice*, 6(6): 22–23.

Edwards, D., Cooper, L. and Burnard, P. (2005), Factors influencing the effectiveness of clinical supervision, *Journal of Psychiatric and Mental Health Nursing*, 12(4): 405–414.

Fowler, J. (1995), Nurses' perception of the elements of good supervision, *Nursing Times*, 91(22): 33–37.

Fowler, J. (1996), Clinical supervision: what do you do after you say hello? *British Journal of Nursing*, 5(6): 382–385.

Gallinagh, R. and Campbell, L. (1999), Clinical supervision in nursing – an overview, *Nursing Review*, 17(3): 52–56.

Gilmore, A. (2001), Clinical supervision in nursing and health visiting: a review of the UK literature, in Cutcliffe, Butterworth and Proctor (eds), *Fundamental Themes of Clinical Supervision*.

Heron, J. (1989), *Six Category Intervention Analysis*, Guildford: Human Potential Resource Group, University of Surrey.

Herron, H. (2000), Supporting health visitors in child protection cases, *Community Practitioner*, 73(9): 751–753.

Ho, D. (2007), Work discussion groups in clinical supervision in mental health nursing, *British Journal of Nursing*, 16(1): 39–46.

Jones, A. (2006), Clinical supervision: what do we know and what do we need to know? A review and commentary, *Journal of Nursing Management*, 14(8): 577–585.

Kelly, B., Long, A. and McKenna, H. (2001), A survey of community mental health nurses' perceptions of clinical supervision in Northern Ireland, *Journal of Psychiatric and Mental Health Nursing*, 8(1): 33–44.

Lyth, G.M. (2000), Clinical supervision: a concept analysis, *Journal of Advanced Nursing*, 31(3): 722–729.

McSherry, R., Kell, J. and Pearce, P. (2002), Clinical supervision and clinical governance, *Nursing Times*, 98(23): 30–32.

O'Riordan, B. (2002), Why nurses choose not to undertake clinical supervision – the findings from one ICU, *Nursing in Critical Care*, 7(2): 59–66.

Padesky, C. (1996), Developing cognitive therapist competency: teaching and supervision models, in P.M. Salkovskis (ed.), *Frontiers of Cognitive Therapy*, London: The Guilford Press.

Pesut, D.J. and Williams, C.A. (1990), The nature of clinical supervision in psychiatric nursing: a survey of clinical specialists, *Archives of Psychiatric Nursing*, 4(3): 188–194.

Price, A.M. and Chalker, M. (2000), Our journey with clinical supervision in an intensive care unit, *Intensive and Critical Care Nursing*, 16(1): 51–55.

Proctor, B. (1987), Supervision: a co-operative exercise in accountability in M. Marken and M. Payne (eds), *Enabling and Ensuring: Supervision in Practice*, Leicester, National Youth Bureau and the Council for Education and Training in Youth and Community Work.

Proctor, B. (2001), The supervision alliance model, in Cutcliffe, Butterworth and Proctor (eds), *Fundamental Themes of Clinical Supervision*.

Rice, F., Cullen, P., McKenna, H., Kelly, B. and Richey, R. (2007), Clinical supervision for mental health nurses in Northern Ireland: formulating best practice guidelines, *Journal of Psychiatric and Mental Health Nursing*, 14(5): 516–521.

Rouse, J. (2007), How does clinical supervision impact on staff development? *Journal of Children's and Young People's Nursing*, 1(7): 334–340.

Severinsson, E.I. and Hallberg, I.R. (1996), Clinical supervisors' views of their leadership role in the clinical supervision process within nursing care, *Journal of Advanced Nursing*, 24(1): 151–161.

Sines, D. and McNally, S. (2007), An investigation into the perceptions of clinical supervision experienced by learning disability nurses, *Journal of Intellectual Disabilities*, 11(4): 307–328.

Sloan, G. (1999), Good characteristics of a clinical supervisor: a community mental health nurse perspective, *Journal of Advanced Nursing*, 30(3): 713–722.

Sloan, G. (2006), *Clinical Supervision in Mental Health Nursing*, London: Wiley & Sons.

Sloan, G., White, C. and Coit, F. (2000), Cognitive therapy supervision as a framework for clinical supervision in nursing: using structure to guide discovery, *Journal of Advanced Nursing*, 32(3): 515–524.

Spence, C., Cantrell, J., Christie, I. and Samet, W. (2002), A collaborative approach to the implementation of clinical supervision, *Journal of Nursing Management*, 10(2): 65–74.

Styles, J. and Gibson, T. (1999), Is clinical supervision an option for practice nurses? *Practice Nursing*, 10(11): 10–14.

Todd, G. and Freshwater, D. (1999), Reflective practice and guided discovery: clinical supervision, *British Journal of Nursing*, 8(20): 1383–1389.

UKCC (1996), *Position Statement on Clinical Supervision for Nursing and Health Visiting*, London: United Kingdom Central Council for Nursing, Midwifery and Health Visiting.

Winstanley, J. (1999), *Evaluation of the Efficacy of Clinical Supervision*, London: Emap Health-care Ltd.

Winstanley, J. and White, E. (2003), Clinical supervision: models, measures and best practice, *Nurse Researcher*, 10(4): 7–38.

Yegdich, T. (1999), Lost in the crucible of supportive clinical supervision: supervision is not therapy, *Journal of Advanced Nursing*, 29(5): 1265–1275.

13 Implementing clinical supervision

Case studies from Leicestershire, United Kingdom

John Fowler

This chapter presents a number of descriptive accounts of how clinical supervision is working in one geographical area. The author has worked in that region for many years and has amassed considerable practical as well as theoretical understandings of clinical supervision. Many accounts and models of clinical supervision, presented in the literature or at conferences, present their way of doing it as the best and only way and at times presented as 'the more complicated the better'. However anyone who has seriously studied clinical supervision working in a variety of different clinical and organisational structures will soon realise that one size does not fit all. Each of the case studies in this chapter gives a very different picture of how the essential elements of clinical supervision were adapted to the needs of each specific environment.

We believe that although there are some core principles of clinical supervision its application to different settings will vary considerably. You may believe that there should only be one model of clinical supervision that is enforced for all nurses. If so, consider the debate developed in this chapter. Currently professional guidelines encourage key principles to be adapted to local needs. This has many advantages in that systems develop to fit specific requirements. A disadvantage however, is that this does not lead to national and international core standards.

Introduction

This chapter is a mini case study looking at examples of clinical supervision within the geographical area of Leicestershire in the UK. Leicestershire is a typical medium-sized county covering 832 square miles and with a population of approximately 950,000. There are three major hospitals in Leicestershire and a number of smaller community hospitals, and a large community-based nursing service. This chapter contains a number of scenarios, each giving a different example of how clinical supervision has been implemented. *Think of this chapter as a number of photographs, each from a different angle. Neither one nor all of the photos give the complete picture of clinical supervision within this one geographical area, but taken as a whole they give a flavour of the diversity of models and styles that typify how clinical supervision has been applied.* It reflects upon the realities of implementation, focusing on the difficulties of combining flexibility of the model to accommodate individual needs with organisational demands for monitoring and governance.

The author has maintained an interest in clinical supervision for over 15 years. This includes academic writing, lecturing, implementation, evaluation and, most importantly of all, hands-on supervision. *There is no truer test of theories or ideas than actually implementing them and trying to get them to work and not just for a few months, but getting them fully embedded in the culture and structure of the clinical area.* The examples of clinical supervision included in this case study are not for the academic purist. The purist will undoubtedly find flaws with the philosophy or model of each or all of the examples and that is their right and probably their duty. Rather, this chapter is a reflection of the realities of taking the relatively simple concept of clinical supervision, which the majority of health care professionals would agree is a 'good idea' and trying to make it work.

There are descriptions of five different scenarios each followed by a short reflection:

1 small closed group – cross geographical boundaries;
2 small group clinical supervision facilitated by a medical consultant as part of a 12-month development programme;
3 clinical supervision within an action learning set;
4 one-to-one clinical supervision;
5 strategic implementation of integrated clinical supervision to all staff.

Small closed group: cross geographical boundaries

This is a small group of six staff, all in middle management positions in different geographical areas of the same employing authority. They are all from different clinical specialities, but have in common a middle management role. They started meeting four years previously after requesting some form of support from the author who was then working in a joint appointment position within the health service and the university. The group commenced meeting monthly, initially with the author acting as a facilitator for the first three months. The author then withdrew and the group continued along the lines of peer group supervision. They had a fairly simple agenda, each member discussing an issue that had occurred during the previous month, with the group offering guidance and support. The author was invited back after 12 months to help the group refocus, particularly in terms of helping one member who was taking on more responsibility for the running of the group than they wanted. The group continued to meet successfully for a further two years. At this time one of the key members retired and another moved authority which resulted in the group gradually ceasing to meet.

> *I found this group extremely valuable. At that time I was working in quite a senior management position in the community. The structure of the organisation meant that I didn't really have any close colleagues of a similar level that I could talk to confidentially. At times I felt quite isolated and just missed that opportunity to talk over things with colleagues. My manager told me about this clinical supervision group that was starting and I was keen to be part of it. There were six of us meeting once a month for about two hours in total. From the first session I knew this was going to be useful to me. It was just so useful meeting with a group of people in a similar managerial position to me. We all had different issues but we learnt so much from each other. Sadly after a few years, a couple of members moved jobs out of the area we sort of fell apart and stopped meeting. But it was a very valuable experience and I would love to be part of another group.*

(Group member)

Discussion

This is an example of an outside facilitator establishing a closed peer supervision group. It then ran successfully for a number of years. The group felt it should remain closed to other staff as a number of management issues they wanted to discuss were sensitive and confidential. This allowed the group to function well and meet their specific needs. However a weakness of a closed group system is that when one or two members leave the group becomes small and often ceases to meet. This should not be seen as a failure: the group successfully served its purpose for a specific group of staff for a number of years. It requires an organic perspective of clinical supervision. This means seeing groups developing, growing and dying according to local needs. The difficulties with this approach are at an organisational and strategic level in terms of trying to monitor, measure and support clinical supervision activity, particularly if some quality audit asks for specific numbers of staff in supervision at any one time.

Small group clinical supervision facilitated by a medical consultant as part of a 12-month development programme

The community matron role was launched in England in 2004. The focus was upon reducing high levels of unscheduled admissions and extended lengths of stay in the acute hospitals. Matrons were recruited to work as generalists addressing the needs of patients with a variety of long-term conditions. In Leicestershire, analysis of community activity over a period of six months showed that a significant number of individuals on caseload were requiring symptom and psychological support related to their entry into the palliative stage of their diagnosed long-term condition. It was identified that the needs of these individuals were often not being met within the current care pathways. The matrons acknowledged that they needed to develop further skills in communication in end of life issues, and the clinical skills required to support this part of the pathway of care. A multi-agency project, funded for one year, was launched to develop collaborative working between community matrons and specialist palliative care doctors with a focus on improving end of life care for patients, particularly with non-malignant diagnoses. 'The Empowerment of Community Matrons in End of Life Care' project incorporated clinical supervision, communication skills training, and joint patient visiting between the consultant doctor and community matron. An important part of this programme was the clinical supervision sessions.

Three clinical supervision groups were established, each facilitated by a palliative care medical consultant. Community matrons were allocated to one of the groups but were free to attend any of the sessions if that was practically more convenient. The groups met once a month for 12 months. In an evaluation of the 12-month programme a number of the CMs spoke about the quiet scepticism with which they commenced the supervision sessions but noted how valuable they soon found the sessions. Of the 35 community matrons attending the sessions only one person did not find the supervision sessions valuable; the majority of CMs found them to be either valuable or very valuable. There was a high attendance with non-attendance normally being due to annual leave and sometimes work commitments. They valued the discussion among peers of the clinical issues relating to palliative care and the specific input that the medical consultant made.

Discussion

This is an unusual example of clinical supervision in three ways: first, it was set up for a fixed term of one year. Second, the facilitators were medical consultants. Third, the supervision sessions were part of a development programme focusing on specialist palliative care. The author, who acted as an independent evaluator of this project, was interested in the community matrons' views regarding a medical consultant acting as a facilitator for the group. The matrons unanimously found this an extremely positive and useful aspect of the supervision. Likewise the consultants valued the opportunity to communicate with non-specialist palliative care practitioners who were at the front line in care delivery. The fixed term nature of the supervision was appropriate to the developmental programme in which the supervision was placed.

Clinical supervision within an action learning set

The author was approached by a service manager with the request to provide some research training and clinical supervision for ten staff, five of which were tissue viability nurse specialists and the other five who were podiatrists who also had a tissue viability specialist interest. It was proposed that the group should meet for a series of six days over 12 months. The group met once every two months and the project was funded for one year as a fixed term project. The first hour was spent in clinical supervision with the author facilitating the meeting. Staff took turns to discuss an area of practice that went well and then an area of practice on which they wanted some advice from their peers. This was followed by an action learning set in which the group of ten subdivided into three sub-groups each working on a clinically orientated project, e.g. evaluating the evidence of the effectiveness of salt on wound healing. The afternoon session was a taught session/seminar on an aspect of the research process.

> *We have only met five times throughout the year, but it has been one of the most valuable ways of using time that I have experienced. The reflective time within the clinical supervision sessions have worked in so well with the learning project and the structured session in the afternoon. I wasn't sure what to expect before the project started, but I am now recommending it to others.*

> (Group member)

Discussion

In a similar way to the previous example of the community matron supervision programme, this application of clinical supervision embeds the clinical supervision within a programme of professional development. Unlike the previous example it was facilitated by a nurse. It has the advantage that the six study days programmed throughout the year are kept as a high priority in the busy clinical diaries of the practitioners because they are part of a 'programme' rather than a collection of disconnected sessions. So often we read of clinical supervision projects failing because staff could or would not prioritise the meetings in terms of their clinical work. The packaging of clinical supervision within a 'programme' seems to overcome that problem. The other interesting feature of this example is the mixing of two quite different clinical professions, those of nurses and podiatrists, each group valuing the experience and contribution of the other. The clinical supervision sessions and the programme as a whole have been highly evaluated by the staff attending and managers are interested in repeating the model for other groups of staff.

One-to-one clinical supervision

One-to-one clinical supervision can be extremely valuable for all clinical situations and all grades of staff. If the supervisee and supervisor are carefully matched for personality, experience and knowledge then the relationship can be transformational. In practice such precise matching is difficult and expensive on people's time and energy. For these practical reasons such one-to-one supervision is often limited to areas of high priority. This may be: supporting new staff for a limited period of time e.g. preceptorship in the UK; staff working often in isolation in particularly demanding situations e.g. child protection; psychotherapy; or those staff with particular needs. An example in which the author has acted in a one-to-one supervisory relationship was with a senior nurse manager who was finding some aspects of staff management a little difficult. I met with the manager monthly for nine months. In the first two meetings I felt the supervisee was coming unprepared, just sitting down and talking almost at random about events. Although cathartic, it was not particularly productive in terms of moving issues forward or a learning experience. I then asked the supervisee to bring a written reflection of one event that she found difficult during the preceding month. This homework seemed to transform the sessions: she became focused and positive. After nine months I was able to withdraw from the relationship and direct the supervisee to a peer group supervision session.

> *Clinical supervision for me has been quite literally a life-changing experience. I was ready to quit my job and leave nursing altogether but then I met up with someone from the local university for one hour a month for clinical supervision. I'm not sure how he did it, but things began to fall into a different perspective.*

Discussion

One-to-one supervision is resource expensive and requires certain skills in the supervisor. As with its counterpart 'mentoring' in the business world, it is of particular value for people at transition points in their career e.g. moving from one role to another, new appointments, people taking on special projects or for those experiencing particular difficulties in their working life. As with any other resource, the human resource is valuable and expensive and should be used efficiently and effectively.

Strategic implementation of integrated clinical supervision to all staff

One of the National Health Service (NHS) Trusts in Leicestershire completed an audit of clinical supervision activity for nursing and allied health care professionals. They found that the implementation of clinical supervision across the Trust varied. Some staff were engaged in one-to-one supervision, more staff were involved in some form of peer group supervision and a number of staff were apparently not involved in any formal clinical supervision. Despite a number of areas of good practice it was difficult to quantify at a strategic level the uptake of clinical supervision and give assurances, in quality audits that *all staff* were actively involved in clinical supervision.

The author was engaged by the Trust to help develop a strategic system of clinical supervision which would be taken up by all staff in a way that was meaningful and quantifiable. The author met with managers and clinicians and, using a modified action learning process, discussed how such a system could be developed. It was important not to damage the variety of clinical supervision activities that were flourishing within the Trust. What was required was a minimum level of activity that was embedded into the Trust's organisational structure, that could be taken up by all nursing and allied health care staff, qualified and unqualified. Finally this activity needed to be undertaken in a way that there was quantifiable evidence that all Trust employees were engaged in it. As well as making it a system that could be measured and recorded at a strategic level, we were committed to making it a meaningful and valuable experience, even for those staff who were entering into formal clinical supervision for the first time, possibly with a degree of reluctance.

Discussions took place with a variety of staff groups and managers and a system of integrated clinical supervision was developed. Workshops were delivered to staff and a simple information package was developed which contained 15 questions and answers about how staff should use integrated clinical supervision (see below for a sample of the information package). In essence, all staff were required to reflect on an activity that involved clinical supervision and complete a short written reflective account. This was to be completed a minimum of four times a year. The line manager is responsible for monitoring and recording that the reflections are completed. This can be reported by the line manager to senior management and can then form a report at a strategic level.

Sample of staff information pack on integrated clinical supervision

Integrated clinical supervision

Clinical supervision is integral to our daily practice: it should be embedded in our routine structures but at the same time we need to make sure we give time to reviewing, discussing, observing, reflecting and recognising our role in supervision. Informal aspects of supervision happen all the time, asking a medical colleague to explain a diagnosis, discussing a care plan with a peer, observing a specialist at work, taking time to explain a procedure to a junior member of staff, are all aspects of clinical supervision.

How does integrated clinical supervision work?

Integrating clinical supervision into our daily professional practice involves:

* *recognising* when elements of supervision are occurring;
* *using* these occasions to the full;
* *reflecting* upon what has happened and how we can learn from it.

    Recognising → Using → Reflecting

Recognising

Integrative clinical supervision is about recognising when these elements are or could be occurring in our routine professional activities e.g. in our handovers, case studies, team meetings, our observation of colleagues, our time out sessions etc.

Using

Whether we are the more experienced person or the less experienced one, we have a duty to make full use of these opportunities. Primarily this will be by asking questions or observing others or fostering discussion.

Reflecting

Reflecting is thinking about why. It means looking for alternative perspectives. It is about discussing, thinking and examining. Often it is aided by writing down our thoughts.

How often should I complete a reflective account?

At certain points in your career you may want to formally reflect at the end of each week. This can be very useful when taking up a new post, or developing a new aspect of your existing role. Once confident in your role, most people find it useful to establish a regular pattern to written reflections, once a month is a good routine (what about the day before payday!). As a minimum the Trust expects you to complete a reflection at least four times a year.

Are these written reflections only for me?

These are not intended to be private reflections. They should be written in a way that allows you to share them with your colleagues and your manager. Write them in the same style you might write in patients' notes or an essay for a professional course. Nothing should be written that breaks confidentiality or is inappropriate regarding colleagues or patients. Periodically, your reflections should form the basis of a discussion with your manager or an appropriate colleague e.g. when discussing your personal development review.

Do I have to do this as well as other forms of clinical supervision reflections that I already do?

Everyone is required to undertake some form of individual reflective writing four times a year. If your current clinical supervision practice encompasses that then carry on with that.

Why do we need to write our reflections down?

Keeping a written record of some of your thoughts and discussions serves at least three purposes:

1   Most professional bodies and employing authorities require some form of written evidence which demonstrates ongoing professional competence and development.
2   The very act of transforming thoughts and discussions into writing makes us think and understand in ways different to just doing or talking about professional practice.
3   Finally at the end of a year we can review our reflections and often surprise ourselves at just what we have covered and learnt during that time.

The principle behind reflection within the context of clinical supervision is to make you think about what you have done or what you might do; explore the options; and identify the best way forward. It should be a positive experience which may lead to further questions, discussions or exploration of the literature.

Figure 13.1 is an example – yours may differ.

Date	1st Jan 2010
Type of clinical supervision	Team meeting ☐ Handover ☐ Case conference ☐ Ward meeting ☑ Observing colleagues ☐ Training session ☐ Professional discussions ☐ Telephone discussion ☐ Email discussion ☐ Self directed enquiry ☐ Other ☐ *(please specify)*
People involved	One to one ☐ Small group ☑ Large group ☐ No-one else ☐ Were they: Nurses ☑ Allied Health Professionals ☐ Medical Staff ☐ Pharmacists ☐ Other ☐ *(please specify)*
Type of clinical area	Community hospital - integrated medicine and rehabilitation.
Main issue thought about	At the team meeting we were discussing discharge planning for Mr X. Staff nurse Y told us how she had contacted social services and arranged for a community OT assessment. I didn't really know what was involved in the home assessment so I plucked up courage and asked if she could explain what it involved. Staff nurse Y explained that as Mr X had to walk with a frame, the community OT needed to check if Mr X could safely manage to get up stairs, make a cup of tea and that there were no hazards in his home.
What are the key points?	First, I learnt about the role of the community OT and what a home assessment was all about. Second, I realised how important it was to book the home visit with the OT in plenty of time, not just wait until the day before we wanted it - the importance of forward planning. Third, I learnt that as a HCA my questions in the team meeting were welcomed and staff nurse Y was happy to explain to me and the other staff.
Is there anything you can take forward from this?	Not to be afraid about asking questions in the team meeting. The importance of a community OT assessment before patients like Mr X can be discharged. The importance of careful planning prior to discharge.

Figure 13.1 Example of reflective writing.

Discussion

This system of integrated clinical supervision aims to establish a minimum standard for all staff that is manageable, useful and measurable. From a strategic management perspective this is essential. It is of limited use to have a few pockets of good examples of clinical supervision in an organisation if that is not replicated, at least to some extent, for all staff. Integrated clinical supervision was developed in partnership with all levels of staff and had senior management support throughout the process, which is essential. This is a relatively new system and yet to be evaluated. However early indications indicate that it is being used and is well integrated into the operational systems.

Conclusion

This chapter has provided a few snapshots of clinical supervision within one geographical area. The scenarios give examples of the variety of ways that clinical supervision is both interpreted and applied within that one geographic area. The first four scenarios typify the implementation of clinical supervision across an employing authority. A number of different styles and philosophies proliferate. The examples of the various styles demonstrate that this variety is not only useful, but essential as the needs of different groups of staff vary and the needs of individuals vary over time.

A weakness of such individualism and flexibility is the lack of a common standard with the option for some individuals to miss or avoid clinical supervision. From a strategic management perspective this is unsatisfactory. One of the responsibilities of a professional nurse at strategic level is not only to give reassurances to appropriate bodies that all staff have a certain standard of clinical supervision, but also to be able to quantify that statement with facts and figures. It is for this reason that integrated clinical supervision was developed and has been included in this chapter. Even the most willing and enthusiastic of us at times need to be told we must do something, sometimes for our own good.

The challenge for the nursing profession regarding clinical supervision is epitomised within this chapter. When there is freedom to develop a system of clinical supervision that is reactive to local needs and builds upon the skills and resources of its key individuals, then clinical supervision flourishes. Individuals feel supported, their practice is positively challenged and innovative, bottom-up developments occur. Sadly however, where this freedom exists, then those staff who do *not* want to be challenged in this way can avoid clinical supervision. Conversely if clinical supervision is imposed, then those who previously avoided it can no longer do so, and those staff who might not fully engage with an imposed system should hopefully achieve at least some of the beneficial outcomes of clinical supervision. However the imposition of a single model may restrict the creativity and individualism of some of the more innovative models we currently witness. The integrated clinical supervision model discussed in this chapter offers a way forward. It brings minimum standards which are quantifiable and the system can be audited. But it hopefully does not inhibit the more creative and innovative structures from continuing to develop. Would it work in your area?

14 Clinical supervision

An overview of the ideas and some requirements for professional practice

Alun Charles Jones

As its title indicates, this chapter offers an overview of clinical supervision and ideas regarding requirements for professional practice. The author discusses the topic by revisiting different formats for supervision and outlining the most common methods and modes. The author draws on varied literature and his own experiences to illustrate the potential benefits and possible pitfalls. The chapter concludes with the suggestion that clinical supervision forms an important part of the framework for clinical governance and, while supervision itself will challenge nurses, there is a need to identify critical elements that help professional practice.

We believe that this chapter presents an interesting overview for all readers. Whether as a supervisor or supervisee, it is important to understand how clinical supervision is linked to professional practice today. We also believe that the author presents an ideal to which the professional can aspire. Clinical supervision can offer the means to achieve a high standard of professional practice.

Acknowledgement

This chapter is an edited version of the author's original article: Supervision for Professional Practice, *Nursing Standard*, 14 (9): 42–44, November 1999.

Introduction

Clinical supervision is a forum that offers nurses guidance, support and education and so enhances and protects the organisation of health care. The Nursing and Midwifery Council (2008) recommends clinical supervision as a way of offering nurses a foundation for professional thoughtfulness and continued education. It is indeed a method of reaching the heart of professional practice. Supervised clinical practice is critical to the advancement of refined, improved and protected caring in professional situations.

Early literature suggested that many nurses viewed clinical supervision as a regulatory tool linked to appraisal, censure and managerial overseeing (Castledine 1994). A further misunderstanding concerning clinical supervision has been that it is a method of counselling or psychological therapy, giving rise to fears concerning personal and professional disclosures. Nevertheless, there are recent reports indicating that nurses are more accepting of clinical supervision (Kilcullen 2007). This may be because of a generation of nurses having become familiar with the ideas during their nurse preparation (Carver *et al.* 2007).

Clinical supervision is concerned with neither management authority nor psychologically therapeutic relationships; although in tangential forms, it encompasses elements of both. It is principally a relationship between respectful colleagues and is concerned with monitoring the progress of clinical work together with nurses' attainments of both safety in practice and excellence in the provision of heath care (Jones 2009). By providing opportunities in clinical supervision to view health care from a distance, a nurse can prepare for, deliver and evaluate clinical practice more effectively. The chance to reflect on nursing work and identify dynamic forces influencing the course of health care is a critical factor in the delivery of an efficient service (Knudsen *et al.* 2009). Supervision of clinical practice should therefore be a planned feature of health care provision.

If, however, clinical supervision is to be meaningful to nursing practice, then the nursing profession must assimilate, modify and individualise the concepts through identifying appropriate methods of practice (Fowler 2006). This requires distinguishing critical elements of support, management and professional education that are helpful to nurses, to define the unique contribution that clinical supervision can make to each specialist area of nursing practice.

Considered support and clinical supervision

Bertman (2005), writing about palliative care, discussed the need for considered support for those who care for patients and their families, suggesting that:

> If to relate on a person-to-person level is of paramount importance, then the atmosphere in which this is possible must be created and incorporated into formal teaching structures.
>
> (Bertman 2005: 7)

Supervised clinical practice can provide such conditions and is critical to the advancement of refined, enhanced and protected caring in professional practice. Research studies concerning supervision and nursing are proving helpful points of reference available to administrators, supervisors and those supervised, who are new to the concepts of supervised professional practice (for example, see Teasdale and Brocklehurst 2008).

Types of professional supervision

In mental health and psychiatric nursing, clinical supervision has traditionally assumed organisational, theoretical or philosophical approaches to complement the delivery of a service. For example, systemic family nursing makes use of a systems-oriented clinical supervision. In like manner, person-centred nursing makes use of person-centred clinical supervision and psychoanalytically informed nursing utilises psychoanalytic ideas in clinical supervision. *Adopting a corresponding framework helps practitioners to think about professional issues in ways that can improve their professional practice.*

Nurses might also usefully develop approaches to clinical supervision that similarly hold up mirrors to their own speciality of nursing practice. In professions other than nursing, practitioners sometimes choose to work with others of a different professional orientation to allow new ways of viewing their work. There are however, both benefits and disadvantages to this approach and usually it is only the most seasoned practitioners that favour it because of the potential for a theoretical muddle. Nevertheless, working with a conceptually naïve practitioner does offer opportunities to look at practice through a fresh pair of eyes, hear with new ears and explain in detail those things that are typically taken for granted (Jones 2009).

Supervision can take place in different formats, including clinical, managerial and training supervision. *Clinical supervision* enables a focus on professional competencies and increases the potential for a high standard of delivery of care to patients and their families. *Managerial supervision* is concerned with accountability and with the monitoring of work commissioned by an organisation. *Training supervision* related to the acquisition of specific skills and competencies and accountability is to the educational establishment.

Clinical supervision can take place before or after an event and can be either planned or ad hoc. In some instances, clinical supervision can be live, and so conducted during an event as in family work where a therapist will have immediate contact with a supervisor outside the therapy session. Supervision can also take place with oneself (Casement 1997), individually and in small groups with peers or a person with greater professional experience or from a different area of speciality. In some instances, supervision can include a team of workers or an organisation.

Particular formats have benefits or otherwise, each requiring different competencies of the supervisor and those supervised. Some nurses might view group clinical supervision, for example, as daunting because of fears of negative evaluations and competition from peers (Jones 2006). Nevertheless, groups offer ways of helping nurses to support themselves and others and to challenge strengths and weaknesses concerned with the delivery of care to patients and their families (Jones 2009).

The benefits of group-format clinical supervision

Working in small groups can be an effective means of managing stress-related difficulties, identifying strengths and supportive networks and so contribute to the maintenance of healthy behaviours (Alleyne and Jumaa 2007). *Group-format clinical supervision can also offer opportunities for nurses to share accounts of professional practice and so learn from the experiences of others (Jones 2009).* Support and learning, offered through groups, can enable adjustments in response to change. Group support can also promote efficient management of crisis and help sustain adaptive behaviours. Nonetheless, group members can become rivals and so groups can present experiences that are unhelpful to members. If conducted insensitively, like all relationships, there is potential for harm to nurses through abuses of power and inappropriate behaviours. There is a need to establish the working conditions that encourage group members to both protect and respect each other's contributions (Jones 2008).

Working arrangements

Whether conducted on an individual basis or in small groups, clinical supervision relationships are both dynamic and collaborative occurrences (Rafferty 2009). *It is a professional necessity that the supervisor and supervisee(s) together define the guidelines within which they are to work and a requirement that they document exchanges appropriately.* Nurses should be mindful that records are sometimes required as legal documents in a court of law (Dimond 1998). Working boundaries, confidentiality, accountability, parameters and limits on discussions are therefore all relevant issues for negotiation. Similarly, choice is important i.e. do we wish to work together, can we work together and do our other roles allow us to work together?

Assumptions can lead to misunderstanding and increase the potential for mistrust or lead to either unhelpful or inappropriate professional practices. It would seem imperative that the benefits or otherwise of supervised professional practice are identified and so supervision can be calibrated to meet the needs of patients and their families together with supervisors, supervisees, colleagues and organisations more generally (Severinsson and Hallberg 2008). In turn, nurses might meet the needs of patients and families in safety and with sensitivity.

The process of supervision

Methods of supervision specific to nursing specialities are still emerging (Carver *et al.* 2007; Rafferty 2009). *Nonetheless, whatever the format of supervision its facilitation can be as either a didactic process, experiential or a mixture of both.* Stuart *et al.* (1995), writing of mental health and psychiatric nursing, note that clinical supervision can be a quasi-therapeutic process because of (arguably) the need to negotiate the psychoanalytic ideas of transference and counter-transference difficulties (psychological processes in which attitudes are passed on, inappropriately, from one relationship to another).

In addition, supervisors need to consider nurses' ways of thinking, learning styles, values and emotional needs in relation to healthcare provision. Nurses might also experience *specific* therapeutic benefits however, through the process of collegiality. A trusting, sharing and mutually challenging relationship can bring about beneficial changes in nurses, both personal and professional (Jones 2009). Stuart (1995) described three modes of the delivery for supervision, which offer guidance to nurses regardless of their chosen branch or speciality.

They are as follows:

Patient-centred supervision

The nurse brings to supervision problems of a technical nature. The supervisor seeks out specific areas of information from the nurse and offers professional advice and guidance, sometimes monitoring events over an agreed period.

Clinical-centred supervision

This method of supervision centres on unseen, unheard or unspoken aspects of professional practice. The supervisor helps a nurse to reflect on events concerned with complex human dynamics and he or she is encouraged to think about factors influencing clinical practice. Working together in this way allows a picture to emerge showing how things might be different.

Process-centred supervision

This is a method of clinical supervision focusing on processes. That is to say of events unfolding between a patient, family members or colleagues, a nurse and the supervisor. Interactions that take place with the nurse and supervisor and interactions between the patients and nurses are analogous, termed as mirroring or paralleling (Hallberg *et al.* 1994).

Caution is needed in that, while all of the methods offer (new) ways of viewing events, they demand specific competencies so that nurses and supervisors do not become emotionally entangled in complex dynamics. It is important not to lose sight of the patient and family or organisational responsibilities. Clinical supervision makes equal demands on both supervisors and supervisees (Nelson *et al.* 2008).

Successful clinical supervision requires that nurses and supervisors are knowledgeable of the fundamentals of building effective relationships. Much of the concern in the nursing literature is with the potential benefits clinical supervision has to offer the organisation of practice. Clinical supervision can, as such, challenge nurses bringing with it additional obligations and responsibilities.

Clinical governance

Clinical supervision formed an important part of the frameworks for clinical governance as originally set out in the government's White Paper, *The New NHS: Modern Dependable* (Department of Health 1997). *Consequently, clinical supervision plays a role in helping NHS Trusts and foundation hospitals to meet requirements to regulate professional practice and ensure the safe delivery of health care.* The complexities of modern professional practice and emotional demands made on nurses through the intimate nature of much of their work means that nurses need a safe and ordered environment to consider how that work is carried out. It is important therefore, that nursing does not become overly preoccupied with issues of guardianship and so lose sight of the many other benefits that professional supervision in its various formats might yield to nurses and their practice.

Conclusion

Clinical supervision, if conducted thoughtfully, has much to offer nurses in their professional development and personal well-being. Moreover, developing methods of supervised practice that complement nursing philosophies of caring would give to nurses an effective means of reflecting on their practice and refining their professional competencies. Whatever the format, supervised professional practice offers nurses, experienced or otherwise, chances to build environments in which healthcare professionals are respected and valued. This is perhaps an ideal, yet one worthy of aspiring to, along with the nursing profession's uncompromising pursuit of professional excellence and safety. Ideas can be shared, colleagues affirmed and supported constructively.

Clinical supervision continues to develop in nursing and the gains for nurses taking part are still emerging. Health policy and empirical evidence obtained from research studies will go on influencing the unfolding, development and evaluation of this still important area of nursing. If carried out thoughtfully, clinical supervision does offer nurses a means of bringing about positive change in many areas of professional practice. It is a method of fostering professional acumen through self-monitoring. Mutually refining and applying nursing knowledge both formal and tacit means that nurses can work in ways that benefit everyone involved in health care.

References

Alleyne, J. and Jumaa, M.O. (2007), Building the capacity for evidence-based clinical nursing leadership: the role of executive co-coaching and group clinical supervision for quality patient services, *Journal of Nursing Management*, 15(2): 230–243.

Bertman, S. (2005), *Facing Death*, New York: Hemisphere.

Carver, N., Ashmore, R. and Clibbens, N. (2007), Group clinical supervision in pre-registration nurse training: the views of mental health nursing students, *Nurse Education Today*, 27(7): 768–776.

Casement, P. (1997), *Further Learning From the Patient: The Analytic Space and Process*, 3rd edn, London: Routledge.

Castledine, G. (1994), Clinical supervision a real aspiration? *British Journal of Nursing*, 3(16): 805.

Department of Health (1997), *The New NHS: Modern, Dependable*, command paper. online, available at: http://www.archive.official-documents.co.uk/document/doh/ newnhs/contents.htm [accessed 21 June 2010].

Dimond, B. (1998), Legal aspects of clinical supervision 2: professional accountability, *British Journal of Nursing*, 7(8): 487–490.

Fowler, J. (2006), The organization of clinical supervision within the nursing profession: a review of the literature, *Journal of Advanced Nursing*, 23(3): 471–478.

Hallberg, I.R., Berg, A. and Arlehanm, L.T. (1994), The parallel process in clinical supervision with a schizophrenic client, *Perspectives in Psychiatric Care*, 30(2): 26–32.

Jones, A. (1999), Supervision for professional practice, *Nursing Standard*, 14(9): 42–44.

Jones, A. (2006), Group-format clinical supervision for hospice nurses, *European Journal of Cancer Care*, 15(2): 155–162.

Jones, A. (2008), Towards a common purpose: group-format clinical supervision can benefit palliative care, *European Journal of Cancer Care*, 17(2): 105–106.

Jones, A. (2009), Fevered love, in L. de Raeve, M. Rafferty and M. Paget (eds), *Nurses and Their Patients: Informing Practice Through Psychodynamic Insights*, London: M&K Publishing.

Kilcullen, N. (2007), An analysis of the experiences of clinical supervision on registered nurses undertaking MSc/graduate diploma in renal and urological nursing and on their clinical supervisors, *Journal of Clinical Nursing*, 16(6): 1029–1038.

Knudsen, H., Ducharme, L. and Roman, P. (2009), Clinical supervision, emotional exhaustion, and turnover intention: a study of substance abuse treatment counselors in the Clinical Trials Network of the National Institute on Drug Abuse, *Journal of Substance Abuse Treatment*, 35(4): 387–395.

Nelson, M.L., Barnes, K.L., Evans, A.L. and Triggiano, P.J. (2008), Working with conflict in clinical supervision: wise supervisors' perspectives, *Journal of Counseling Psychology*, 55(2): 172–184.

Nursing and Midwifery Council (2008), *Clinical Supervison for Registered Nurses*, online, available at: www.nmc-uk.org/Nurses-and-midwives/Advice-by-topic/A/ Advice/Clinical-supervision-for-registered-nurses/ [accessed 2009].

Rafferty, M. (2009), Using Winnicott (1960) to create a model for clinical supervision, in L. de Raeve, M. Rafferty and M. Paget (eds), *Nurses and Their Patients: Informing Practice Through Psychodynamic Insights*, London: M&K.

Severinsson, E. and Hallberg, I.R. (2008), Clinical supervisors' views of their leadership role in the clinical supervision process within nursing care, *Journal of Advanced Nursing*, 24(1): 151–161.

Stuart, G.W. (1995), Actualising the psychiatric nurse's role: professional performance and standards, in G.W. Stuart and S.J. Sundeen (eds), *Principles and Practice of Psychiatric Nursing*, 5th edn, St. Louis, MI: Mosby.

Teasdale, K. and Brocklehurst, N. (2008), Clinical supervision and support for nurses: an evaluation study, *Journal of Advanced Nursing*, 33(2): 216–224.

15 Introducing clinical supervision in a rural health care organisation

An Australian experience

Lisa Lynch, Brenda Happell and Kerrie Hancox

This chapter features a summary of the process of implementing clinical supervision in an Australian rural healthcare organisation. After describing the method for the study, the five key categories or stages of the implementation process are outlined. Following this the Lynch Model of the implementation of clinical supervision is described according to its six main steps.

One of the advantages, allegedly, of globalisation, the creation of the World Wide Web and the corresponding 'shrinking' of the world is the swift access to valuable sources of information from all around the globe. By comparison, consider for a moment that the reporting of one of the most important scientific discoveries – namely confirmation of Einstein's Theory of General Relativity by Arthur Eddington[1] – didn't occur until one year following the observations and measurements. Whereas in a world with a 'www:' prefix, experiences that occur in one corner of the globe can sometimes show up within hours of their occurrence all over the rest of the world (assuming one has Internet access!) This has, arguably, also contributed to the increasing realisation that lessons learned in one corner of the world can have utility and application in other (sometimes far away) parts of the world; particularly if there are case related (idiographic) commonalities. So while the lessons learned in rural Australia may seem esoteric to some, the editors encourage readers to look for the commonality between the experiences reported and their own, and thus transferability of the findings from one corner of the globe to another.

Introduction

Increasingly, the benefits of clinical supervision (CS) are being recognised not just for nurses but for the quality and integrity of nursing practice. CS is not without considerable economic cost and given the increasing fiscal constraints affecting health care, the health and well-being of the professional and the quality of care provided may not be sufficient justifications in themselves; cost effectiveness of CS should also be demonstrated. It might therefore be reasonable to expect that CS has been and continues to be carefully implemented, through a process based on policies and procedures to enhance the likelihood of success and the ability to demonstrate positive outcomes. However, a review of the literature does not support this assumption; rather it suggests a lack of guidance and leadership from government and nursing professional (registration) bodies who have been relatively silent on the issue of implementation. This relative absence of policy direction has been highlighted as one factor that has contributed to the many difficulties associated with the implementation of CS (Mullarkey and Playle 2001; Clifton 2002; Riordan 2002; Lynch *et al.* 2008).

Guidance for the implementation of CS has primarily been included in some text books (see, for example, Butterworth and Faugier 1992; Bond and Holland 1998; Driscoll 2000); and these texts offer some useful suggestions regarding the implementation of CS. Driscoll (2000)[2] for example, highlighted the need to assess the culture of the health service prior to undertaking a structured and staged approach to implementation. This assessment involves identifying the strengthening and weakening factors inherent in the organisation, and identifying strategies to promote the strengths and overcome and minimise the weaknesses. Cultural assessment was also a feature of the work of Clifton (2002) and Lynch *et al.* (2008), whereas Bond and Holland (1998) articulated five necessary stages in the implementation process: developing a definition of CS; promoting staff involvement; providing education and training for supervisors and supervisees; ensuring CS for the supervisors; and, finally, developing a framework for evaluation monitoring and support. Successful implementation, according to this approach, involves specific staff assuming responsibility for specific roles. These roles should be supported by working groups of staff with specific interest in and/or experience with CS (Bond and Holland 1998). As valuable and/or useful as these suggestions may be, for the most part they lack detail and moreover, would perhaps benefit from experiential evidence to support the proposed process of implementation. As a means to help strengthen this body of work and provide a robust account, this chapter accordingly offers a summary of the process of implementing CS in an Australian rural health-care organisation.

Implementation in action: the case of one mental health service

In 2000 the Victorian government made a significant investment in CS in the form of the creation (and appointment) of a number of senior educational and professional development positions in nursing. In the absence of guidelines and protocols, mental health services were responsible for their own CS implementation process. In our case, an exploratory research method was used to examine the process and journey of the CS implementation strategy for one mental health service in rural Victoria, Australia. This service took on the introduction of CS with enthusiasm and determination. An unintended consequence of this experience was the development of mechanisms and strategies that formed the basis of a model to guide the implementation of CS.

Methods

A mixed methods approach (Greene 2007) was adopted, utilising a combination of qualitative exploratory interviews and a documentation audit. The study setting was selected for two main reasons: first, the organisation was acknowledged by others as having achieved successes in implementing CS; and second, as a rural service, there would be additional complexities to those encountered in a metropolitan service, most notably the problems created by distance. The research included an audit of all documentation (including minutes of meetings and the strategic plan) associated with the implementation process and in-depth interviews with seven members of the implementation team. The initial stage of data analysis was largely analogous to the force field analysis described by Driscoll (2000). This approach facilitated the identification of the main strengths and weaknesses of the organisational culture and the approach(es) taken in response to these. The interviews were recorded and transcribed verbatim to provide a full account of the interviews (Patton 1989). The transcripts were read and reread searching for broad categories. Significant phrases or statements were identified from the transcripts. Similarities and differences were then identified as a way to begin to interpret the initial data. These areas were then coded in readiness for the analysis process.

Findings

Analysis of the data revealed five main stages in the implementation process. These five stages articulated the timeline or sequence of implementation and provided a framework for their implementation process. Each stage was characterised by specific factors and influences, a number of which extended across more than one stage. These stages are presented in Table 15.1.

Stage 1: assessing the culture

Knowing the culture, through assessment, of the organisation emerged as a core theme. Although identified as the preliminary stage for this research, assessing and reassessing the culture was characteristic of most of the stages. This stage was similar to that described by Driscoll (2000) as part of his field force analysis with a view to identifying strengths and weaknesses and responding accordingly. The culture prior to the implementation of CS was described as largely negative, with strained

Table 15.1 Implementation process: stages and influencing factors

Stages	Influencing factors
1 **Exploration: assessing the culture**	Organisational culture Exploring the possibilities
2 **The initial implementation strategy**	Leadership Organisational culture Education and training The Project–Strategic Plan
3 **Strategic planning**	Reflection Clinical Supervision Implementation Committee The Project–Strategic Plan
4 **Implementing the strategic plan**	Clinical Supervision Committee Education and training Organisational culture
5 **Reflecting on the past and moving forward**	Organisational culture – culture change Sustainability On reflection

Source: Reproduced with permission from Lynch *et al.* (2008). *Clinical Supervision for Nurses.*

relationships between management and clinicians. Clinicians described a distrust of management, which was expressed through a general dissatisfaction with the work environment and high levels of stress and burnout.

CS was not automatically identified as the strategy to address these issues, but emerged as the preferred option after other ideas such as educational support, staff/peer support and structural and system changes were considered. After making this decision to implement CS, the team recognised the need for a structured approach.

Stage 2: the initial implementation strategy

Leadership was identified as a crucial ingredient for success to champion the successful introduction of CS (see also Clifton 2002). A leadership group was formed and quickly took on the task of restoring confidence amongst the staff. The organisational culture continued to be an important consideration. Addressing this required a concerted effort as many nurses believed that this would be another 'new thing' that would not be sustained by management in the long term.

The team contracted an external organisation to provide education and training for both supervisors and supervisees. The training programmes were written and developed by the Directors of Clinical Supervision Consultants (www.clinicalsupervision.com.au). The rationale was to promote quality, by providing supervisors adequately prepared for the role, educate supervisees about the CS, and demonstrate commitment to the initiative. The primary benefits of external training were seen as independence; promoting engagement with other organisations, and providing a clear distinction between clinical supervision and management.

The first course was evaluated favourably by all participants including the leadership group, the management group, and potential supervisors and supervisees. The participants valued the flexibility of the programme. Rather than undertake a traditional piece of assessment such as an essay or examination, the participants were able to work together collaboratively to develop a strategic plan. This facilitated a sense of group cohesion towards a common goal and left them with a tangible product as an outcome. Indeed this process led directly to the third stage of implementation.

Stage 3: strategic planning

This stage involved the formalisation and finalisation of the strategic planning approach. This began with a process of reflecting or 'taking stock' of the progress to date. The leadership group felt confident that they had been successful in obtaining organisational support, securing leadership, and facilitating training and education through an external provider. Through these initiatives a subtle change in the culture was being observed with more enthusiasm and less scepticism from the nursing staff.

At this point, the group recognised the need to formalise the leadership group and the Implementation Committee was formed to complete the strategic plan. Members were allocated clear roles and responsibilities, including writing: the project background and overview; the vision values and mission statement; projects aims and objectives; information about the implementation strategy; and an information package including articles on models, examples of CS agreements, record forms and other references articles.

At an individual or small group level, specific tasks were allocated such as marketing, policy writing, and evaluation. The opportunity to self-select in areas of interest or ability was available to members. This had some advantages but also led to some conflict, reflecting the individual styles and personalities of members. At this stage in the process there was not one recognised leader and no formal process for making decisions, which often led to circular and repetitive meetings. Nevertheless, the group members were able to complete a strategic plan and present this plan as their course assessment and to senior management. In addition to the formal strategic plan, smaller groups were allocated responsibilities within the following three areas: communication and marketing; policy and procedures; and evaluation. Communication and marketing was considered essential in promoting ownership of the initiative throughout the organisation rather than the protégé of the implementation committee.

The communication and marketing process was taken very seriously. The committee (and organisation) wanted to develop something that would be both meaningful and attract attention. Ultimately they chose the theme 'Growing Together'. This was later decorated with art work that was used on a poster; the committee also produced a folder with information about CS and potential supervisors. An official launch was held to promote the importance of the initiative and its relevance across the whole service. All staff received personal invitations from management and the event was teleconferenced to remote sites.

With the support and guidance of the course facilitators one small group took carriage of developing the policies and protocols required to ensure a clear and consistent approach to the implementation process. These individuals produced a draft of relevant documentation that was subsequently distributed to the broader team for comment and amendment. Another group took carriage of the evaluation, assisting the organisation to participate in an internal and an external evaluation.

Stage 4: implementing the strategic plan

With the groundwork completed, Stage 4 became the action-oriented phase. The major features at this time were: the establishment of the CS committee; meeting the ongoing need for education and training; and maintaining organisational culture and support. At this point the Implementation Committee was renamed the Clinical Supervision Working Party and its activities and status became more formalised. A call for membership was made to senior nurses, nurse managers and other nurses with experience in CS. A chair and a minute taker were appointed. Discussion on items of interest was encouraged, but now with an emphasis on actions. Specific members were allocated specific actions and given deadlines to complete the required work. This change was viewed as an important part of group maturation, particularly the transparency of leadership and the formalised process to ensure that ideas led to outcomes.

The ongoing need for education and training was a major consideration at this stage. The provision of education and training for managers became a priority as a means to securing their support and commitment, and to increase their understanding of CS and the role it could play within the organisation. There was a mixed reception, varying between appreciation of management commitment and concern that CS would ultimately be overseen or even controlled by management. This led to a change in approach to the participants for future training. A letter was sent from the committee to each nurse who had completed the one day training pro-gramme aimed at potential supervisees. The letter sought the names of five nurses they would feel confident and comfortable to enter a supervisory relationship with. Those receiving the greatest number of nominations were contacted and informed of their nominations and were asked if they were interested in undertaking the training. Not only did this approach ensure that the people trained as supervisors would be sufficiently valued by their colleagues, it also enhanced the esteem and confidence of those who had been nominated. Most agreed to participate and indeed completed the training. From the perspective of potential supervisees, this restored CS within the clinical domain and allayed concerns that this would become another tool of line management.[3]

Stage 5: reflecting on the past and moving forward

The last stage focused on reflection and consideration of the future. *Organisational culture remained an important focus but there was stronger consideration of how the implementation of CS had impacted on the organisation rather than vice versa.* The participants described their perceptions of a change of culture that had influenced far more broadly than just CS itself. Nurses had become notably more responsive to, and less suspicious of, the idea of CS. This had spin-off effects and had been seen to have improved the relationships between clinicians and managers across the board.

At the time that this research was conducted, almost three years had passed since CS had been introduced into the organisation, and participants were pleased that it had continued this long. However, concerns about the ongoing sustainability remained. The team saw that research, evaluation and quality assurance activities would be imperative to demonstrating tangible outcomes and therefore supporting the sustainability of this initiative. In addition to outcomes, the team recognised the importance of maintaining the drive and passion, not only of the working group, but for all nurses within the organisation.

The team also reflected on the process that had led them to this point. There were certain aspects that some would change if they were able to start again with the benefits of hindsight. These included: identifying leadership at an earlier stage; and considering more than one leader to avoid the one person being charged with much of the responsibility and accountability. Some concern remained about the training of senior managers and it was suggested that a shorter course, specifically tailored to the role that management should play in ensuring the successful implementation of CS, without controlling and directing the process. The reflections led to some other practical ideas that might have improved the process including: calling for expressions of interest from potential clinical supervisors; ensuring enough supervisors were trained and available across the region; and lobbying for specific funding to be earmarked for research and evaluation.

Key aspects of our process of implementation

The implementation of CS was a fluid process rather than following specific rigid guidelines. Nevertheless five main stages were identified:

1   assessing the culture;
2   the initial implementation plan;
3   strategic plan;
4   operationalising the strategic plan; and
5   reflection and evaluation.

Although presented in a linear format, there was considerable blending across stages. It was also noted that a number of the influencing factors such as organisational culture, leadership, and education and training occurred across stages. *A group of individuals recognised a number of organisational problems that resulted, at least in part, from low morale and a strong disconnect between clinical practice and management. CS was identified as a potential strategy to overcome some of the issues identified: the task then was to make this happen.* The process began relatively informally and became more structured over time, largely in response to difficulties encountered or issues that emerged, based on the recommendations.

As is so often the case, this group of individuals had to find their own way in order to realise a goal they thought was worth pursuing. They had no formal guidelines to follow and were not privy to the lessons learned by others who had embarked on the same venture. Of course guidelines alone are not a measure of success, and no doubt the passion, commitment, skill and expertise of these nurses constituted an irreplaceable aspect of the successful outcomes. However, lessons were learned that could prove invaluable for others who wish to follow a similar path. This recognition led to the development of a model for the implementation of CS: the Lynch Model (named after the principle researcher and first author) (Lynch and Happell 2008a, 2008b, 2008c).

The Lynch Model for the implementation of clinical supervision

Introduction

The Lynch Model is based on six main steps. Having been developed directly from the research findings, its focus is practical with the primary aim of facilitating implementation. The model is presented in Figure 15.1.

Step One: clinical supervision or?

The myths and misconceptions surrounding CS are widely documented (see, for example, Mackereth 1997; Mullarkey and Playle 2001; Lynch *et al.* 2008) as are the difficulties that ensue from such confusion (Mackereth 1997; Yegdich 1999; Cutcliffe and Hyrkäs 2006). It is therefore important to have clarity that CS is the most appropriate intervention to meet certain specific (and identified) needs of the organisation at that time. The starting point should be with what the organisation

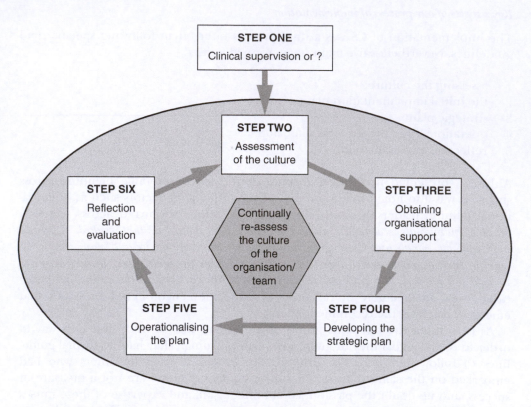

Figure 15.1 The Lynch Model of implementation (source: reproduced with permission from Lynch *et al.* (2008) *Clinical Supervision for Nurses*).

Note
The circle around Steps Two to Six reflects the dynamic nature of the implementation process indicating that you can repeat these stages or variations a number of times throughout the implementation process in a circular manner.

wants/needs for its staff and whether CS is the most appropriate initiative to meet some of those needs. This will require defining or coming to a shared understanding of what CS is and how it intersects with existing structures, such as line management, mentorship and preceptorship. Remembering that CS is not a panacea for every ill that avails an organisation should help in judicious choices about when and where CS would be an appropriate development. The example provided earlier in this chapter clearly demonstrates the complexity of introducing CS. It is inevitably a time-consuming process requiring energy, passion and high levels of motivation. To give every chance of success it is essential to be confident that the expected outcomes are worth the effort.

Step Two: assessment of the culture

Organisational culture is a key ingredient for successful implementation (Handy 1993). It is important that an accurate picture of the strengths and weaknesses is undertaken. Driscoll (2000) recommends that a force field analysis be undertaken to identify both the strengthening and resisting forces. This process provides an indication of the degree of readiness of the organisation as well as providing a springboard for the subsequent steps in the implementation process. While Driscoll's (2000) concept of a force field analysis is a useful starting point, it does not readily distinguish between levels of strengths and barriers; inevitably some forces will be stronger than others. For example, lack of funding is likely to be a greater barrier than lack of availability of appropriate training opportunities as solutions for the latter are likely to be found more easily than the former. Once the force field analysis is completed the pushing and resisting forces should therefore be ranked or prioritised.

With this priority list in mind the next step is to develop an action plan to address the pushing and resisting forces in order of importance and level of influence (Driscoll 2000). Additionally it is important to identify the roles and responsibilities that individuals have within the initial action plan (Bond and Holland 1998). This enables a more informed approach to the resources available and the problems likely to be encountered.

Step Three: obtaining organisational support

Without organisational support, the authors would argue that the successful implementation of CS is virtually impossible. Given the likelihood that some of the needs will vary from one organisation to another, it is important to understand the specific needs of the particular organisation.[4] After completing Steps One and Two, the extent of the organisational support required will become more apparent. This enables a more organised approach to underpin any requests for resources.

Step Four: developing the strategic plan

The next step following support is strategic planning. Leadership and consultation become pressing concerns at this stage. The success of CS requires active engagement with a variety of key stakeholders including: management and administration; nurse educators; nurse managers and senior nurses; clinicians at varying levels; other collaborating agencies; and key individuals or groups within the organisation. Leadership is necessary to ensure that consultation initiatives are carried through and the momentum for the initiative is maintained. The content and structure of the strategic plan should be directly influenced by the information gathered during the consultation process. Although the structure should be tailored for each specific organisation, the following information should be included:

- the vision, mission, goals and the overall aims and objectives for the implementation of CS;
- a brief background of the rationale for the introduction of CS (based on data collected during the consultation phase);
- an agreed definition of CS;
- implementation strategy – a clear plan identifying tasks, roles and timelines, including:
  - education and training;
  - communication and marketing;
  - policies and protocols;

- plan for research and evaluation;
- relevant documentation including copies of agreements and record forms;
- any other information relevant to the individual organisation.

Step Five: operationalising the plan

At this stage the CS committee or working party should be formalised in order to focus on operationalising the strategic plan. At this stage education and training and communication and marketing are likely to be the priorities. There are a number of factors to consider when deciding the most appropriate approach to training. Providing training/education internally ('in house' – using the educational resources already in existence within the organisation) is likely to be less expensive and easy to organise, but may not be embraced if a negative attitude prevails towards the organisation, and internal trainers would be part of the broader culture. External training/education potentially has a greater sense of independence. However, external trainers may lack sufficient knowledge of the organisational culture to deliver the education and training that reflects the specific needs of that organisation. Lynch and Happell (2008b) suggest a hybrid model that involves an internal and external trainer to maximise the benefits and minimise the disadvantages of both approaches.

The idea of communication and marketing is not always recognised within the health care sector. However, it may be instrumental in determining the success or otherwise of an initiative such as clinical supervision. At the very least, communication and marketing provides the opportunity to draw attention to, and create an interest in, the new strategy. The data collected in Step Two should directly influence the strategy adopted and Step Three data will highlight the resources available to support it. Documentation is valuable at this stage to keep the process on track, set timelines and measure achievements against goals (see also Cutcliffe 2000).

Step Six: reflection and evaluation

Sustainability should be an inherent consideration for the implementation of any new strategy. Any plan for sustainability should be informed by both formal evaluation and informal reflections on the problems and successes encountered during the journey. The culture of the organisation must be re-assessed (as in Step Two) to once again identify the strengthening and resisting forces. Findings from the evaluation should assist in determining the success of the project according to the original aims and objectives. Where the aims and objectives have not been met in either full or part, the implementation committee should consider re-examining the model and repeating Steps Three, Four and Five. For example, if the uptake of CS is significantly lower than expected, the committee would need to investigate possible reasons, such as the lack of protected time to attend sessions, and develop approaches to overcome these problems. Other strategies should be things such as training for supervisees, or a boost to the communication and marketing. This stage also provides an ideal opportunity for dissemination of the knowledge gained through the implementation process. In addition to dissemination within the organisation, this can also involve publications in nursing or health journals and conference presentations. Ideally, further research and evaluation activities would be planned at this time.

Maintaining the dynamics

The circle around Steps Two to Six of the model reflects the dynamic nature of the implementation process: there is a continuing need for revision and reassessment. Even where the implementation process is considered successful, the organisation itself will not be static. Changes in structure, leadership and other personnel will impact on the broader organisational culture, and changes to the strengthening and resisting forces must be attended to in order that clinical supervision is sustainable.

Conclusion

Clinical supervision was successfully implemented into a mental health service in rural Victoria. This outcome reflected the passion and commitment of a small group of senior nurses. They achieved results in the absence of guidelines and direction. During the implementation process, they developed a structure that responded to the specific nature of the organisation, building upon its strengths and addressing its weaknesses. This approach was revealed through analysis of the research findings, and directly influenced the development of the Lynch Model of implementation (Lynch and Happell 2008c). It is intended that the articulation of this model will provide a framework to guide the implementation of CS in other organisations.

Notes

1 See Dyson, F.W., Eddington, A.S. and Davidson, C.R. (1920), A Determination of the Deflection of Light by the Sun's Gravitational Field, from Observations Made at the Total Eclipse of May 29, 1919, *Philosophical Transactions of the Royal Society A*, 220: 291–333 (doi:10.1098/rsta.1920.0009), online, available at: www.adsabs. harvard.edu/ abs/1920RSPTA.220..291D.
2 Clearly drawing on the seminal work of Lewin (1946).
3 As concerns about the inappropriate conflation between managerial and CS continues to be shown to be one of the principal reasons for resisting CS (Yegdich 1999; Cutcliffe and Hyrkäs 2006; Lynch *et al.* 2008) this is a very good example of using the existing evidence base to inform how CS can be implemented.
4 Though there is also likely to be some commonality across the needs of the organisation and therein lies some of the value of experiential evidence such as provided in this chapter.

References

Bond, M. and Holland, S. (1998), *Skills of Supervision for Nurses*, Oxford: Open University Press.
Butterworth, A. and Faugier, J. (eds) (1992), *Clinical Supervision and Mentorship in Nursing*, London: Chapman & Hall.
Clifton, E. (2002), Implementing clinical supervision, *Nursing Times*, 98(9), 36–37.
Cutcliffe, J.R. (2000), To record or not to record: documentation in clinical supervision, *British Journal of Nursing*, 9(6), 350–355.

Cutcliffe, J.R. and Hyrkäs, K. (2006), Multidisciplinary attitudinal positions regarding clinical supervision: a cross-sectional study, *Journal of Nursing Management*, 14(8), 617–627.

Driscoll, J. (2000), *Practicing Clinical Supervision: A Reflective Approach*, London: Balliere Tindall.

Greene, J.C. (2007), *Mixed Methods in Social Inquiry*, San Francisco: Wiley & Sons.

Handy, C. (1993), *Understanding Organizations: How Understanding the Ways Organizations Actually Work can be Used to Manage them Better*, Oxford: Oxford University Press.

Lewin, K. (1946), Action research and minority problems, *Journal of Sociological Issues*, 2(4): 34–46.

Lynch, L. and Happell, B. (2008a), Implementing clinical supervision: Part 1: Laying the ground work, *International Journal of Mental Health Nursing*, 17(1): 57–64.

Lynch, L. and Happell, B. (2008b), Implementing clinical supervision: Part 2: Implementation and beyond, *International Journal of Mental Health Nursing*, 17(1): 65–72.

Lynch, L. and Happell, B. (2008c), Implementing clinical supervision: Part 3: The development of a model, *International Journal of Mental Health Nursing*, 17(1): 73–82.

Lynch, L., Hancox, K., Happell, B. and Parker, J. (2008), *Clinical Supervision for Nurses*, Oxford: Wiley-Blackwell.

Mackereth, P. (1997), Clinical supervision for potent practice, *Complementary Therapies in Nursing and Midwifery*, 3(2): 38–41.

Mullarkey, K. and Playle, J. (2001), Multi professional clinical supervision: challenges for mental health nurses, *Journal of Psychiatric and Mental Health Nursing*, 8(3): 205–211.

Patton, M. (1989), *Qualitative Evaluation and Research Methods*, 1st edn, Beverly Hills, CA: Sage.

Riordan, B. (2002), Why nurses choose not to undertake CS: the findings from one ICU, *Nursing in Critical Care*, 7(2): 59–66.

Yegdich, T. (1999), Clinical supervision and managerial supervision: some historical and conceptual considerations, *Journal of Advanced Nursing*, 30(5): 1195–1204.

Part III

The practice and experience of clinical supervision

16 Clinical supervision

My path towards clinical excellence in mental health nursing

Paul Smith

This chapter focuses on the experiences of a registered mental nurse (RPN) of receiving and engaging in clinical supervision. From early experiences of and exposure to clinical supervision during a formal programme of study, to engaging in clinical supervision as a staff nurse on an inpatient unit and then as a community psychiatric nurse attached to a general practitioner's surgery, this chapter provides a window into the lived world of the supervisee (in various settings and stages of one's career). The chapter advances the argument how engaging in clinical supervision helped the author develop his skills and knowledge, which in turn improved the care he offered to clients and maintained his health and clinical effectiveness. Drawing on specific examples of problems and/or challenges he encountered in his practice, the author shows how these real issues were brought into the supervision sessions and how they were faced, considered and subsequently addressed. The chapter also draws attention to some of the practical disadvantages that can occur if certain principles are overlooked.

While the editors are mindful of the evidence-based movement and the need for evidence to support the widespread introduction of clinical supervision, they are less comfortable with (artificial) so-called hierarchies of evidence and the almost inevitable low 'ranking' of qualitative evidence. Such hierarchies of evidence are by no means universally accepted. An alternative view posits that research methods within quantitative and qualitative paradigms can be regarded as a toolkit; a collection of methods that are purposefully designed to answer specific questions and discover particular types of knowledge. To attempt to place these designs (and the evidence they produce) into some artificial and linear hierarchy only serves to confuse and obfuscate. If what is needed to answer a particular problem (e.g. the comparison of the therapeutic effects of two approaches to the organisation/delivery of CS) is a meta-analysis of the current studies in this area, then for that particular problem, that is clearly the best form of evidence. Concomitantly, if what is required to answer a particular problem (e.g. what are the lived experiences of experiencing effective CS) is deep, thorough, sophisticated understanding, then for that particular problem, qualitative findings are the best form of evidence. Both types of evidence are needed, both types of evidence are valuable: the discovery of both types of evidence should be encouraged.

Introduction

In this chapter I am going to make the argument that clinical supervision (CS) is effective in developing skills and knowledge, improving care delivered to patients/clients and maintaining the clinical effectiveness and health of the supervisee. I achieve this by describing my experience of CS, using specific examples of problems or challenges I faced in my own clinical practice. I will also draw attention to some of the practical disadvantages that can occur if certain principles are overlooked.

The examples are loosely arranged in three, chronologically correct, stages namely:

1 my introduction to CS while studying for a post-registration diploma titled 'Understanding Therapeutic Relationships' which was run by clinical psychologists and validated by Nottingham Trent University;
2 my experience of CS provided by a nursing colleague as we worked on an inpatient unit for people with enduring mental health problems; and
3 latterly in my role as staff nurse in an acute, general practitioner-attached community mental health team.

While this chapter may not be overly academic and is descriptive and discursive, I believe it is scholarly and persuasive nonetheless. My gratitude goes to my supervisors, who here remain anonymous, for the love, patience and support they have shown me. I hope and believe that they would agree with me when I suggest that at least some of the time spent in providing me supervision has resulted in valuable (and even measurable) gains for the people we claim to care for.

Early experiences of clinical supervision

For the first six years of my nursing career I was not given CS in the form I recognise as relevant and necessary today. As a student nurse (RGN, 1984 syllabus) I was allocated to registered nurses while on clinical placement, some of whom were bemused or threatened by the frequent questions I had, and some were tolerant of my striving to do and know the right way to do things. As a junior staff nurse I was extremely fortunate to have experienced colleagues who forgave me my sometimes insensitive challenges of not only procedures and routines but also their clinical practice. During this time I frequently received critical, balanced feedback about my technical skills, my application of knowledge to clinical situations and developments in my own practice, much of which was helpful and constructive. Indeed it continued through further training which led to me becoming a Registered Nurse (Mental Health) and a staff nurse on a rehabilitation/challenging behaviour/continuing care unit for people with 'severe and enduring' mental health needs. But in all this time I had little guidance to help me examine, analyse, explore the reasons as to why I did what I did, said what I said, and/or behaved the way I behaved. It is reasonable to suggest that I gained insights through reflection upon and within my practice, by discussions with peers and colleagues, and from being exposed to praise, criticism and indifference by others. But I was frequently aware that there was something missing from the picture although, I did not know what.

After nine months of working in the inpatient unit, I commenced a course in 'Understanding Therapeutic Relationships'. An integral part of this was a module that involved receiving CS from a psychologist with the aim of participants learning more of the processes that occur in their interpersonal therapeutic relationships with clients. Throughout the course participants brought issues from their clinical practice to the supervision group. We alternated the sessions between participants, which generally lasted between an hour and ninety minutes. We had received teaching as to the purpose of the sessions, which were not specifically to address issues of technique or clinical knowledge but to gain an understanding about *process*. This meant that our descriptions of interactions between us and our clients were less valuable than the exploration of what we thought were going on while the interaction or events occurred.

Formative group supervision sessions

The issues I brought to the group were to do with the difficulties I was experiencing in developing a therapeutic interpersonal relationship with a resident upon the unit of which I was a staff member. I had been allocated as the key worker to a male resident, Dave, who had been an inpatient for several years within various mental health facilities. The difficulty that I was experiencing was how to stop Dave from interrupting conversations with noisy demands for staff to listen to what he wanted to say about his voices. A nursing care plan had been in force which reflected the general perception of staff that Dave was behaving without reasonable consideration for accepted social norms, as well as a clinical view which did not consider engagement in discussion about the content and meaning of auditory hallucinations as being therapeutic. Dave often became more insistent in his demand to be listened to, leading to mutual frustration, anger on his part and no successful resolution to his requests.

As I described what I thought was a reasonable therapeutic approach, i.e. to reinforce generally accepted social norms in line with the prevailing philosophy of the unit, my supervisor asked me to reflect on what could be happening in the interpersonal dynamics between Dave and members of staff. She asked me directly how I felt while Dave was demanding attention from me. She asked me to speculate how Dave was feeling when he was told he could not talk about something he thought was very, very important. I realised we both felt powerless, angry, ignored, devalued.

I have never forgotten the impact of realising that, for what had seemed good reasons, I was colluding in a system that was resulting in anger and frustration for both Dave and members of staff. *Through these CS sessions I became aware that I had no conceptual justification for refusing to listen to Dave talk at me about his voices other than I did not know what to do to help him if I did.* I also became aware of my emotional response to Dave which was interfering in the therapeutic interpersonal relationship (Peplau 1988). For example, in recognising and admitting to my own sense of irritation, indignation, or anger when Dave confronted me or colleagues, I was able to ask myself whether my response was justified (in the context of being therapeutic). To my discomfort I was able to identify that some of my reaction was because I felt and thought that I, a staff nurse, should be shown more respect, perhaps more gratitude, from this rude, thoughtless, demanding man! I had become an authority figure who Dave was challenging as he had challenged his father since he was a child, although for years I would have espoused the idea that a nurse should work co-operatively with the patient, promoting their sense of independence and challenging passivity and dependence.

Through this CS, I now understood how Dave's expectations of me (and others) were based on experience of previous relationships when he had taken a subordinate but rebellious role. I now had an experience of working with transference and counter-transference (see Brown and Pedder 1991). I had discovered what transference felt like and, once enlightened, was able to respond to his behaviour in a way that did not confirm unhelpful thoughts and feelings that he had towards authority figures but in a way that empowered him and affirmed him as an individual. For example, when Dave did or threatened to do something which was potentially problematic, such as go to the pub to get drunk, he was no longer told he could not. Instead I discussed with him what his wants were, what the organisational requirements were and together a mutually beneficial solution was reached. What was avoided was an unhelpful reprise of an authoritarian father figure and a rebellious child (Harris 1973). The outcome of this was that Dave reduced the number of assaults he made on staff for the next two years and felt able to arrange sessions when he and I would talk about his voices.

By bringing more examples of my interaction with Dave to CS I was able to gain a deeper understanding of nature and quality of the transactions between us. More importantly I was able to change and adapt my own practice to the benefit of Dave. Instead of attempting to control Dave's demands for attention I began to seek actively opportunities for him to ventilate his frustrations and fears about the voices that caused him distress. It became possible to reject a view, which had not been challenged throughout my training, that voices were symptoms and not to be encouraged and which led me to the developments in Cognitive Behavioural Therapy (Kingdon and Turkington 1991; Alford and Beck 1994; Birchwood and Tarrier 1992; Chadwick *et al.* 1996; Sanju *et al.* 2004) to 'treat' hallucinations and delusions.

My continuing experience of CS has been with my line manager. I agree with the well documented view that difficulties arise when line managers offer CS supervision because the focus of the supervision can easily move from the needs of the supervisee to those of the manager and the employer (see Butterworth and Faugier 1992; Cutcliffe and Proctor 1998a, 1998b; Stevenson 2005). *The truth is that there were some issues I felt unable to take to my formal supervisor for different reasons. One was that in admitting to some thoughts and feelings, I was concerned that this would prejudice my professional standing with my manager. A second reason, closely related to the first, is that there are some issues which practitioners are not comfortable about in exploring even with themselves, and to do so with someone in authority is even more problematic.* In my own case this has included feelings of anger towards a resident of whom I was becoming frightened. Fortunately I was able to take this issue (and others) to someone who I implicitly trusted and who did not feel obligated to inform my employer of our discussion. Because I had a place of safety I was able to express raw feelings, thoughts and emotions without fear of censure. In return I was relieved of the guilt and shame I had for merely experiencing human emotions, and was thereby empowered to change some of my own thoughts and beliefs, change my working practice and to develop strategies for working with the behaviour of the resident involved. This shows that CS allows us to be human and professional. In my case it permitted me to continue working in a homely environment with people who had or were likely to assault or threaten me and to do so in a therapeutic way without resorting to authoritarian attitudes. I believe that this example also illustrates a danger of receiving CS from a line manager, no matter how strong the professional or personal ties are. Regrettably, I could provide testimonies from dozens of colleagues whose 'clinical supervisors' consider CS sessions to be about their own issues, about caseload management or about control. This is not CS and can only be detrimental to patient/client care and the professional development of the nurse being supervised.

While the CS took place over several years there are specific examples that illustrate the effectiveness and value of the supervision I received. One example involved a resident who had recently been admitted to the unit after a period of time on an acute psychiatric admission ward which had followed deterioration in his relationship with his parents. Jack was resentful of not being allowed to live with his parents due to his disturbed and aggressive behaviour. He expressed bizarre ideas about being influenced by aliens and the occult in the past and thought his real mother had been replaced by the present woman who looked like her and sounded like her but could not be her because his mother would have him to live at home. He was disturbed by some of these ideas and even more troubled by the sense of abandonment he felt. Jack was skilled in many activities of daily living although chose not to attend to his hygiene or grooming and was careless with personal possessions.

As an individual I occasionally felt a responsibility for Jack. Through several CS sessions I was able to recognise that I was emotionally responding to Jack's explicit and implicit demands to be mothered, to be nurtured, to be rescued from the consequences of his own choices and actions. My supervisor facilitated this understanding by asking me how I felt or what I thought was being demanded from me by Jack when he behaved in ways which were apparently careless or rebellious. It was not that I was unaware of what Jack was doing, but by exploring the transference and counter-transference I was able to respond with greater self-awareness. I was able to recognise the unhelpfulness of my own unconscious desire to help, to nurture and to parent. Identifying the transference/counter-transference that was present meant that I was able to act in a way that was to eventually result in an increased sense of personal autonomy and responsibility for Jack. I gained a sense of empowerment through CS and felt increasingly able to empower Jack in having an expanding area of choice and responsibility. We were able to revisit parenting issues that he had experienced in ways that were more appropriate to our ages and abilities, and Jack was able to describe these issues as he gained an understanding of them.

Growth of self-awareness

It is not accurate to suppose that I brought all issues to CS knowingly. While I gave thought to what I wanted to talk about beforehand, invariably I would incidentally describe, with some emotion, an event that had occurred, without immediately realising its significance. When I talked of being confused or angry or sad it became apparent that Jack or whoever was experiencing similar or the same emotions. As I became more self-aware I could then reflect back to a client/resident that emotion, albeit in a tentative way, and encourage awareness-raising of their own mood states.

For example, this was particularly helpful in developing my therapeutic relationship with Jack, as he was not skilled in recognising and adapting to rising levels of anger or sadness. One evening Jack had become angry when a member of his family had made comments which Jack had difficulty in 'hearing', and he assaulted his family member. It was distinctly possible that further assaults were going to occur and that Jack was past the point at which he could be talked down or the situation de-escalated (Maier 1996). He was informed of our next response, which would be to 'hold him' until the threat of violence was withdrawn. Jack was also reminded that we recognised that neither he nor the nurses would like this; we had no wish to harm him and would prefer for him not to have to endure the holding. The situation eventually required a physical intervention that within a minute resulted in Jack saying he was calm and that he would go to his room. (An interpretation of this rapid reduction in Jack's emotional arousal could be that there had been a resolution of the bind he was in. He had been angry but did not have the skill to express this more effectively. Nor was he able to back down in that situation without losing face. Intervention by nursing staff conformed to past interventions he had experienced in previous establishments, including hospital environments, and so he was able to follow the part he had played on numerous occasions. Significantly there was a difference in the part played by the nursing staff, in that throughout the incident dialogue was maintained in a way that did not emphasise a need to control Jack but to manage the situation.)

It was as Jack returned to his room I felt an almost overwhelming sense of sadness and loss and instead of interpreting this as my own personal response to a violent incident I decide to check out with Jack how he felt. A few minutes later, with his permission, I was sitting on his bedroom floor, drinking a cup of tea and describing how I felt to Jack, and speculated that I was not the only one who felt sad. Instead of denying he felt bad and saying he was all right, a habitual shorthand way of avoiding any difficult discussion or realisation, Jack acknowledged sadness and we sat and cried together. He was able to own his emotion in that situation and showed some empathic understanding of others as well. He also was able to appreciate that his actions had resulted in unpleasant consequences for lots of people, and was able to accept responsibility for his part in the incident. A further benefit was that he did not get his revenge on anyone involved in the restraint procedure, which was also a departure from the norm.

Reflecting on critical incidents

I have found that the effectiveness of 'Critical Incident Analysis' (Minghella and Benson 1995) is also increased if carried out in the context of ongoing, skillful CS. That is to say the process(es) by which an incident can be analysed by gathering information to establish what happened, how it happened, why it happened and thereby gaining some insight into any lessons that could be learned from the incident are greatly enhanced if all participants can contribute freely to the process. This premise can be borne out by focusing on two violent incidents in which I was involved. The first involved my mishandling a situation and the second where, even in hindsight, it seems there was nothing that I could reasonably have done differently that would have prevented the assault. The first occurred when I entered, with permission, a resident's bedroom, to discuss something that was causing him some distress and about which he was beginning to get agitated. Missing the danger signals, I overstayed my welcome and had a shoe thrown at me. I was saved from further assault by the timely intervention of another member of staff. Team members provided a debriefing that shift but it was during a CS session I was able to explore my reasons for staying in the bedroom. I am certain without the safety of CS and supervisor that I trusted, I would not have had the opportunity to examine the intrapersonal process I was going through in that bedroom. We were able to identify the technical mistakes I made: e.g. allowing an increasingly agitated patient get between me and the door, not leaving the room earlier. We also explored how I felt at the time, why I did what I did and what I was hoping to achieve by acting the way

I did. The CS did not result in self-condemnation but in self-realisation and the opportunity to change my practice.

The second incident involved a resident who, with no warning, made an aggressive demand that something of his be given to him. Despite following an approach that was the optimum for de-escalating the situation, I was subjected to a bodily assault, which resulted in a period of sick leave. It was CS that enabled me to acknowledge my true thoughts and feelings to the assailant as I prepared to return to work. I had adopted an attitude which was admirable had it been true, that of understanding and forgiveness (as a result of my personal theological views/beliefs and personal philosophy). In addition, I have been exposed to a great deal of nursing literature which uncritically exhorts nurses to have unconditional, positive regard for patients/clients (e.g. Rogers 1952). In truth I did bear feelings of anger, betrayal, sadness and fear. What I was able to do was own up to these feelings in CS, secure in the knowledge that, barring confessions of illegality or gross professional misconduct, I could admit to perceived failure or weakness and not fear censure.

A need for caution

I remain surprised and saddened when I hear of colleagues who are suspicious about the intro-duction of CS to their practice. I suppose it is with some justification that nurses are cautious or sceptical when they see a hastily developed policy implemented with no consultation and little thought given to the training of supervisors. I have heard many stories of how managers use CS sessions as a management tool; supervisors who appoint themselves, dictate the agenda of the supervision sessions, and who verbalise their belief that it is all a waste of time anyway. I have worked with colleagues who are offended or frightened by the suggestion that they open their practice up to the gaze of anyone else. *But I have experienced how, when done adequately, CS is about growth and development not about censure.* Further, it has enabled me to improve my service to residents/clients and they have directly benefited by changes in my clinical practice.

Towards clinical excellence

When I moved jobs to work as a community psychiatric nurse (CPN) (attached to a general practitioner practice) I experienced a culture shock. While I was used to individual work with clients, I was not fully prepared for the implications of having no one to take over at the end of a shift. The most pressing need is the requirement to carry out assessments as to the risk of suicide, significant self-harm or risk to others within a limited time period. I was also faced with the different demands and opportunities presented by a different client group, and how to apply existing knowledge to different clinical problems. At my job interview I was assured that CS was considered to be part of normal working practice, and this has been the case. I was able to access informal supervision on an ad hoc basis, discussing difficulties and successes as we met coincidentally within the office. Formal CS sessions were planned, noted in our diaries and given priority over other meetings and appointments. As a result of the emphasis given to CS in the CPN team, a culture of support has developed that encourages a sharing of experiences. The team has acknowledged the importance of the opportunities to have colleagues listen to one another, ventilate feelings, help explore and resolve technical or practical difficulties and also be free to pass their own reflections upon issues raised. It is not a replacement for CS but a helpful addendum.

The issues I bring to CS continue to involve transference and counter-transference. It has been of considerable help to bring to CS situations where clients have adopted roles which do not permit therapeutic nursing to occur (Peplau 1988). For example, I have seen numerous clients who are referred not because they themselves want help but because a partner or parent has insisted they see a doctor. However, while I can know this I do not always feel comfortable discharging a client when I believe there is real potential for change. CS gives me the opportunity to express this discomfort and in doing so I usually recognise that my feelings have to do with my agendas, to be seen as effective, to help people whether they want it or not. My supervisor can sometimes enable this process by allowing me to continue talking, sometimes it involves questioning. *My assertion is that in receiving CS from skilful, knowledgeable, compassionate supervisors I was allowed to gain insights into my own practice that had direct benefits to the clients I was working with.*

Similar situations have also occurred when I have mistaken my agenda for the client's need. An example of this was while I was still seeing Bob. He had lost his job as a heavy goods vehicle driver two years previously due to arthritic changes in several joints, which continued to cause him physical discomfort despite the prescription of strong analgesia. He had developed severe depression to the extent he paid no attention to personal hygiene and was at risk of severe neglect without the support of close family. He expressed a sense of hopelessness about the future and a belief there was nothing left to live for. My difficulty was that he was not interested in engaging in a process to challenge the thoughts that were exacerbating the hope-lessness and depression. He was only bothered how I could help him get to an out-patient's appointment to see an orthopaedic consultant without him 'cracking up'. I took my frustrations to CS. By being asked what it was that Bob wanted I was able to see my error. I agreed it was not wrong for him to have an agenda that was different to mine. He had to cross a hurdle before he could give attention to the problem he thought I had invented for him. My frustration evaporated as I decided to work with Bob instead of deciding that he needed my nursing care. I subsequently discovered that when our agendas coincided, he quickly came to understand how changing his thinking would enable him to adapt to his changed circumstances. Within a short time he was both depression- and pain-free.

Final thoughts and reflections

My assertion is that in receiving CS from skilful, knowledgeable, compassionate supervisors I was allowed to gain insights into my own practice that had direct bene-fits to the clients I was working with. It could be argued that as I was someone who habitually reflected upon his own practice, I would have worked much of this out anyway (though I do not agree with that position). My point is that it was especially valuable for the few issues that got under my radar that I needed CS. I have found out that a view from outside oneself is frequently necessary. *The craft of psychiatric/ mental health nursing is such an all-embracing human activity that it is too easy to be caught up in the doing and to lose sight temporarily of the processes that we are involved in.*

I also believe that CS has an equally important benefit: I have been able to chart my development. I have had the opportunity for someone I trust to acknowledge the changes, the successes that have arisen out of my clinical development. I have had a regular opportunity not only to let off steam but also to act constructively as a result. And I remain as hungry to develop myself and clinical services to benefit resident/client care as ever after 22 years of nursing. I do not believe my experience is unique. There are many people who could write persuasive arguments to support the use of CS and I have read many others. The disappointing thing is that the nursing discipline still seems to be deciding whether it is worth the effort. I hope my experience, outlined in this chapter, will help convince nurses that CS is indeed worth the effort.

References

Alford, B.A. and Beck, A.T. (1994), Cognitive therapy of delusional beliefs, *Behavioural Research and Therapy*, 32(3): 369–380.

Birchwood, M. and Tarrier, N. (1992), *Innovations in the Psychological Management of Schizophrenia*, Chichester: Wiley & Sons.

Butterworth, A. and Faugier, J. (1992), *Clinical Supervision and Mentorship in Nursing*, London: Chapman & Hall.

Brown, D. and Pedder, J. (1991), *Introduction to Psychotherapy: An Outline of Psychodynamic Principles and Practice*, 2nd edn, London: Tavistock/ Routledge.

Chadwick, P., Birchwood, M.J. and Trower, P. (1996), *Cognitive Therapy for Delusions, Voices and Paranoia*, Chichester: Wiley and Sons.

Cutcliffe, J.R. and Proctor, B. (1998a), An alternative training approach in clinical supervision, part one, *British Journal of Nursing*, 7(5): 280–285.

Cutcliffe, J.R. and Proctor, B. (1998b) An alternative training approach in clinical supervision, part two, *British Journal of Nursing*, 7(6): 344–350.

Harris, T.A. (1973), *I'm OK–You're OK*, New York: Harper & Row.

Kingdon, D.G. and Turkington, D. (1991), The use of cognitive therapy with normalizing rationale in schizophrenia, *Journal of Nervous and Mental Disease*, 179(4): 207–211.

Maier, G.J. (1996), Managing threatening behaviour, *Journal of Psychosocial Nursing*, 34(6): 25–30.

Minghella, E. and Benson, A. (1995), Developing reflective practice in mental health nursing through critical incident analysis, *Journal of Advanced Nursing*, 21(2): 205–213.

Peplau, H.E. (1988), *Interpersonal Relationships in Nursing*, 2nd edn, Basingstoke: Macmillan.

Rogers, C.R. (1952), *Client-Centred Therapy*, London: Constable.

Sanju, G., Bandopadhay, S. and Cowan, C. (2004), A case report of informal cognitive therapy of delusions by a carer: a novel treatment paradigm? *European Psychiatry*, 20(1): 80–81.

Stevenson, C. (2005), Postmodernising clinical supervision in nursing, *Issues in Mental Health Nursing*, 26(5): 519–529.

17 Supporting palliative care nursing

The roles of clinical supervision

Alun Charles Jones

In this chapter, the author shares his experiences as a researcher and clinical supervisor with palliative care nurses. Alun refers to published accounts of his research studies with community palliative care nurses and hospice nurses throughout the chapter. This research and clinical work has led him to believe that sharing an experience, without concern for negative judgement, but with prudence, supports palliative care nurses. This helps to make sense of care provision, and so events become more understandable and accessible.

We believe this chapter acknowledges the particular and complex needs of palliative care nurses. It shows clearly how these nurses can benefit from clinical supervision in their daily contacts with people suffering serious illness, their families, and also managing relationships with colleagues and people outside of work. Beyond this specific population of nurses, though, this chapter may also be interesting and enlightening for those whose work is with patients who have chronic illnesses and are in long term care facilities. These nurses have a similar need for support and encouragement.

This chapter is an edited version of the author's original article "Clinical supervision in promoting a balanced delivery of palliative nursing care" (Jones 2003a).

Introduction

Repeated contact with illness, death and grief can challenge the resources of palliative care nurses. Working with patients who have serious illness and who need palliative care can be difficult for all health care professionals because of the poignancy of many situations. Nonetheless, with appropriate preparation and support, palliative care nurses and other health care professionals can gain opportunities for personal and professional growth while developing better self-understanding (Monroe and Oliviere 2007; Jones 2009a).

Palliative care

Providing palliative care to people with serious illness and their families is both complex and demanding. The World Health Organization (WHO 2009) illustrates this complexity of the demands placed on health care professionals in the definition of palliative care as follows:

> Palliative care is an approach that improves the quality of life of patients and their families facing the problem associated with life-threatening illness,

through the prevention and relief of suffering by means of early identification and impeccable assessment and treatment of pain and other problems, physical, psychosocial and spiritual.

Health care professionals therefore need to feel supported in order to counterbalance the difficulties and demands of providing palliative care. Subsequently, it is important that appropriate support mechanisms are available to palliative care nurses who can pass on feelings such as fear, anxiety and ultimately their values, beliefs and attitudes to patients and families (Jones 2006).

It is important due to the nature of work with seriously ill patients and their families that palliative care nurses gain a genuine sense of hope, and so recognise what is realistically achievable in their personal and professional lives, enhancing feelings of meaning and purpose (Palsson and Norberg 1995). Speaking together about experiences of illness might foster the idea in nurses that many achievements are gained with the collaboration of others. Moreover, disappointments are an inevitable part of life. With support, such as clinical supervision, palliative care nurses might become better able to contain the fears and anxieties of patients and their families, allow greater feelings of personal autonomy so those in their care will be better able to tolerate uncertainty and strong feelings of concern.

Clinical supervision and palliative care

Clinical supervision is a professional arrangement, which offers supervisees opportunities to think about managerial issues, educational needs and secure periods of calm and recuperation from the effects of the workplace (Jones 1997, 2008). These are arguably some fundamentals of balanced professional relationships.

Early on, Inskipp and Proctor (1994) referred to these important aspects of clinical supervision as *normative, formative* and *restorative* functions. Various authors, in relation to clinical supervision and nursing practice (Bowles and Young 1999; Kilcullen 2007), have discussed these functions. Palliative care nurses report that because of judiciously carried out supervision, worry and concerns are better contained and addressed constructively, while permitting opportunities to affirm strengths and achievements in context (Jones 2009b). This method of supporting professional practice can therefore offer nurses a chance to step out of the cauldron of health provision and think about what is going on before acting.

Experiences of research and clinical practice lead me to believe that clinical supervision is a professional format that offers personal insights and professional benefits to nurses of all specialties (Jones 2006). My supposition has been that work discussions about the management of serious illness, death, dying and bereavement and the feelings invoked can help nurses to think about events and assist in more discriminating communications with themselves and others. Caring for people with serious illness can be debilitating and cause difficulties, the source of which might not be readily appreciated or easily communicated. Clinical supervision is therefore a potentially useful medium for palliative care nurses to discuss their work.

The opportunity to reflect on practice and identify dynamic forces of health care influencing the course of a person's health and illness is perhaps a most critical factor in the delivery of an efficient human service (Corner 2002). *My work with palliative care nurses is based on the belief that clinical supervision allows nurses to untangle and address complex issues regarding the safety and effectiveness of professional practice in an atmosphere of personal regard and respect for others* (see Rafferty 2009).

In addition, we might better understand, through undertaking clinical supervision, personal and professional issues that influence each other by allowing palliative care nurses to balance their work with appropriate periods of rest. Clinical supervision might allow nurses to think about events without decontextualising the experience, permitting new ways to consider personal management of organisational difficulties including relationships with others (Jones 2009b).

By speaking about their experiences, palliative care nurses can begin to gain confidence in their abilities and affirm themselves for their many competencies and embedded knowledge and wisdom (Jones 1997). In some instances, however, competency can mean recognising when periods of tiredness and tension suggest a need for changing aspects of work organisation. Some issues, which can bring about pronounced feelings of stress to palliative care nurses, include the following: *managing relationships with colleagues and people outside work, feeling isolated, searching for meaning, strong positive and negative feelings aroused by work, and repeating behaviours which are unhelpful* (Jones 2009b).

The literature shows that there are likely to be many other concerns and issues that the health care professionals and nurses face in their day to day practice (Benner *et al.* 2009). However, in this chapter I want to focus on palliative care and nurses working with serious illness, death and bereavement from a psychological point of view. This is arguably different from other types of work and so raises specific concerns (Jones 2003b). I will also examine some areas of work that palliative care nurses have typically reported as stressful and describe the ways that clinical supervision helped each nurse manage work-related difficulties.

Managing relationships with colleagues and others

In the following example, a palliative care nurse shares with a supervisor her concern about her relationship with a manager:

NURSE: I cannot get on at all with my nurse manager these days. We both seem so stressed that we just do not seem to agree on anything. I really respect her and I know she has a difficult job to do but find it hard to contain my feelings.

SUPERVISOR: Yes, I can see that it troubles you. I also realise that managing your feelings constructively is important as is maintaining good relations with your manager. I wonder if you could tell me what sort of situation you find difficult. Do you think we might get a clearer idea of the problem?

In this account, the supervisor confirms the importance of the nurse's feelings without suggesting right or wrong and so maintains a supportive stance. The supervisor invited the nurse to explore the difficulties in an atmosphere of understanding. This permitted opportunities for thinking about events in new and constructive ways. Together the supervisor and nurse worked towards maintaining good relationships in times of difficulty.

The work of palliative care nurses can also influence other important relationships outside work. Palliative care nursing to some can represent unacceptable aspects of living and dying. Many palliative care nurses tell anecdotally that others attribute to them almost pernicious, magical powers because of their closeness to cancer-related illness. Images of violation and decline typically stigmatise associations with cancer. Palliative care nurses, while caring for people with other serious illnesses, to many represent cancer. Some view palliative care nurses as a metaphor for cancer and the author Susan Sontag (2001) described this phenomenon in some detail in her book *Illness as a Metaphor*. Sontag argues that illness becomes identified with particular psychological traits. That is to say, some people believe that the nature of an illness conveys the character of a person. Others stigmatise palliative care nurses, because of their affiliation to people with cancer and serious illness more generally.

Feeling isolated: death's companions

Anxieties about illness and death can show as others' fears of palliative care nurses because of the nature of their work (Jones 1999). One nurse recalled in clinical supervision how others viewed her as 'death's companion' and the sense of isolation that it brought about for her:

NURSE: Sometimes I will say to someone … a friend perhaps, you look poorly have you a cold? The response is amazing. It is seen as a pronouncement of impending death. Often, people will say to me 'don't *you* ever say that I look unwell'.

This example illustrates how professional identities can be from time to time unhelpful and sometimes isolate a nurse outside work. Rather than feeling affirmed for her chosen work, the nurse felt shunned because knowing of her work reminded others of their human vulnerability and the natural conclusion of life. In this instance, it was required that the nurse separated herself from her professional role as a palliative care nurse guided by the questions from the supervision and then her roles outside work, identifying supportive networks appropriate to each.

Palliative care nurses can gain a greater sense of empathy for colleagues. The observations from my research studies (Jones 1998, 1999, 2006, 2009b) have shown that clinical supervision can help nurses recognise ways in which others might attempt to shield themselves from the pain of serious illness and death.

One palliative care nurse recognised how difficult the work could be for other professionals and in doing so, reduced his sense of anger. The nurse had been troubled by events and explained to me:

NURSE: It used to make me so angry when a doctor would visit the house and spend what seemed like relatively little time with the patient. It appeared that he would just prescribe medication and leave me to get on with the difficult and messy stuff. Sometimes, I feel so angry, that I go home and I am unable to think of anything for the whole evening, weekend, whatever. Through thinking now in supervision about ways in which I protect myself, I can see that is, maybe, what they are doing … [protecting themselves]. If curing someone judges success and there just is not a cure, then I suppose, it means looking failure in the face. Death is a doctor's failure. It helps to know that … the problem is theirs to deal with and not mine. Although understanding what that means, I will do more to understand [other professionals] in future.

He realised a burden that he had carried belonged in part to others and that illness and death influence others in different ways. By thinking about his feelings and exploring attitudes and values, he freed himself from troubling feelings of guilt. The nurse also gained a greater regard for the difficulties faced by other professional groups, in this instance a medical doctor, and was better able to address issues of concern responsibly yet with sensitivity for the doctor's fears.

A good example of developing mutually supportive relationships because of supervision is illustrated in the next account of a palliative care nurse's work. A community mental health nurse working with a dying person had requested the palliative care nurse's professional support. The nurse assumed overall responsibility for the management of care. Clinical supervision, however, allowed the nurse time to consider the likely outcome of, and an opportunity to think about strategies that were likely to be more appropriate. Subsequently, the nurses foresaw difficulties regarding taking on too much so encouraging other professionals to withdraw defensively. A dying person and the family might perceive such withdrawal as abandonment. A more appropriate strategy, we decided, would be for the nurse to support the community mental health nurse throughout the episode of care, so forging a creative partnership between disciplines. Heightened professional empathy and teamwork permitted them to share the responsibility and support each other. Care became meaningful and manageable.

The nurse later commented:

> Normally, I would have taken over responsibility for all of the care and found it burdensome. Initially the community mental health nurse wanted me to assume responsibility. Although later, she explained that she did not want to say so at the time. Working together though has been a good experience. At first, I suppose, I was a bit wary of her ... you know professionally. Working together made me realise the knowledge that I have gained over the years. I could use that knowledge to guide and inform the community mental health nurse in her care planning. I must admit I enjoy our working together.

Addressing strong feelings

Sometimes recurrently facing issues concerning serious illness can lead to strong feelings and impulsive activities such as buying expensive clothes, holidays and gifts for oneself (Jones 1998). This might be because working with serious illness challenges values and meanings concerning life and notions of death. Untimely or unsatisfactory deaths can cause emotional upheavals in nurses and other health care professionals and contest with ideas of a consummate end to life.

Palliative care nurses have told me that buying new things helps ease a transient sense of nothing in life being important. This is not because they are fundamentally spendthrifts but rather facing serious illness and death repeatedly can lead to extremes of feelings, both positive and negative. In some instances, a strong sense of futility can colour a nurse's life with a need for counterbalances.

A palliative care nurse captures these feelings very well in the next statement:

> Sometimes, I just spend like there is no tomorrow. The nature of this work sometimes makes me feel that I should not feel any pleasure. Still, if I overspend

I feel guilty later, as if I am bad in some way. I do it impulsively and then I feel ashamed.

Typically, statements like these reflect the need for restoration, personal death awareness, and not being able to feel pleasure suggests weariness with issues concerning serious illness. It might of course also be the case, that sometimes nurses feel a pervasive sense of guilt. This occurs because they are healthy and without illness and constantly in the presence of others who are not. In this instance, a response was required from me that emphasised significant parts of the content of the statement. Care was needed to respond accurately, so as not to flood nurses with strong or unmanageable feelings:

SUPERVISOR: I am wondering how this might relate to your work situation?

NURSE: Oh yes ... ha! I had not really thought of the meaning of that when I said it.

SUPERVISOR: Shall we, consider how you are feeling in the context of your work?

NURSE: Yes, all right (*pause*) well I think that knowing that there might be no tomorrow (*pause*) well perhaps makes us want to feel alive today (*pause*) maybe. So impulsive buying is a way to care for me I suppose (*sigh*) hmm! Nevertheless, there is also some thing about the idea of having new things. Like starting again, out with the old and very definitely in with the new.

SUPERVISOR: We have discussed similar issues previously: people you care for dying and, almost without respite, your concern for a new referral. So buying, you are suggesting, is a way to protect you from feeling overwhelmed with sickness and death (*pause*) but somehow leads to feelings of guilt. Do I have that right?

NURSE: Hmm (*long ponder*). I think now we are talking about it in this way (*pause*) thinking about such trivial things in the face of so much misery seems wrong and yet, well I do my best to help. Perhaps I should not be so hard on myself ... or maybe find ways to treat myself ... support myself in work ... ways that do not arouse guilt..... However, it is like the work ... replacing the old with the new (*sigh*) continually. I think that causes me quite a bit of guilt.

SUPERVISOR: So perhaps we could consider your workload and ways that you might manage aspects of it differently or vary your work to allow you periods of rest.

It is worthwhile thinking about what might be discussed in clinical supervision and how seemingly unconnected statements can relate to the workplace. For example, a nurse might be feeling angry, distressed or pressured by events that do not appear to be directly concerned with work. Whenever this happens, the supervisor can choose to invite the nurse to ventilate his or her feelings before beginning supervision and so clear the air or think about how statements reflect issues concerning supervision or the workplace.

There are no formula answers and much will depend on the relationship between the supervisor and nurse and the agreed working boundaries. There is of course a need to be mindful that clinical supervision should not slide over into psychological therapy for the nurse because this is not its purpose. In the above example, the supervisor wondered aloud, allowing the nurse to make her own links and connections with areas of her work. A conversation followed which helped the nurse think constructively about balancing her working week.

Repeating unhelpful behaviours

Occasionally a need to care for others can show as repeated feelings of ownership for patients and families (Jones 2009b).

This is evident in a palliative care nurse's account of her feelings:

> Oh yes, I do become a bit jealous when someone else becomes involved (other professionals). They are all my patients. You can get a buzz from nursing you know. They need you ... It's adoration I suppose. There is no point in pretending that it does not give you a high. It is as a drug ... strange to think you can be addicted to death.

Another nurse similarly reported:

> Yes, I realise that I get a sense of excitement when everything is busy around me. I can see that ways I organise work sometimes mean that I am taking on too much. It is as if I cannot help it. When I think about it though, it probably means that I do not feel guilty ... about what, I do not know. Nevertheless, I feel myself taking on too much and then I can rather say, well, you deserve this weekend, new dress, whatever.

When there is a strong desire to give to others, nurses can take on too much responsibility and then are unable to manage. The gap between what we might wish were possible and what is realistically achievable can cause feelings of guilt.

A palliative care nurse explains:

> I am always left feeling that I should do more. I rarely derive a feeling of satisfaction. I often know what could be achieved for the patients but I am limited by others. How can I care properly without control over others? In most instances, others exert power over me, in many different ways. I am just left feeling guilty.

In the above account, a nurse relates her feelings of powerlessness. She feels swamped by a sense of contradiction. Strong internal motivations cause her to try to achieve more than is possible within the confines of alliances with other members of the health care team but also the realities of life.

In the nurse's account, internal configurations of the world and outside pressures complement each other to the extent that a person can feel driven to achieve more than is possible. In this instance, clinical supervision provided the environment within which to challenge established ways of viewing the world. Removing barriers to change allowed the nurse to think about new and creative ways to structure work.

Balancing work and affirming professional practice

Palliative care nurses should work within clearly identified professional frameworks encouraging all professionals to view their roles realistically. The roles of palliative care nurses might also encompass periods away from clinical work allowing perhaps projects to be undertaken to successful conclusion and perhaps providing positive feelings of accomplishment. This would offer important balance and calming periods for nurses to restore their energies and combat feelings of burnout (Jones and Cutcliffe 2009).

Burnout is a term used to describe a syndrome of emotional and psychological fatigue. A person experiencing burnout can experience feelings of depersonalisation along with low or changeable mood. Burnout can negatively affect personal and professional attainments. It commonly occurs in professionals who work in human service (Maslach *et al.* 2001). Palliative care nurses could be actively encouraged to undertake professional development and research directly concerned with the delivery of palliative care.

It also seems important that sensitive appraisal systems fulfil a justifiable human need for affirmation and confirm the value of palliative care nurses' contributions to services. Appraisals would offer a means through which to identify professional pathways that allow the productive realisation of knowledge gained from working with the seriously ill, the dying and bereaved. Nurses generally need reference points and opportunities for benchmarking their work (Billings *et al.* 2001).

Safe and effective clinical supervision

Palliative care nurses undertaking clinical supervision need to forge creative environments to address the complexity of being human and caring for others. Choice, professional safety and therapeutic effectiveness should therefore be prominent in the minds of the supervisor, supervisee and organisation. Because of the responsibilities they carry, some roles, such as line manager, hinder the supervisory process and so nurses need to give this careful consideration before agreeing to work together as supervisors or supervised (Jones 2001).

Clinical managers, while typically experienced nurses, might experience discomfort arising from listening to conflicts and tensions, which are a natural part of the delivery of human service. Because of responsibilities concerning the delivery of a clinical safe service, it could be difficult for a manager to work with a nurse in clinical supervision on his or her own directorate. However, this might work across directorates.

It is therefore important that supervisors and supervisees consider whether they are best suited to work together (Jones 1996). Fundamentally, clinical supervision should be creative, allowing nurses to realise talents and abilities as well as ensuring safe professional practice. Furthermore, we all have different ways of learning and this will conceivably colour our view of the world and events. It is perhaps necessary to identify learning styles and ways they may be best harnessed in clinical supervision to learn about professional practice.

Within a necessary uniformity, nurses can make unique contributions to nursing work. An inventory of supervisors such as Supervisor e-Network might go some way to achieving the right match between palliative care nurses. This could contain professional biographies including personal and professional interests and experience and make available within organisations e.g. within and between hospitals and hospices or other agencies. It might also be possible to identify which professional roles would reduce or enhance the effectiveness of clinical supervision and protocols developed by including an evaluation system in this network. Working models or frameworks for recognising situations in which supervisors and those supervised working together could promote effective relationships.

Sometimes there are simply no satisfactory solutions to life's problems. In many instances, we will not help patients and their families in ways that they would choose in an ideal world (Jones 2009b), in which case, palliative care nurses might not receive the depth of approval they need to carry out much of what is difficult and demanding work. *Supervisors can help by encouraging palliative care nurses to ponder on, speak about their achievements, and affirm the good in their work. Supervisors can also moderate pressures to achieve perfection by asking nurses to consider both positive and negative aspects of their professional practice and to view them as part of the totality of health care.* Working in this way attends to the *normative, formative* and *restorative* elements of supervision as described by Inskipp and Proctor (1994). Palliative care nurses can manage professional relationships appropriately; learning follows, restoring balance to nursing practice.

Conclusion

If we establish and develop approaches to clinical supervision thoughtfully, nurses can gain from a hope-inspiring means of addressing the complexities of palliative care. They can move from the inside of nursing practice and look afresh at the care they offer to the seriously ill, the dying, bereaved and the environments in which they work. Clinical supervision can give to nurses an experience that brings about positive change and encourages an ability to adjust to alterations in organisational life. We might also help each nurse to learn from examples how to create similar conditions for others.

References

Benner, P., Tanner, C.A. and Chesla, C.A. (2009), *Expertise in Nursing Practice: Caring, Clinical Judgment and Ethics*, New York: Springer.

Billings, D.M., Connors, H.R. and Skiba, D.J. (2001), Benchmarking best practices in web-based nursing courses, *Advances in Nursing Science*, 23(30): 41–52.

Bowles, N. and Young, C. (1999), An evaluative study of clinical supervision based on Proctor's three function interactive model, *Journal of Advanced Nursing*, 30(4): 958–964.

Corner, J. (2002), Nurses' experiences of cancer, *European Journal of Cancer Care*, 11(3): 193–199.

Inskipp, F. and Proctor, B. (1994), *The Art, Craft and Tasks of Counselling Supervision: Making the Most of Supervision*, London: Cascade.

Jones, A. (1996), Clinical supervision: a review and commentary, *Journal of Psychiatric Nursing Research*, 3(1): 220–229.

Jones, A. (1997), Clinical supervision in moderating organisational conflict and preserving effective relationships, *International Journal of Palliative Nursing*, 3(5): 293–299.

Jones, A. (1998), Clinical supervision with community Macmillan nurses: some theoretical suppositions and casework reports, *European Journal of Cancer Care*, 7(1), 63–69.

Jones, A. (1999), The 'heavy and blessed experience': how can psychoanalytic ideas inform the delivery of care to the seriously ill? *Journal of Advanced Nursing*, 30(6): 1297–1303.

Jones, A. (2001), The influence of professional roles on clinical supervision, *Nursing Standard*, 15(33): 42–45.

Jones, A. (2003a), Clinical supervision in promoting a balanced delivery of palliative nursing care, *Journal of Hospice and Palliative Nursing*, 5(3): 168–175.

Jones, A. (2003b), On projective identification, containment and feeling special: some thoughts about hospice nurses' experiences, *American Journal of Hospice and Palliative Care*, 20(6): 441–446.

Jones, A. (2006), Group-format clinical supervision for hospice nurses, *European Journal of Cancer Care*, 15(2): 155–162.

Jones, A. (2008), Clinical supervision is important to the quality of healthcare provision, *International Journal of Mental Health Nursing*, 17(5): 379–380.

Jones, A. (2009a), Returning meaning to palliative care staff, editorial, *European Journal of Palliative Care*, 16(4): 161.

Jones, A. (2009b), Fevered love, in L. de Raeve, M. Rafferty and M. Paget (eds), *Nurses and Their Patients: Informing Practice through Psychodynamic Insights*, Keswick: M&K Publishing.

Jones, A. and Cutcliffe, J.R. (2009), Listening as a method of addressing psychological distress, *Journal of Nursing Management*, 17(3): 352–358.

Kilcullen, N. (2007), An analysis of the experiences of clinical supervision on registered nurses undertaking MSc/Graduate Diploma in renal and urological nursing and on their clinical supervisors, *Journal of Clinical Nursing*, 16(6): 1029–1038.

Maslach, C., Schaufeli, W.B. and Leiter, M.P. (2001), Job burnout, *Annual Review of Psychology*, 52: 387–422.

Monroe, B. and Oliviere, D. (2007), Unlocking resilience in palliative care, in B. Monroe and D. Oliviere (eds), *Resilience in Palliative Care: Achievement in Adversity*, Oxford: Oxford University Press.

Palsson, M.B. and Norberg, A. (1995), District nurses' stories of difficult care episodes narrated through systematic clinical supervision sessions, *Scandinavian Journal of Caring Science*, 9(1): 17–27.

Rafferty, M. (2009), Using Winnicott (1960), to create a model for clinical supervision, in L. de Raeve, M. Rafferty and M. Paget (eds), *Nurses and Their Patients: Informing Practice through Psychodynamic Insights*, Keswick: M&K Publishing.

Sontag, S. (2001), *Illness as Metaphor and AIDS and its Metaphors*, New York: Picador.

WHO (World Health Organization) (2009), *WHO Definition of Palliative Care*, online, available at: www.who.int/cancer/palliative/definition/en/.

18 Clinical supervision for United Kingdom medical professionals

Helen Halpern

Until recently, doctors in the United Kingdom have had little formal experience of clinical supervision. However, there is a new requirement for regular, formal educational and clinical supervision for all doctors in training grades. Therefore, the topic of clinical supervision for general practitioners is timely in the UK today. Over the last few years, the author and her colleagues have pioneered a framework for supervision skills which has been taught in workshops for medical educators in primary and secondary care. The author has found that experienced clinicians value this model as a facilitator to useful conversations with colleagues about workplace dilemmas, difficult cases, team interactions, problems with trainees and help with career decisions. The author introduces, in this chapter, the model which is based on ideas drawn from a variety of sources, including family therapy, systemic approaches and narrative ideas. She also outlines some of the main theoretical ideas drawn upon and the means by which these have been introduced to clinicians.

We believe that this chapter is very important to educators and clinical supervisors who are providing or have been invited to provide clinical supervision to doctors or to interprofessional teams which include doctors. In addition to the education model, the author also introduces a selection of valuable readings around the topic.

Introduction

Until recently doctors in the United Kingdom had little formal experience of supervision, at least not in a form that might be familiar to most mental health care professionals. Although clinicians in training receive technical supervision and experienced professionals seek opinions from peers, there is no culture of routine reflection on practice with a regular supervisor. However, this is changing as clinicians become aware of the rich tradition that exists in many professionals who work alongside them. In addition, a number of public and regulatory bodies have emphasised the need for new practitioners to receive more systematic supervision and there is now a requirement for regular educational and clinical supervision for all doctors in training grades.

Over the last few years a group co-ordinated by Dr John Launer and myself (Dr Helen Halpern) has pioneered a way to teach supervision skills in workshops for medical and dental educators in order to meet the changing culture and requirements of practice. The model was developed at the Tavistock Clinic in London where both of us, who have a background as general practitioners (GPs), had also been trained as systemic family therapists. Originally the model was created by Dr

Caroline Lindsey and Dr John Launer, to offer training in systemic practice for GPs and others working in primary care to use when seeing patients or working with teams. Over time it became clear that skills for working with families could also be relevant for supervising peers and trainees. We therefore started to focus on training in supervision skills and this model rapidly caught on, especially within GP training. We now deliver a wide range of training workshops in supervision skills for primary and secondary care educators at the London Deanery (the organisation responsible for postgraduate medical and dental training in London). Our trainings range from one-day workshops for hospital consultants to a year-long part-time certificate course for clinical teachers who want to acquire proficiency in the model and teach it themselves.

Our theoretical base comes from various sources, particularly systemic and narrative ideas, and we aim to develop a culture of supervision which involves a circular process of learning and teaching. In this chapter I will outline some of the theoretical background that informs our ideas and the ways we put this into practice to make it clinically relevant. I will give a flavour of the training workshops we offer and discuss some of our thoughts for future development.

Challenges

Professional conversations in medicine move between two overlapping domains performance-related (duties of a clinician) and developmental (duties towards the clinician) as shown in Figure 18.1.

The performance-related part fits with the 'normative' aspect of supervision suggested by Proctor (2001) while the developmental part fits with the 'formative and restorative' aspects. We recognise that supervision in medicine should provide support, deal with essential technical competence and also provide help with a review of the contexts that influence work, team interactions and communication skills. All these features appear to be linked with safer professional practice (Long *et al.* 2009) and fewer complaints (Kinnersley and Edwards 2008).

By teaching generic conversational micro-skills and helping clinicians to find an appropriate balance of support and challenge in their conversations, we hope

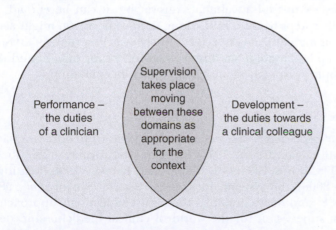

Figure 18.1 The domains of supervision.

to provide them with techniques that promote both patient safety and reflective practice so that they can develop new ways of thinking about their work. Taking a systemic view that people, contexts and actions are interlinked, small shifts in perspective have the potential to open whole new vistas. We recognise how difficult it can be for busy clinicians to find protected time for reflection and how educational and developmental work has to be balanced with time for service provision.

Many people attending our courses are concerned about how to supervise trainees and come expecting to talk about difficulties with learners. Some are initially sceptical about the usefulness of supervision skills beyond supervising trainees. Even in this area they felt that supervision was often mainly technical e.g. explaining how to carry out a procedure. We hope that the skills acquired on the course help them to think about their work in a new way. Even with technical problems, as long as it is clinically safe, it may be more beneficial for supervisors to support trainees to work out what to do for themselves, rather than taking over. Trainees may lack confidence and need the assurance of a more experienced colleague so that sometimes simply speaking about the problem will generate a solution without the supervisor having to provide an answer. We hope that in addition to addressing these issues they leave with skills that are transferable to conversations with patients and their families, with colleagues and wider networks, as well as valuing their own supervision. Indeed a supervisor in one situation may be a supervisee in another. Clinicians from different specialities have found that they can successfully supervise each other. This often comes as a revelation to those involved. They discover that it is not always necessary to know the technical details of a case in order to provide useful supervision. The skill is in asking questions that can draw out thinking, ideas and resources to move the supervisee forward. We teach the value of a 'not knowing' approach (Anderson and Goolishian 1992) where the supervisor can ask apparently naive questions and challenge the jargon and assumptions that sometimes accompany expertise in a particular clinical area.

Some supervisors feel isolated, with limited peer support and little value placed on this kind of work by managers, but supervision does not always have to be time-consuming; a few words with a colleague can be effective. Indeed it is possible that professionals waste time by avoiding the discussion of difficult topics or dilemmas. Sometimes it is not necessary to find an ultimate answer but it can be enough to develop ideas about the first steps to take. In the long term, supervision might actually save time through helping clinicians to acquire their own 'internal supervisor' (Casement 1985). This implies an ability to observe and reflect for oneself and the capacity to consider multiple perspectives, imagining what others might say.

Theoretical framework

The unique feature of our approach is that we have taken ideas from different paradigms, particularly narrative (e.g., Geertz 1973; Ricoeur 1984; Bruner 1986; Riessmann 1990; Mattingly 1998; Brody 1994; Greenhalgh and Hurwitz 1998; Mattingly and Garro 2000; Charon 2006) and systemic ideas (e.g. Palazzoli Selvini *et al.* 1980; Cecchin 1987; Tomm 1988) and have combined these with educational approaches to create a framework of supervision for the world of clinical medicine and dentistry, training clinicians to supervise other clinicians.

The premise of our systemic theoretical approach is that the world is composed of complex interactions and patterns between people and contexts. We use this framework to think about processes in supervision itself and also within the groups we are training. We use questions to understand meanings, to bring out relationships and differences over time and from differing perspectives. The questions arise from taking a position of curiosity to generate hypotheses (Palazzoli Selvini *et al.* 1980; Cecchin 1987). Interventive interviewing (Tomm 1988), which we call 'conversations inviting change', is a useful framework for asking different kinds of questions. However, these therapy-based ideas do not always fit well with clinicians and some of the material has been adapted to be more relevant and accessible (Halpern 2009).

Another important theoretical foundation is that of narrative, which suggests that people make sense of their experiences through the telling and re-telling of stories (Churchill and Churchill 1982). In supervision, conversations are used to tease out how clinicians relate their story; the language they use and how they process their thinking, in order to offer an opportunity for change. This is helpful in the kinds of scenarios which people often present where they feel stuck. In a stuck story (Andersen 1987b) thoughts and ideas go round and round without making progress. Un-sticking a story often begins when people verbalise their thoughts; simply hearing these spoken aloud can affect how things are understood. Part of the process of supervision involves interrupting the repetitive, rehearsed stories and challenging assumptions and prejudices to provide an opportunity to discover new thoughts and ideas which can contribute to more helpful understanding. We therefore develop supervisors' skills in observing and questioning non-verbal cues and emotions, listening to the nuances of words and carefully tracking language to question supervisee's narratives. We bring these theoretical threads together in the framework of the Seven Cs (Launer 2006) which we propose as concepts to hold in mind during supervision:

1 *Conversation.* The dialogue between supervisor and supervisee focuses on the needs of the supervisee using a questioning approach to provide an opportunity for the supervisee to rethink and redefine their stories and to bring about change.
2 *Curiosity.* Questions are usually more effective than statements, suggestions or advice. Curiosity can help to make hypotheses on which to base further questions, in addition to establishing what the supervisee already knows, what options they have already thought of, or want to explore further.
3 *Contexts.* It is often more important to discover the contexts for a problem rather than focusing on the content. The meaning of what people say is determined by a wide variety of contexts including the supervision relationship itself and the ways that power is perceived. Other contexts include beliefs, values and preferences, and organisational pressures.
4 *Complexity.* Most problems brought to supervision are inherently complex. Supervision offers opportunities for supervisees to enrich their understanding of what is going on, to find a way forward. Getting away from simple cause and effect explanations may facilitate the development of more sophisticated options. Small changes in one area can also lead to new outcomes in other parts of a complex system.

5   *Creativity.* Supervision requires imagination and risk-taking on both sides. It can help people to think 'outside the box'.
6   *Caution.* Supervision requires an ability to work with respect; operating within the limits of the supervisee's capacity to tolerate anxiety, while not avoiding an appropriate level of challenge that can help develop their thinking.
7   *Care.* Supervision requires thought about confidentiality and must include an ethical commitment from both supervisor and supervisee.

We could well add 'confusion' as this is often an aspect of any process of change. The Seven Cs are not intended to be an exhaustive list or a recipe and we encourage people to use the framework in ways that suit them within their own work setting.

We believe that a technique based on asking questions is a powerful tool for the creation of new thinking. This way of working is new to most of the people who attend our workshops. Asking questions has many other advantages:

- They signal interest and can help set the scene and clarify beliefs and understanding.
- They 'foster an attitude of curiosity, of eagerness to learn more' (Freedman and Combs 1996: 6).
- They can help the supervisor and supervisee calibrate where they are in their conversation.
- In contrast to statements, questions can help the supervisor and supervisee avoid making assumptions.
- They can trigger new thinking, increase complexity and promote creativity for problem solving.
- They encourage supervisees to think. This means that the supervisor does not necessarily need specialised knowledge in order to be helpful.
- By asking questions which address the views of others (triadic questions) it is possible to extend perspectives on a particular issue.
- Asking questions in a non-judgemental way can help overcome defensiveness and resistance.
- Good questions make a link with the supervisee's own experience and can help reflection.
- Supervisors working in this way are likely to be less paternalistic and the supervisee can own the solution.
- They help to develop solutions that fit the particular context so that if any advice is offered it is likely to be more appropriate.

When training people in our model, we ask supervisors learning the technique to confine themselves to asking questions and to withhold giving advice unless there are ethical or clinical governance concerns which need to be addressed. When they are in the position of being supervisors many doctors and dentists tell us that they find this very difficult. Some feel that providing rapid solutions and giving advice is exactly what they have been trained to do. However, as supervisees they report that they are much more likely to change if ideas come from themselves. People who are used to a more didactic style can find it difficult to adapt and the process can take time. We offer the technique as another skill that can be integrated with existing practice.

We acknowledge that this questioning approach does not always fit. There are circumstances when a supervisor has to give immediate advice without inviting any element of choice or reflection; a surgeon supervising a trainee in the operating theatre may need to be directive and didactic, allowing other aspects of supervision to take place at a different time or in a different context.

Implementation in practice

Courses were originally set up in the 1990s for professionals working in primary health care teams. A narrative and systemic-based approach was used to teach about the consultation and to develop skills in working with patients, families and teams (Launer and Lindsey 1997). People on these courses wanted to talk about cases and situations which were troubling them. It seemed to be more effective for them to supervise each other about these real-life situations rather than through role-plays. It became apparent that the same skills could be extended to include conversations about teamwork and careers, with some overlaps with mentoring and management. As education became further professionalised within medicine and dentistry a variety of new workshops were developed.

Short courses

The people who attend short courses (half-day, one-day and three-day) include doctors from both primary and secondary care and also nurses, dentists, practice managers, medical educators and other allied professionals. Some courses are held at a central London location, others take place at Hospital Trust Postgraduate Centres for local clinical staff. The three-day workshops are held at fortnightly intervals so that participants can try out their skills and reflect on their learning between sessions.

At these courses we give a brief overview of the background of supervision, including the framework of The Seven Cs. We demonstrate 'Conversations Inviting Change' by inviting a course participant to be supervised on a live issue by one of the facilitators in front of the group. We believe that it is invaluable for participants to have as much experience as possible in giving, receiving and observing supervision in facilitated small groups of between three and five members. This allows people to practice with the support of a few colleagues and with a facilitator who can coach all the group members and give focused feedback. We slow down the supervision by freeze-framing, pausing to tease out the process and to generate opportunities for thinking about how best to ask the next question. We ask supervisors to work to three guidelines while they are learning the new skill, recognising that this may be different from their usual style. These guidelines are:

1   only ask questions;
2   make the next question follow on from something that has already been mentioned;
3   save any advice to the end.

The three guidelines map onto theoretical ideas from the Milan group of family therapists (Palazolli Selvini *et al.* 1980). The supervisor works by making hypotheses which generate questions. They maintain their curiosity by following the supervisee's narrative and must be prepared to change their hypothesis and questions if they do not seem to fit or to be helpful for the supervisee. By withholding advice to the end the supervisor is more able to remain curious and therefore also maintain a state of neutrality.

In the small groups we use the observers as a reflecting team (Andersen 1987a). We ask them to observe the supervision process and to use their curiosity to help generate observations and questions. This has a number of benefits:

- It develops people's capacity to observe both content and process.
- It actively engages the observers but in a position of being one-removed. This can free their thinking and help them to formulate hypotheses and questions that are not available to the supervisor.
- It generates wider perspectives and offers new angles for enquiry.
- In certain cases the group can act as bench-markers and as an information resource.
- An additional spin-off is that the observers pay close attention to the process and are able to give very astute and focused feedback to the supervisor.

People attending our courses have brought a huge range of issues for supervision. These include:

Issues with trainees e.g. health problems, attitude problems including lack of insight, difficulties in engaging with others, underperformance, career choices, stretching excellent trainees.

Issues with patients e.g. patients whom the doctor dislikes, patients who will not take advice, lack of clarity about what patients want, managing patient expectations, patients who admire the doctor too much, talking about technically difficult situations so that patients can understand, consultations which did not seem to go well, grey area diagnoses, dissatisfied patients and 'heart-sinks', difficulties with confidentiality, ethical issues such as end-of-life decisions especially when there is lack of agreement amongst colleagues about how to proceed, and emotional aspects of consultations: sadness, anger, frustration.

Teamwork issues e.g. managing colleagues who seem to be undermining/bullying/playing people off against each other, how to say 'no', whistle-blowing, allegations of harassment or bullying, concerns about members of other teams, working with people who do not get on with each other/people who seem to be unapproachable.

Management issues e.g. developing leadership and negotiation skills, managing some of the difficulties involved in running a business, employment issues and staff disciplinary procedures, handling complaints, difficulties related to appraisal.

Supervision workshops for clinical teachers

This is a series of three-hour workshops at fortnightly intervals for people who want a regular opportunity to bring cases for supervision by their peers and to enhance their own supervision skills.

Professional certificate in supervision skills for clinical teachers

This course is run by the London Deanery together with the Tavistock Clinic to become teachers of supervision skills in medical and dental settings. We aim to provide a safe place for learning so that participants can explore new ideas, where curiosity and challenge are actively encouraged and people's differences are valued as a potential for creativity. The facilitators attend a year-long course of 15 half-day

Table 18.1 Examples of the reading

Topics	References
Education theory and practice	• Cantillon, P. and Sargeant, J. (2008), Giving feedback in clinical settings, *British Medical Journal*, 337(a1961): 1292–1294. • Connolly, B. (2008), *Adult Learning in Groups*, Maidenhead: McGraw-Hill Education. • Harden, R. (2008), Death by PowerPoint: the need for a fidget index, *Medical Teacher*, 30(9–10): 833–835. • Jaques, D. (2003), ABC of learning and teaching in medicine: teaching small groups, *British Medical Journal*, 326(7387): 492–494. • Kaufman, D. (2003), ABC of learning and teaching in medicine: applying educational theory in practice, *British Medical Journal*, 326(7382): 213–216. • Marshall, R., and Bleakey, A. (2009), The death of Hector: pity in Homer, empathy in medical education, *Journal of Medical Ethics: Medical Humanities*, 35: 7–12.
Systemic theory and practice	• Asen, E., *et al.* (2004), Ingredients of the systemic approach, Chapter 2 in *Ten Minutes for the Family: Systemic Interventions in Primary Care*, London: Routledge. • Burr, V. (1995), Does language affect the way we think? Chapter 2, in *An Introduction to Social Constructionism*, London/New York: Routledge. • Campbell, D. and Groenbaek, M.(2006), Ideas that underpin the model, Chapter 2 in *Taking Positions in the Organization*, London/New York: Karnac.
Narrative theory and practice	• Kalitzkus, V. and Matthiessen, P. (2008), Narrative-based medicine: potential, pitfalls and practice, *The Permanente Journal*, 3(1): 80–86. • Launer, J. (1999), Narrative-based medicine: a narrative approach to mental health in general practice, *BMJ*, 318(7176): 117–119. • McCarthy, J. (2003), Principalism or narrative ethics: must we choose between them? *Journal of Medical Ethics: Medical Humanities*, 29(2): 65–71.
Narrative-based medicine	• Charon, R. (2008), Narrative evidence based medicine, *The Lancet*, 371(9609): 296–297. • Greenhalgh, T. (1999), Narrative based medicine: narrative based medicine in an evidence based world, *British Medical Journal*, 318(7179): 323–325. • Greenhalgh, T. and Hurwitz, B. (1999), Narrative based medicine: why study narrative? *British Medical Journal*, 318(7175): 48–50.
Supervision theory and practice	• Launer J. (2003), Practice, supervision, consultancy and appraisal: a continuum of learning, *British Journal of General Practice*, 53(493): 662–665. • Long S., Neale G. and Vincent C. (2009), Practising safely in the foundation years, *British Medical Journal*, 338(b1046): 887–890. • Proctor B. (2001), Training for the supervision attitude, skills and intention, in J.R. Cutcliffe, T. Butterworth and Proctor, B., (eds.), *Fundamental Themes in Clinical Supervision*, Routledge, London. • Scaife J. (2001), Frameworks for supervision, Chapter 5 in J. Scaife, *Supervision in the Mental Health Professions: A Practitioner's Guide*, Hove, Brunner-Routledge.

workshops held at fortnightly intervals. Theoretical reading is set for each workshop to cover the following topics: (1) Education theory and practice, (2) Systemic theory and practice, (3) Narrative theory and practice, (4) Narrative-based medicine, and (5) Supervision theory and practice. Examples of the readings are presented in Table 18.1.

The theory is presented by the course members themselves. The style is interactive and is founded on the learning needs of the group. The course tutors contribute to the theoretical ideas and help with the group process. Understanding family and team interactions informs thinking about systems in supervision as well as the factors which may influence how supervisors respond to issues and feelings raised by supervisees. Because of this we include work on personal genograms and the organisational relationships of the certificate course participants. Course members practise giving and receiving supervision with immediate feedback on skills development from their peers and course tutors.

In addition to these workshops, participants are expected to gain ten days of experience in facilitating supervision skills workshops and to keep a portfolio to illustrate evidence of reflective learning. Learner facilitators start as observers and gradually take on a more active role as they become more proficient and confident. They also contribute to planning the workshops and to debriefing afterwards. The course tutors deliver some parts of the course as well as supporting and coaching those learning to facilitate. This includes interventions such as modelling ways of working with the group, encouraging reticent facilitators to interrupt and providing feedback afterwards. The model of learning to facilitate supervision is summarised in Figure 18.2.

We explain the process of continuing educational development taking place so that people attending workshops know that although all the facilitators are experienced supervisors they in turn are being supervised on their facilitation and supervision skills.

Continuing development

We continue to think about how to refresh learning, to increase our range of resources and to address the needs of people who have different learning styles. To reinforce the skills learnt on our courses there is an e-learning module which is freely accessible on the London Deanery website (www.faculty. londondeanery.ac.

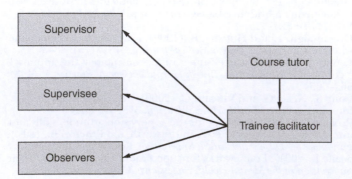

Figure 18.2 Model of learning to facilitate supervision.

uk/e-learning), local groups have been set up across London so that clinicians can continue to develop their skills and practise peer supervision and we have launched a training DVD.

We have set up a monthly support group for facilitators where they can share good practice, learn from things that have not gone smoothly, develop new ideas and thinking about theory and practice, and continue reflective learning. We would also like to develop supervision skills training for trainees as a potentially fruitful way to reach the senior clinicians of the future. Introducing supervision skills early in clinical training links with the idea that there is also a need to teach clinicians how to be supervisees (Cutcliffe 2001). There is not necessarily a difference in levels of sophistication; learning the skills to become a supervisor is likely to make someone a better supervisee and experiencing good supervision is likely to both make someone a better supervisee and, in turn, a good supervisor. As our cohort of facilitators grows there will be more capacity for disseminating this way of working.

In addition we are keen to make cross-links with other related training courses so that we can learn from each other.

Conclusion

Supervision skills are at the heart of professional conversations. Clinicians need time and training to develop the attitudes and skills for working in this way and for a change to come about. Within medicine and dentistry, although there is an increasing amount of supervision for trainees, there is still great variability in its frequency and quality (Grant *et al.* 2003) and whether it simply addresses technical issues or promotes reflective practice. We believe that the skills we teach are not only appropriate for working with trainees but have the potential to be useful at all stages of professional development. There is not yet a culture of ongoing peer supervision and some consultants report that their experience on our course was the first supervision they had received since they were appointed. We hope that this may change as clinical teaching becomes more professionalised.

Questions that continue to occupy our thoughts are:

- How much training do clinicians need to develop and retain skills for supervision?
- How to ensure that our method of training remains relevant and appropriate for the needs of clinicians working in primary and secondary care?
- How does supervision make a difference to patient care?
- Does it protect clinicians from complaints and burnout?
- Is the provision of supervision cost effective?

Up to now most research has been about supervision within nursing and psychological therapies. Intuitively it makes sense that offering clinicians these skills and techniques should improve their job satisfaction, support their ability to work in teams and provide better patient care. There is some limited evidence to support these assertions (Lloyd and Becker 2007; Kilminster *et al.* 2007) but more is certainly needed. As Karl Lewin (cited in Cooperrider and Srivasta 1987: 150) said, 'We should consider action, research and training as a triangle that should be kept together.' In an evidence-based clinical world, in order to secure funding and contracts we must provide concrete proof that this method of supervision is effective, to assure clinicians that they are getting the best possible training and that patients will benefit from this.

References

Andersen, T. (1987a), The reflecting team: dialogue and meta-dialogue in clinical work, *Family Process*, 26(4): 415–428.

Andersen, T. (1987b), The general practitioner and consulting psychiatrist as a team with 'stuck' families, *Family Systems Medicine*, 5(4): 468–481.

Anderson, H. and Goolishian, H. (1992), The client is the expert: a not-knowing approach to therapy, in S. McNamee (ed.), *Therapy as Social Construction*, Thousand Oaks, CA: Sage, pp. 25–39.

Brody, H. (1994) My story is broken: can you help me fix it? Medical ethics and the joint construction of narrative, *Literature and Medicine*, 13(1): 79–92.

Bruner, J. (1986), *Actual Minds, Possible Worlds*, Cambridge, MA: Harvard University Press.

Casement, P. (1985), *On Learning from the Patient*, London/ New York: Tavistock Publications, pp. 29–56.

Cecchin, G. (1987), Hypothesizing, circularity and neutrality revisited: an invitation to curiosity, *Family Process*, 26(4): 405–412.

Charon, R. (2006), *Narrative Medicine: Honoring the Stories of Illness*, New York: Oxford University Press.

Churchill, L. and Churchill, S. (1982), Storytelling in the medical arena: the art of self-determination, *Literature and Medicine*, 1: 73–79.

Cooperrider, D. and Srivastra, S. (1987), Appreciative Inquiry in Organizational Life, in, R. Woodman and W. Pasmore (eds), *Research in Organizational Change and Development, Vol. 1.*, Maryland Heights, MO: Elsevier Science/JAI Press.

Cutcliffe, J.R. (2001), An alternative training approach in clinical supervision, in J.R. Cutcliffe, T. Butterworth and B. Proctor (eds), *Fundamental Themes in Clinical Supervision*, London: Routledge, pp. 47–63.

Freedman, J. and Combs, G. (1996), *Narrative Therapy: The Social Construction of Preferred Realities*, New York/London: W.W. Norton and Co., p. 6.

Geertz, C. (1973), *The Interpretation of Cultures*, New York: Basic Books.

Grant, J., Kilminster, S., Jolly, B. and Cottrell, D. (2003), Clinical supervision of SpRs: where does it happen, when does it happen and is it effective? *Medical Education*, 37(2): 140–148.

Greenhalgh, T. and Hurwitz, B. (1998), *Narrative Based Medicine: Dialogue and Discourse in Clinical Practice*, London: BMJ Books.

Halpern, H. (2009), Supervision skills for clinicians and the Johari Window; a framework for asking questions, *Education for Primary Care*, 20(1): 10–14.

Kilminster, S., Cottrell, D., Grant, J. and Jolly, B. (2007), AMEE Guide No. 27: Effective educational and clinical supervision, *Medical Teacher*, 29(1): 2–19.

Kinnersley, P. and Edwards, M. (2008), Complaints against doctors, *British Medical Journal*, 336(7649): 841–842.

Launer, J. (2006), *Supervision, Mentoring and Coaching: One-to-one Learning Encounters in Medical Education*, Edinburgh: Association for the Study of Medical Education.

Launer, J. and Lindsey, C. (1997), Training for systemic general practice: a new approach from the Tavistock Clinic, *British Journal of General Practice*, 47(420): 453–456.

Lloyd, B. and Becker, D. (2007), Paediatric specialist registrars' views of educational supervision and how it can be improved: a questionnaire study, *Journal of the Royal Society of Medicine*, 100(8): 375–378.

Long, S., Neale, G. and Vincent, C. (2009), Practising safely in the foundation years, *British Medical Journal*, 338(b1046): 887–890.

Mattingly, C. (1998), *Healing Dramas and Clinical Plots: The Narrative Structure of Experience*, Cambridge: Cambridge University Press.

Mattingly, C. and Garro, L. (2000), *Narrative and the Cultural Construction of Illness and Healing*, Berkeley/Los Angeles, CA: University of California Press.

Palazzoli Selvini, M., Boscolo, L., Cecchin, G. and Prata, G. (1980), Hypothesizing, circularity, neutrality: three guidelines for the conductor of the session, *Family Process*, 19(1): 3–12.

Proctor, B. (2001), Training for the supervision alliance: attitude, skills and intention, in J.R. Cutcliffe, T. Butterworth and B. Proctor (eds), *Fundamental Themes in Clinical Supervision*, London: Routledge, pp. 25–46.

Ricoeur, P. (1984), *Time and Narrative, Vol. I*, Chicago: University of Chicago Press.

Riessmann, C. (1990), The strategic uses of narrative in the presentation of self and illness, *Social Science and Medicine*, 30(11): 1195–1200.

Tomm, K. (1988), Interventive interviewing Part III: intending to ask lineal, circular, strategic or reflexive questions? *Family Process*, 27(1): 1–15.

19 Providing cross-discipline group supervision to new supervisors

Challenging some common apprehensions and myths

Paul Cassedy, Mike Epling, Liz Williamson and Gale Harvey

This chapter was originally presented in *Fundamental Themes in Clinical Supervision* (Cassedy *et al.* 2001: 198–209). Due to the importance of the topic and the timelessness of the content, the editors have chosen to include the chapter in this book as well. The authors focus on discussing cross-discipline group supervision. They describe how, at the request of their local NHS Trust, two mental health nursing tutors provided a series of group supervision sessions to general registered nurses who were about to take on the role of clinical supervisor for the first time. They show how the groups were established, illustrate some of the experiences of being in these groups, and identify some of the issues that arose, primarily during the early stages. The chapter draws attention to one particularly important issue, which is that some novice supervisees may be discouraged from participating in supervision if their supervisor is from a different discipline. However, exposure to and experience of supervision provides such novices with an awareness that the supervisor's skill in providing supportive, reflective and challenging supervision is more important than sharing the same discipline.

This chapter is particularly useful for supervisors and supervisees. It is a classic piece of work and, therefore, important for educators, administrators and researchers. Because this supervision was successful, it can provide valuable information for those endeavouring to develop cross-disciplinary supervision and, potentially, also for those interested in the growing field of interdisciplinary and interprofessional collaborations.

Setting up the supervision groups

Back in 1997 clinical supervision was a new concept for the majority of the 1,500 registered nurses in the large teaching hospital where two of the authors were employed. They had the task of implementing a pilot project to introduce supervision within the Trust. Volunteers were asked to be trained as supervisors and 18 registered nurses came forward. The supervisees were drawn from six areas which volunteered for the pilot project, but the supervisors came from all across the hospital.

Purposeful time had been spent by a working party to consider and provide a framework for implementation that would be carefully planned, covering as many aspects as possible to establish a culture and provide high quality clinical supervision. In keeping with the structures suggested in the relevant literature (Hawkins and Shohet 1989; Butterworth 1992; Bond and Holland 1998), and since this was to be a new experience, supervision for the supervisors was identified as essential within this framework, providing the much-needed support.

Links had been established with the local education provider in particular through the supervision course that was offered to the Trust. As the facilitators of that course, the first two authors were therefore approached by the second two authors to facilitate group supervision to these new supervisors for the duration of the pilot study (six months).

In addition to providing this learning experience, the group was viewed as valuable for the new supervisors in providing an experience of what it feels like to be a supervisee. Participation in the group offered a unique means of learning, enabling empathic qualities to develop as more insight and respect can be gained as one begins to value the whole process of supervision.

The first two authors accepted this invitation with a mixture of enthusiasm and anxiety. Although both these authors have many years of experience facilitating groups in practice and educational settings, this was the first time they would be formally supervising general nurses in a setting and environment that is alien to their own. Both these authors have a background in mental health, human relations, counselling and training. Each of these subjects can be regarded as somewhat 'mystical' to those unfamiliar with the idiosyncrasies of the subject and as a result, may have caused a degree of caution in the potential group members. These anxieties existed on several levels. First, there was the initial anxiety of the supervision itself. The authors felt that they would be focusing on their role of supervisor rather than the role of general nurse, but concerns existed regarding the possibility that issues could arise about practice that was beyond their understanding and experience. Second, the authors had anxieties that mental health backgrounds might prove to be an issue in facilitating group supervision for general nurses.

Supervisors and supervisees sharing the same discipline

It is the authors' experience from running training courses in clinical supervision that when first embarking on the concept, the supervisee initially wants someone from the same discipline and background to supervise him or her. There is probably an element of safety here, in that potential supervisees do not want to feel vulnerable and exposed and they have always previously gone to a colleague for support. *However, as knowledge and experience is gained supervisees gradually realise that there is a greater opportunity for development in choosing someone, irrespective of his or her background, who will stretch them and be more challenging.*

The fact that the facilitators were from different backgrounds did not manifest itself as a significant issue for the group members. When the initial arrangements were being formulated and during the preliminary sessions, the new supervisors welcomed the opportunity of working with someone with more experience in supervision. The potential supervisors suggested that they were concerned with the skills the facilitators exhibited as supervisors rather than their clinical backgrounds. *It is the authors' belief that it is more important for the supervisor to be competent in and understand the process of supervision, than it is to share the same clinical background as the supervisee.*

The new supervisors were divided into three groups of six members each; there was a considerable range of specialties and grades within each group. Only two had received supervision before and there was an even mix of those who knew one another and those who did not. There was apprehension about taking part in group supervision alongside the anxiety of taking on the role supervisor for the first time. Page and Wosket (1994) allude to the notion that becoming a supervisor is rather like learning to swim. Although the new supervisors would be getting their feet wet by going in at the shallow end there was also the opportunity of taking lessons and learning alongside a more experienced swimmer. The facilitators felt qualified to take on the role of group supervisor as Carroll (1996) and Scanlon (1980) suggest, having previous supervision experience and the transferable skills of teaching and facilitating, so this was about to be put to the test.

The group experience

There were no pre-conceived ideas or guidelines about how to use the sessions, only that these supervisors would need considerable support as this new role was in its infancy. As in any new role or setting the nurse may find herself in, there needs to be a period of mentorship and nurturing. To help safeguard this new journey, it was considered important to create a contract for the supervision group to enable some degree of control over the experience. A good starting point for encouraging empowerment and ownership is to discuss the very issues that may cause concern to the individuals involved (Hawkins and Shohet 1989; Bond and Holland 1998). Airing these anxieties provided a forum to share and explore a range of issues which are not only important to the supervisor in the group, but may also parallel the very same concerns of the supervisee in the work setting.

The group decided that the time allowed for each member would be divided equally but urgent matters would take precedence. As status within the group was diverse, it was considered to be important to address this and the group wanted to ensure that it was put to one side to create an egalitarian approach. The authors attempted to create a level playing field to provide supportive challenge that would avoid competitiveness and encourage reflection, exploration and sharing. Each member agreed to be prepared for supervision, and the group would decide the agenda on the day.

Confidentiality was discussed; the decisions reached were analogous to the agreements that were stated between supervisors and supervisees. Revisiting the United Kingdom Central Council guidelines for professional practice (UKCC 1992) proved to be a good starting point. A breach of this code, a breach of law or serious exploitation or endangerment to others would normally be occasions to disclose information to another source (Morton-Cooper and Palmer 2000).

Concerns of disclosure, which would involve reporting serious malpractice and how these could be dealt with in the supervisory alliance, were aired, but also what-if scenarios were brought to the fore (see Cutcliffe *et al.* 1998a, 1998b). Many issues are not easily answered; reminding the group that they were also in a supportive relationship and would not be left isolated calmed anxiety about the possibility of serious disclosure. An issue that was related to confidentiality emerged in one group and had an effect on both the attendance and dynamics. Feltham and Dryden (1994) point out that group supervision does have its drawbacks; notably the group dynamics can be a complicating factor.

Blurring of relationship boundaries

A member of the group had a close friendship with another group member's supervisee. This was not disclosed or picked up by the facilitator at first, but there was some absenteeism and when all were present some hesitance and holding back of material. A group member finally revealed this in a group evaluation round. Although the names of the supervisees were not used in the group, identities in this small world can be recognised so anonymity cannot be maintained, only the conditions of confidentiality can be provided. This was explored and discussed with the group with the conclusion that it would be more therapeutic to be open and honest about such matters and that we as a group needed to establish strategies to overcome such issues. Many staff, even within large hospitals, are going to have some awareness or acknowledgement of one another. Even if not, certain persons still may be able to be identified from the material the supervisor is working on. The issue here for the group and subsequent supervision arrangements is to maintain the boundaries and responsibilities of clinical supervision. Some group members will know one another and their supervisees; a group member may have a different role over another member's supervisee, which could cause a blurring of boundaries or conflict of roles.

Power (1999) argues that a supervisor should not agree to supervise anyone that he or she has a close relationship with. Bond and Holland (1998) state that it is the responsibility of the supervisor to hold tight boundaries and keep any other role outside the supervision sessions. Perhaps both of these views can be substantiated, but when a supervision group finds itself with such issues, practical measures may be needed. One such method would be for group members to disclose a supervisee's first name and then perhaps his or her area of work. If any group member recognises the supervisee as someone well known to him or her, he or she should acknowledge this and leave the room whilst this supervision work is being presented. Another method would be, following negotiation with the group, to have the last ten minutes of session for an individual to work alone with the supervisor if his or her supervisee was well known to another in the group. By making every effort to respect confidentiality, this would help maintain objectivity and avoid potential damages of avoidance or collusion.

The early stages: finding our feet

Attendance of one group was spasmodic in the early stages, which could have had a number of contributing factors. Some will always drop out for unplanned unexpected reasons, e.g. leaving the area. There is also the notion that in the initial stages of implementing supervision, anxiety levels of staff will be raised, in particular if it is to be group supervision (Hawkins and Shohet 1989). This could result in absenteeism either from the supervision sessions or from work itself, as staff are apprehensive and uncertain of attending. It is well documented that receiving supervision can reduce stress levels in the supervisee (Butterworth *et al.* 1997). However, undertaking the role of supervisor for the first time can have the opposite effect and increase the supervisor's level of stress.

This, in some small way, seemed to be the case here. In the pilot evaluation supervisors did admit to some anxiety about the size of the group and they felt uncomfortable with self-disclosure, which affected levels of reflection. A few supervisors found the whole process too much and opted out while for some others the group size created some reticence. One supervisor during the evaluation stated that 'it wasn't until my group reduced to three supervisors that I really felt comfortable and was really able to reflect on my performance.' Another mentioned that 'it wasn't that I didn't trust all the group members, although I did feel some concern about the makeup of the group and possible impact on outside working relationships. The group felt too big and a little intimidating,' then went on to add, 'I never felt sufficiently at ease to want to address important issues, especially due to the fragmented nature of the group in the early sessions.'

A delicate balance is needed here, as Charleton (1996) points out that supervision is approached with a mixture of anxiety and relief: anxiety at the thought of exposing their clinical practice and relief that there is someone who will really listen and provide support. It can be a problem to maintain attendance and keep commitment and motivation high, in particular in the early stages of the group when only meeting once a month in what can be a disquieting experience. Support and encouragement is certainly needed but what also needs to be built in is a professional approach to value the whole process of supervision, and a responsibility to make and keep that commitment. If we do not take that personal responsibility, then we are not only letting ourselves and our profession down, but arguably our patients or clients as well.

The supervision sessions themselves were also fragmented at the start of the pilot in the work setting. Some found it hard to meet regularly; there were cancelled appointments and when some meetings did occur, there were perceived to be no major issues to discuss or explore. So for some new supervisors the relationship with the supervisee was difficult to get going and the alliance slow to develop. This meant that those supervisors who had not met with their supervisees felt inhibited or even embarrassed about attending the group sessions. Further exploration with the group revealed that some form of parallel process might have been occurring. Although this is a very complex phenomenon, a simple definition would be that at times the dynamics of the relationship between client and nurse become paralleled or mirrored in the relationship between nurse and supervisor. Carroll (1996) gives a comprehensive overview of this phenomenon from a psychoanalytical and counselling perspective, while Power (1999) goes into some detail from a nursing perspective. Therapeutic relationships do take time to grow and develop, even more so when the meeting is only for one hour a month. So the rather fragmented start to the supervision process for some in the work setting appeared to mirror that of one of the supervision groups in the pilot project. Perseverance, commitment and enthusiasm were needed by all those concerned in the process as well as the full backing and co-operation of those on the periphery. The supervision group needed to become aware of this so that they could address the issue and work on their own group co-operation.

An advantage of group supervision over individual supervision is that participants can share their abilities and resources for a common purpose. Listening to other group members presenting their supervision work can help others in the group to identify and express issues in their work setting. This is particularly valuable, as new supervisors may well experience similar difficulties (Bond and Holland 1998). There are developmental opportunities as each member can be a co-supervisor for one another, enabling reflection and supervision skills to develop. Creativity has an opportunity to be rediscovered and developed for the task in hand. The authors needed to remind themselves to take risks and were eventually rewarded with a greater richness of learning and experience. Tuckman's model (1965) of group development suggests there will be confusion and conflict in the early stages but if successfully managed, it will lead to a successful performance of the task.

Themes arising from the group

There were common themes of material that emerged from the group supervision sessions. Rather than the supervisee focusing on his or her clinical practice, it tended to be relationships with other members of staff or his or her own personal development issues. It seemed that at least initially most supervisees needed to focus on the formative and restorative aspects of supervision rather than on the normative function. There could be several reasons for this; it would seem that there is little already available in terms of support systems to focus on personal issues related to teamwork and professional development. *Such issues may therefore have been stored away or built up over a period of time leading to a backlog of concerns or issues needing to be addressed before the supervisees could move on to examining their own practice in more depth.* This is not to suggest that there is no need for supervision in the normative function for general nurses.

Bond and Holland (1998) propose that the focus of supervision leads from the restorative to the formative and finally to the normative when safety in relationship and process has been established. The experiences the group reported in the nature of the material brought to supervision can therefore be viewed as following such a pattern and process, which needs to be worked through in the development of the supervisory relationship. Progressing onto exploring issues relating to practice would be the next phase of the process.

It is possible that initially the supervisees need to feel fully supported to reflect more in depth on their care and relationships with patients. There is a misconception that it is only when nurses are working with patients intensively over a long period that there is need to reflect on that work and the relationship. Nurses working in areas with a rapid turnover of patients often underestimate the significance of their relationship with patients and families for the patients and themselves. Even brief relationships may leave unresolved issues for the nurse, which could be explored in supervision. The supervisors new to their role may have allowed some supervisees to keep their focus on familiar issues as this gave them an opportunity to build up their own confidence in their role before having to face more demanding situations that may raise anxiety, e.g. dealing with uncertainty.

A common theme also emerged in how the supervisors tackled these issues and the types of interventions they used. Perhaps because the supervisors were apprehensive of this new role and of being viewed in a position of responsibility, they tended to be rather prescriptive and solution-focused in their interventions. This tendency to focus on the actions and activities of the supervisee with problem solving in mind was seen to be a measure of success. There was also the misconception on the supervisors' part that solutions to problems identified in supervision could be written up for the evaluation in order to demonstrate its value to the organisation. Indeed, following the pilot and evaluation a number of supervisors reflected that this was primarily a symptom of their lack of experience with supervision and that it fitted more comfortably with their more familiar nursing role.

What emerged from the group sessions and proved to be valuable learning were the ways the new supervisors perceived their authority and how comfortable they felt with it. Pickvance (1997) states that new supervisors will bring to the role their own feelings and experiences regarding authority. The facilitators felt that it was paramount that the supervisors did not over-identify with an authoritarian role by being too prescriptive and being seen to have all the answers. Conversely there should not be denial of the role by an avoidance of challenging supervisees and leaving sessions without clarity or focus. Both these characteristics appeared in the supervision sessions as some supervisors found it easier to stay purely supportive while others wanted to focus intently on outcomes. This will have the effect of undermining the supervisee and the whole purpose and process of supervision. What needed to be established in the supervision relationship was a genuine space for reflection, thinking and development, not only for the supervisee but also the supervisor.

Seeing the big picture

This ability did develop during group supervision and the supervisors were able to work with their supervisees in a different style from any previously experienced. This was not only to be more facilitative in their approach but also to have a wider vision. Hawkins and Shohet (1989) refer to this as helicopter vision, which is the ability of the worker to switch perspectives at various times. The purpose is to help the supervisor to take a broader perspective on the supervisee. This is not only to focus on their practice and work setting but also to consider their (the supervisors') own behaviour and experience and the reasons for acting as they do.

One supervisor presented a case where the supervisee felt left out and not part of the ward team. What they both initially began to explore was to find a solution to the problem and how to resolve it. This was in part due to the supervisor's desire to problem solve as this was her usual way of working. During group supervision this was processed and other possible interventions and ideas reflected upon. Following this exploration, the supervisor felt more able and thus competent to utilise facilitation skills and help the supervisee to reflect more deeply. When the case was next presented in supervision, it surfaced that the supervisee felt more isolated with herself rather than with others and a broader picture emerged. She worked part-time, was caring for an elderly relative and had just returned to practice following maternity leave. She now lacked confidence in herself and questioned her ability in a changing ward environment.

The supervisor had helped the supervisee to focus more on how to build up her self-esteem and confidence, what she actually wanted for herself and how to develop more supportive relationships in her team. Eventually there was more insight and understanding and the supervisee felt more able to disclose her feelings to others. She began to update herself with practice issues which enabled her once again to feel involved. Hawkins and Shohet (1989) point out that the skill of seeing things in a wider context is difficult at first and can only fully be developed during the actual supervision process. This was also our experience as the skills began to emerge and then develop during the life of the group.

Moving towards supervisee-centred skills

Perhaps also due to a lack of skill or experience, there was some initial anxiety of utilising more the catalytic or facilitative type of intervention and its links to helping in a counselling type of role. Supervision is not counselling, although many of the skills and certainly the qualities that make the working alliance are transferable. The overall intention and purpose of each is different: counselling is focused solely on the person being counselled while the focus of supervision is primarily on issues that ultimately affect the supervisee's practice. However, this should not discount the need for support for the supervisee as a person and in his or her emotional and psychological development. As Bond and Holland (1998) argue, support is open-ended. Good supervisors need to develop their use of counselling skills as well as feeling confident and comfortable with that process. There needs to be an ability to be aware of their appropriate and inappropriate use as well as to recognise when they may need to refer elsewhere. The supervisor needs at least to be able to contain any emotional material the supervisee brings to supervision and have at least some understanding of the psychological processes that may be occurring. A fear that new supervisors may often have is saying the wrong thing or not wanting to put their foot in it. However, if they truly are actively listening and communicating their empathic understanding there needs to be no such fear. Communication skills such as paraphrasing and reflecting back key words or feelings are very powerful in enabling the supervisee to be really heard and understood. But what the new supervisor will need is to feel supported in this different way of working and have a forum, such as their own supervision, to explore any issues that may arise.

The essential ingredients of good communication, learning and supervision are Rogers' core conditions of warmth, genuineness and empathy (Rogers 1962). It is important for us all to re-establish this at times, in particular when the relationship is difficult or demanding and when rapport is hard to establish. We endeavoured to create these conditions in the group to create a climate and culture to serve as a good model for relationships.

Final reflections

Overall, the involvement in group supervision for the new supervisors was a positive experience. Although it took some time for trust to develop with the facilitators we all felt the benefits by the end of the pilot project. The facilitators have learned that there is a fine balance of support and challenge needed at the start of a group, alongside being able to keep the balance of commitment, enthusiasm and responsibility to the task. Perhaps the facilitators did not successfully juggle all the aspects together at the beginning. The facilitators have also gained a wider experience in group facilitation and felt it is successful to supervise others of a different discipline in this capacity. We are also indebted to the various group members for providing us with material and valuable learning that we can take back into our educational setting and the supervision course.

The group members report that they will take away the experience of being supervised, in that levels of self-awareness regarding the role of supervisor have increased significantly. The development of facilitation skills and the ability to view the supervisees' work in a wider perspective have also been fostered. The supervisors reported that it was important that they were supported and nurtured through this beginning process of being a guardian to another (their supervisees). The analogy of parent and grandparent that Page and Wosket (1994) refer to is a useful one to use here. If the supervisor is acting as a 'parent-type figure' to the supervisee then the supervisor of the supervisor is similar to a 'grandparent figure'. The supervisor who is new to the role will need fostering for some time while he or she becomes more effective and competent in that role. This analogy also addresses the question of where the continuous line of supervision ceases. The supervisor of the supervisor (grandparent) can eventually withdraw as they place more trust in their supervisors. However, they can be a reassuring figure in the background for welcome support when needed or at times of emergency. Grandparents will occasionally seek out help and support from other adults or peers in a similar role; the facilitators certainly did this at times, with certain colleagues and ourselves. They would share some of our ideas or findings or check out with one another some small detail.

Through their development and learning most group members felt they had now reached a stage where they could function more autonomously as a supervisor. Some have arranged to meet in small peer groups while others can utilise their own clinical supervision at times to reflect on their supervision role. The arrangements for providing support for the supervisors will inevitably vary. This will depend on the overall amount of supervision work the nurse is undertaking, but will need to be monitored. All the supervisors will however, continue with their own clinical supervision. As the UKCC (1996) position statement proposes, this will assist lifelong learning, as indeed, some will eventually step into the role of 'grandparent' and become a supervisor of supervisors themselves.

References

Bond, M. and Holland, S. (1998), *Skills of Clinical Supervision for Nurses*, Buckingham: Open University Press.

Butterworth, T. (1992), Clinical supervision as an emerging idea in nursing, in T. Butterworth and J. Faugier (eds), *Clinical Supervision and Mentorship in Nursing* London: Chapman & Hall.

Butterworth, T., Carson, J., White, E., Jeacock, J., Clements, A. and Bishop, V. (1997), *It is Good to Talk. Clinical Supervision and Mentorship: An Evaluation Study in England and Scotland*, Manchester: University of Manchester, The School of Nursing, Midwifery and Health Visiting.

Carroll, M. (1996), *Counselling Supervision, Theory, Skills and Practice*, London: Cassell.

Cassedy, P., Epling, M., Williamson, L. and Harvey G. (2001), Providing cross discipline group supervision to new supervisors, in J.R. Cutcliffe, T. Butterworth and B. Proctor (eds), *Fundamental Themes in Clinical Supervision*, London: Routledge, pp. 198–209.

Charleton, M. (1996), *Self-Directed Learning in Counsellor Training*, London: Cassell.

Cutcliffe, J.R., Epling, M., Cassedy, P., McGregor, J., Plant, N. and Butterworth, T. (1998a), Ethic dilemmas in clinical supervision, part 1 – need for guidelines, *British Journal of Nursing* 7 (15): 920–923.

Cutcliffe, J.R., Epling, M., Cassedy, P., McGregor, J., Plant, N. and Butterworth, T. (1998b), Ethic dilemmas in clinical supervision, part 2 – need for guidelines. *British Journal of Nursing* 7 (16): 978–982.

Feltham, C. and Dryden, W. (1994), *Developing Counselling Supervision*, London: Sage.

Hawkins, P. and Shohet, R. (1989), *Supervision in the Helping Professions*, Milton Keynes: Open University Press.

Morton-Cooper, A. and Palmer, A. (2000), *Mentoring, Preceptorship and Clinical Supervision*, 2nd edn, Oxford: Blackwell Science.

Page, S. and Wosket, V. (1994), *Supervising the Counsellor*, London: Routledge.

Pickvance, D. (1997), Becoming a supervisor, in G. Shipton (ed.), *Supervision of Psychotherapy and Counselling*, Buckingham: Open University Press.

Power, S. (1999), *Nursing Supervision: A Guide for Clinical Practice*, London: Sage.

Rogers, C. (1962), *On Becoming A Person*, London: Constable.

Scanlon, C. (1980), Towards effective training of clinical supervisors, in V. Bishop (ed.), *Clinical Supervision in Practice*, London: Macmillan.

Tuckman, B.W. (1965), Developmental sequences in small groups, *Psychological Bulletin* 63 (6): 384–399.

UKCC (United Kingdom Central Council) (1992), *Code of Professional Conduct*, 3rd edn, London: UKCC.

UKCC (1996), *Position Statement on Clinical Supervision for Nursing and Health Visiting*, London: UKCC.

20 The realities of clinical supervision in an Australian acute inpatient setting

Michelle Cleary and Jan Horsfall

This chapter draws on the findings of an ethnographic study of Australian acute inpatient mental health settings, which sought to better understand the cultural realities of clinical supervision (CS) for this culture/population (see Cleary and Freeman 2005). Having outlined the research design and key findings, this chapter then discusses the findings in light of current literature and highlights some future considerations/issues that will need resolving, if CS is to become a widespread reality in Australian acute inpatient mental health settings. It is noteworthy that this chapter shows how many of the mental health nurses in acute inpatient mental health units, when asked, formally agree that clinical supervision is important, but informally regard it as having a limited experiential value. This may in part be attributable to many nurses believing that they are already involved in CS, though these experiences do not correspond with established definitions of formal CS.

In the view of the editors this chapter, as with some others in this book, offers further evidence of the miscomprehension and misunderstanding that many still have regarding the nature and purpose of CS. This consequently further underscores the need for a shared nomenclature; given that (all) sciences need understandable, stable and internationally-accepted systems for naming and categorising phenomena within the boundaries of the disciplinary area. It can be argued that CS needs this list of agreed names, definitions, principles, rules and recommendations that govern its formation, use and application. Until we have this, there is little surprise that the outcomes of engaging in a variety of practices that share only some (if any) of CS's rudiments, principals and practices bear little or no resemblance to those outcomes which are more commonly encountered when one engages in real, high quality CS. As the authors point out, the belief that existing structures inherent to nursing practice already convey the benefits of CS may contribute to the culture of passive resistance to it.

Acknowledgements

This chapter is based on the following paper published in *Issues in Mental Health Nursing*: Cleary, M. and Freeman, A. (2005), The cultural realities of clinical supervision in an acute inpatient mental health setting, *Issues in Mental Health Nursing*, 26(5): 489–505.

Introduction

There is extensive published literature on the topic of clinical supervision (CS), but despite decades of discussion about its potential benefits, there is confusion about nurses' understanding of CS and the pragmatics of implementing appropriate models (Cleary and Freeman 2005, 2006). For example, in a recent systemic literature review and methodological critique of empirical studies of clinical supervision, Buus and Gonge (2009) concluded that there was limited empirical evidence to support the claim that clinical supervision is a good thing, and does what the promoters claim it does. There is also limited evidence that CS enhances supervisee knowledge and skills, or improves nurse–patient effectiveness (Bradshaw *et al.* 2007; Hines-Martin and Robinson 2006; Scanlon and Weir 1997; Sloan and Watson 2001). Hence, as well as ambiguity, there are disagreements over issues of CS theory, practice and research (Buus and Gonge 2009; Rizzo 2003). This confusion could be seen as mirroring that of mental health (MH) nurses working in acute inpatient units, and there is unlikely to be further clarity until nurses' perceptions are more fully understood. In this chapter, we commence by presenting an overview of findings from an ethnographic study that sought to better understand the cultural realities of clinical supervision in acute inpatient mental health settings (Cleary and Freeman 2005). We then discuss these findings in light of current literature and provide some future considerations if CS is to become a widespread reality in acute inpatient mental health settings.

Cultural realities of clinical supervision: an overview of the findings

Research respondents identified CS as a 'supportive' forum for nurses to 'ventilate concerns/problems' in a non-judgemental, collegial, confidential way, as well as discuss practice issues with peers. The 'exchange of ideas' and access to peer 'support' provided an opportunity to explore 'clinical strategies' and 'reflect on and develop clinical skills' and some nurses indicated that they would 'like to continue with clinical supervision'. CS has been promoted as a way of increasing 'self-awareness' and 'confidence', thus leading to greater job satisfaction. One participant reiterates the value of reflection on practice for the present and the future:

> I think reflection is very important … we're going to experience lots of things and being able to honestly reflect on how we handled the situation or how we saw somebody else handle the situation is the best way.

Some nurses, particularly those newer to the setting, discussed over-identification with patients as potentially problematic. Reflective practices provide an opportunity to explore feelings, and commonly nurses do this with colleagues through peer review, preceptorship programmes and discussion. If boundary transgressions are made by novices, more experienced nurses or peers would take the individual aside and have an impromptu talk for the benefit of nurse and patient. Sometimes nurses are convinced it is 'your colleagues who know you best … who'll come up and say "Just sort of step back for a while".' Thus, informal approaches to preventing boundary transgressions were viewed by nurses to be more relevant to current clinical circumstances despite the promotion of CS as a means of ensuring that staff practise in an 'ethical manner'. Overall, reflection on practice was identified by many participants as providing a level of transparency in the negotiation, delineation, and management of boundary issues, resulting in greater confidence and self-awareness.

Thus, nurses are certainly aware of many of the advantages conveyed by CS but many prefer ad hoc coping methods such as informal sharing and eliciting the support of trusted colleagues, rather than more formal approaches. The need to 'take time out and ventilate' with caring colleagues was believed important with discussion occurring in the privacy of staff offices away from patient care areas. Although this option was not available when patients were acutely disturbed or distressed and/or required a high level of observation, informal support with one's peers was seen to be more flexibly responsive to the clinical realties of everyday work as, generally, colleagues were available and accessible.

The findings clearly demonstrate a strong team culture and nurses described colleagues as being 'really supportive'. Teamwork and collegial relationships were considered part of the 'nature of the work' and provided opportunities for peer review and supervision. There were a number of formal strategies in place to facilitate good communication within the team including: informal consultation; nurse-multidisciplinary team handover; case review; multidisciplinary team meetings; nursing handover; and staff meetings. In addition, collegial relationships encouraged the sharing of nursing workloads, helping nurses to cope and manage competing demands. The notion of 'teamwork' (amongst nurses and other health professionals) was also believed necessary for 'effective' care, and therefore a worthwhile goal in itself.

Respondents considered it to be particularly important for experienced staff on the team to spend time with less experienced nurses or nurses 'new to the ward' to provide education, support and opportunities to evaluate practice and interactions with consumers. This was commonly referred to as preceptorship or CS. Preceptorship can be helpful for more experienced nurses too by giving them access to different perspectives and challenging accepted yet possibly outmoded nursing interventions or approaches.

> ...when you're in the system for a long time, you tend to get into a routine but when you have someone fresh ... say, '...I don't really feel comfortable with the way you do that' ... It makes you think, perhaps I've been doing it for so long I think it's perfect, but it's not.

Discussing the complexities of practice with colleagues and finding solutions to nursing problems was considered essential, and many nurses told how their confidence in their practice had grown and developed through 'reflective practice', the passing of time, 'day-to-day encounters' and 'experience'.

Ward peer supervision and other informal supports identified by nurses may account in part for the perception that CS was already occurring (or was about to) when in fact it was not. This belief may be further reinforced by an awareness that all clinical staff 'are expected or required' by management to receive CS. However, the lack of emphasis placed on CS by nurses may also be attributed to some of their more generic beliefs about the profession of nursing itself. Nurses believed patients were well looked after, the unit was 'effective', worked 'very well' and was 'a good place to work'. There was a sense that the only people who can really appreciate the subtleties and complexity in the unit are other mental health nurses: 'you can sort of stand back and debrief with other people who understand ... the only people that can really understand are the people who work alongside you'.

Paradoxically, what respondents liked about their work were the things they found frustrating. This included the challenging, hectic and unpredictable nature of acute care, and the constant pressure and demands. They described each day as 'different' with the work characterised by 'uncertainty' and 'crisis'; to the extent that almost everything was 'urgent'. One-to-one CS was considered impossible due to unit constraints but group supervision had previously been established. The CS group was open which meant those nurses on duty on the day of the group supervision attended. The pragmatics of rotating rosters (e.g. leave, night duty, days off, staffing and skill mix) meant it was difficult to organise dates that suited the same group of staff. This reportedly led to difficulties with 'rehashing' of the same topics with different nurses and everybody wanting to 'talk at once'. Whilst it was deemed important to have a focus for the group, some nurses believed that issues discussed were 'not resolved' and that for clinical supervision to be useful, the 'concerns' of staff must be acted upon. There was a generally held belief that CS should not be mandatory, particularly group supervision.

Most nurses had a clear understanding of supervisee and supervisor roles and responsibilities, but there were differences in opinion regarding how clinical supervision could be improved. Some would prefer one-to-one CS, others believed that the time of day the supervision was scheduled (at the end of the shift when nurses are tired) was an issue. If held outside of work hours, there was a general belief that 'time in lieu' should be granted. Participants did not actively pursue individual CS opportunities and questioned its feasibility, identifying 'time and staffing levels' as constraints. Thus, despite a unit policy of offering CS, 'in reality it just isn't feasible and doesn't work'.

Discussion

CS was nominally endorsed but in reality, other informal means of acquiring professional support and guidance inherent in mental health nursing provided many of the benefits usually ascribed to formal supervision. This may explain the absence of a commitment to clinical supervision as the other informal and formal support strategies identified by participants were possibly more naturalistic and accessible. They also provided a daily opportunity to reflect on reactions to the patient, the nature of professional relationships, and nursing strategies, without creating extra stress due to time taken away from unit and work building up. As nursing has become more complex and demanding, reflective strategies are essential to acknowledge experiences, process responses, question practices, refine problem solving, and develop acceptable professional parameters.

Supportive nursing relationships can provide a sense of belonging and an opportunity to learn in a respectful manner from senior staff, particularly for nurses newer to mental health. Taking time out to discuss problematic situations, accessing senior nurses, role models and ad hoc supervision is helpful for professional reflection, stimulating a sense of security, providing guidance, and offering a new perspective. This approach may also have been preferred as it is difficult for nurses to overtly identify themselves as stressed or not coping and formal attendance at CS could be perceived as an admittance of this. Complementary literature also recognises that support is crucial for busy mental health nurses working in stressful environments to contain anxieties, and prevent fatigue and stress (Flood *et al.* 2006; Hummelvoll and Severinsson 2001).

In the current study a strong team culture was important and existing team strategies (e.g. nurse-multidisciplinary team handover and team meetings, nursing handover etc.) convey some of the benefits of CS and could possibly be considered a form of peer supervision. The cultivation of an environment where nurses feel comfortable talking about daily concerns contributes to safe and therapeutic practice, whereas formal CS is reliant upon honesty and self-disclosure by the supervisee, however skilled the supervision.

Non-formal CS activities fostered mutual respect and trust as well as good and easy communication, aspects essential for effective clinical teaching and learning. Some senior nurses questioned their own practice in response to 'left-field' comments from more junior staff, thus the relationship was rendered more reciprocal and fluid, adapting to the exigencies of 'here-and-now situations'. Daily access to peer supports may have contributed to the belief held by many nurses that they were already undertaking CS, despite these informal approaches not fitting with established practices of formal clinical supervision. However, this is not an uncommon scenario. In another study, supervisees confused CS with de facto clinical supervision, time out and common sense; in fact many understood they had been partaking in clinical supervision for years (White *et al.* 1998). Further, the positives of this informal approach such as flexibility, a focus on support, and familiarity with colleagues, may limit impartiality and make discussions vulnerable to the personal agendas of the staff involved.

The pragmatics of rotating rosters in this setting necessitated an open clinical supervision group, and changing participants undermined group cohesion and trust. The disadvantages of the open CS group format included a reluctance to self-disclose, an absence of focus and repetition of content. The diverse, unpredictable clinical demands inherent in everyday work inevitably limited access to group CS and, potentially, nurses' preparedness to invest their time and energy in it. Supervisee anxiety, issues regarding confidentiality, the professional background and experience of supervisors, and the demands that management might place upon accessing information discussed during supervision are recognised elsewhere (Jones 2003; Nicklin 1995). These issues may be tempered by using experienced external supervisors which has the advantage of being perceived by staff as impartial with clear delineation between the needs of management and the role of the supervision.

To summarise, whilst some participants were positive about CS in theory, in reality, cultural beliefs about its role, structural barriers, and the perceived effectiveness of informal supports meant many nurses did not perceive a need for formal CS. Thus, implementing CS requires the consideration of multiple factors including the definition of CS, existing nursing culture, resourcing issues, expansion of the evidence base, and ensuring CS models are tailored to the real vagaries, urgency and diverse ongoing pressures in acute mental health inpatient units.

Further considerations

In nursing, models of CS are often trumpeted without consideration of the facility characteristics or the everyday reality of the work environment. There is limited empirical evidence to unequivocally support CS's contributions to practice improvement, let alone better patient care, but the literature conveys the impression that our knowledge on this topic is more robust and trustworthy than it actually is (Buus and Gonge 2009). Despite extensive unequivocal discussion on CS, the reality is that there are very few published examples of its successful implementation in acute inpatient mental health facilities. Although it is claimed that there are efforts currently underway to build clinical supervision into normal mental health nursing practices (Brunero and Stein-Parbury 2008; Edwards *et al.* 2006), others note this as an aspiration rather than a reality (Grant and Townend 2007) and there are clearly problems with its implementation (Rice *et al.* 2007). It is also unlikely that large-scale investment of funds will be allocated until there is unequivocal evidence of a causal relationship between clinical supervision, improved patient care and better nursing care (White and Roche 2006). White and Roche's (2006) recent study showed that clinical supervision is not embedded in the culture or routines of most Australian mental health facilities (see also Cleary and Freeman 2006).

Limited attention has been given to the cultural and organisational context that shapes the CS practice (Grant and Townend 2007). Research has revealed concerns from nurses about the practical benefit of clinical supervision, the time taken away from patients when attending, the additional burden placed on colleagues while they are undertaking supervision and the potential for the supervisor to judge or criticise (Arvidsson *et al.* 2000; Fowler 1996a, 1996b). In order to prevent clinical supervision being viewed as an additional burden to acute inpatient mental health practice, it is important to clarify its aims, benefits, and most effective models. CS should also be clearly defined with specific roles and responsibilities. In addition, preceptoring and mentorship programmes are often already established in inpatient settings and encompass many elements of clinical supervision.

Further challenging the development of a culture of clinical supervision in inpatient settings is that nurses tend to work from a common diary which determines their daily activities making it difficult to prioritise time for CS. In allied and medical professions CS has evolved mainly because of the autonomous nature of the work but mental health nursing often has a strong interactive and mutually supportive culture (Cleary and Freeman 2005).

This variation in the conceptualisation of CS and its operationalisation has led to questions being asked as to whether it is foolhardy to force the same CS model upon all supervisees without considering the differences and variations in the care context (Cutcliffe 2005; Stevenson 2005). It should also be noted that the development and success of models is dependent on the appropriateness to the profession and its speciality and locality (Butterworth *et al.*1996; Fowler and Chevannes 1998; Scanlon and Weir 1997). Clinical supervision will continue to be viewed ambivalently whilst clinicians are unclear about its ambit and without this evidence base the introduction of CS will be hampered.

Learning from our mistakes via case studies in which CS was unsuccessfully introduced may be helpful according to Grant and Townend (2007) who posit the following two questions. The first, how can organisation and clinical supervision champions develop appropriate structures and processes to achieve a balance between time spent on effective clinical supervision and that engaged in clinical practice with clients? The second, how can the practice of clinical supervision be encouraged sensitively that takes into account the stresses of contemporary mental health nursing practice? If clinical supervision is needed, then it should be defined by the mental health nurses who will partake of it.

Finally, Rice and colleagues (2007) provide an extensive set of recommendations which may assist organisations and clinical supervision champions to develop sustainable contemporary, relevant and sustainable clinical supervision practises. Lynch and Happell (2008a, 2008b, 2008c) also present a model for the implementation of clinical supervision that considers the complex factors that are likely to influence the uptake of supervision, including organisational culture, leadership, education and training, sustainability and evaluation.

Conclusion

The rhetoric of excessive claims for CS in the face of acute mental health units characterised by pressure, urgency and chaos only serves to devalue a potentially useful process. Ad hoc CS only serves to reinforce cautious attitudes towards supervision and supports the cultural belief that it has limited value in-practice. Nurses are more likely to pursue and persist with CS when a constructive environment is established that supports CS. Even though these findings were originally published in 2005, they resonate with current literature and the realities of present day practice. Given the substantive literature on this topic – is perhaps too much is being asked of this one process, especially in acute inpatient settings? CS will continue to be viewed with suspicion if its introduction is top-down and the orientation is that of quality control; or managers are allowed to pass themselves off as impartial confidantes and teachers. Acute care nurses have limited time and for them to commit to any process of supervision it must be meaningful, user friendly and relevant. As it stands, many nurses believe that CS has limited experiential value and are therefore cautious towards its wholesale adoption in practice. This culture will not be overcome easily. Further exploration of viable models consistent with the setting and the diverse needs of nurses are required.

References

Arvidsson, B., Löfgren, H. and Fridlund, B. (2000), Psychiatric nurses' conceptions of how group supervision in nursing care influences their professional competence, *Journal of Nursing Management*, 8(3): 175–185.

Bradshaw, T., Butterworth, A. and Mairs, H. (2007), Does structured clinical supervision during psychosocial intervention education enhance outcome for mental health nurses and the service users they work with? *Journal of Psychiatric and Mental Health Nursing*, 14(1): 4–12.

Brunero, S. and Stein-Parbury, J. (2008), The effectiveness of clinical supervision in nursing: an evidence-based literature review, *Australian Journal of Advanced Nursing*, 25(3): 86–94.

Butterworth, T., Bishop, V. and Carson, J. (1996), First steps towards evaluating clinical supervision in nursing and health visiting I: Theory, policy and practice development, a review, *Journal of Clinical Nursing*, 5(2): 127–132.

Buus, N. and Gonge, H. (2009), Empirical studies of clinical supervision in psychiatric nursing: A systematic literature review and methodological critique, *International Journal of Mental Health Nursing*, 18(4): 250–264.

Cleary, M. and Freeman, A. (2005), The cultural realities of clinical supervision in an acute inpatient mental health setting, *Issues in Mental Health Nursing*, 26(5): 489–505.

Cleary, M. and Freeman, A. (2006), Fostering a culture of support in mental health settings: alternatives to traditional models of clinical supervision, *Issues in Mental Health Nursing*, 27(9): 985–1000.

Cutcliffe, J.R. (2005), From the guest editor – clinical supervision: a search for homogeneity or heterogeneity? *Issues in Mental Health Nursing*, 26(5): 471–473.

Edwards, D., Burnard, P., Hannigan, B., Cooper, L., Adams, J., Juggessur, T., Fothergil, A. and Coyle, D. (2006), Clinical supervision and burnout: the influence of clinical supervision for community mental health nurses, *Journal of Clinical Nursing*, 15(8): 1007–1015.

Flood, C., Brennan, G., Bowers, L., Hamilton, B., Lipang, M. and Oladapo, P. (2006), Reflections on the process of change on acute psychiatric wards during the City Nurse Project, *Journal of Psychiatric and Mental Health Nursing*, 13(3): 260–268.

Fowler, J. (1996a), The organization of clinical supervision within the nursing profession: a review of the literature, *Journal of Advanced Nursing*, 23(3): 471–478.

Fowler, J. (1996b), How to use models of clinical supervision in practice, *Nursing Standard*, 10(29): 42–47.

Fowler, J. and Chevannes, M. (1998), Evaluating the efficacy of reflective practice within the context of clinical supervision, *Journal of Advanced Nursing*, 27(2): 379–382.

Grant, A. and Townend, M. (2007), Some emerging implications for clinical supervision in British mental health nursing, *Journal of Psychiatric and Mental Health Nursing*, 14(6): 609–614.

Hines-Martin, V. and Robinson, K. (2006), Supervision as professional development for psychiatric mental health nurses, *Clinical Nurse Specialist*, 20(6): 293–297.

Hummelvoll, J.K. and Severinsson, E. (2001), Coping with everyday reality: mental health professionals' reflections on the care provided in an acute psychiatric ward, *Australian and New Zealand Journal of Mental Health Nursing*, 10(3): 156–166.

Jones, A. (2003), Some benefits experienced by hospice nurses from group clinical supervision, *European Journal of Cancer Care*, 12(3): 224–232.

Lynch, L. and Happell, B. (2008a), Implementing clinical supervision: Part 1: Laying the ground work, *International Journal of Mental Health Nursing*, 17(1): 57–64.

Lynch, L. and Happell, B. (2008b), Implementing clinical supervision: Part 2: Implementation and Beyond, *International Journal of Mental Health Nursing*, 17(1): 65–72.

Lynch, L. and Happell, B. (2008c), Implementing clinical supervision: Part 3: The Development of a Model, *International Journal of Mental Health Nursing*, 17(1): 73–82.

Nicklin, P. (1995), Super supervision, *Nursing Management*, 2(5): 24–25.

Rice, F., Cullen, P., McKenna, H., Kelly, B., Keeney, S. and Richey, R. (2007), Clinical supervision for mental health nurses in Northern Ireland: formulating best practice guidelines, *Journal of Psychiatric and Mental Health Nursing*, 14(5): 516–521.

Rizzo, M.D. (2003), Clinical supervision: a working model for substance abuse acute care settings, *Health Care Manager*, 22(2): 136–143.

Scanlon, C. and Weir, W.S. (1997), Learning from practice? Mental health nurses' perceptions and experiences of clinical supervision, *Journal of Advanced Nursing*, 26(2): 295–303.

Sloan, G. and Watson, H. (2001), Illuminative evaluation: evaluating clinical supervision on its performance rather than the applause, *Journal of Advanced Nursing*, 35(5): 644–673.

Stevenson, C. (2005), Postmodernising clinical supervision in nursing, *Issues in Mental Health Nursing*, 26(5): 519–529.

White, E. and Roche, M. (2006), A selective review of mental health nursing in New South Wales, Australia, in relation to clinical supervision, *International Journal of Mental Health Nursing*, 15(3): 209–219.

White, E., Butterworth, T., Bishop, V., Carson, J., Jeacock, J. and Clements, A. (1998), Clinical supervision: insider reports of a private world, *Journal of Advanced Nursing*, 28(1): 185–192.

21 Clinical supervision for nurse educationalists

Personal perspectives from a postgraduate mental health nursing course

Peter Goward, Joe Kellett and John Wren

This chapter considers clinical supervision for nurse educationalists. It sets such practice within the context of a postgraduate mental health nursing course. It provides some background to the development of the course, identifies the nature of the supervision provided and goes on to discuss the value of supervision for nurse educationalists. The chapter also points out the differences in the organisational structure between universities and the NHS. As a result, the well-documented problems that arise from a person having the dual roles of clinical supervisor and line manager may not be as significant an issue for university staff as they could be for NHS staff.

We believe that if practitioners are providing clinical supervision, then it would be prudent (if not necessary) for them to also receive clinical supervision. This position applies equally to clinicians and educationalists. Indeed, many nurse educationalists continue to practice as clinicians, which adds further weight to this argument. Clinical supervision, we believe, should be a career-long activity, and the authors of this chapter provide further evidence to support this position.

Introduction

During the latter part of the 1990s local and national commissioning intentions have responded to the need to increase the number of qualified nurses who are capable of meeting the increasingly complex needs of mental health care provision. The move from a predominantly NHS-based setting into Higher Education Institutions encouraged the deliverers of educational programmes to think more closely about the nature and level of such provision.

Our local analysis resulted in the development of the Pre-registration Postgraduate Diploma in Health Care Studies with professional registration as a mental health nurse. This two-year programme is designed for those who hold a first level or higher degree in a health related subject such as psychology or sociology in accordance with Statutory Instrument 1456, Rule 14A(8)(c)(i). Successful students are able to access an option to continue in pursuance of a master's degree. In keeping with most current thinking (Sainsbury 1997; Norman *et al.* 1996) the course development team were very clear that the programme needed to be primarily skills-based with the underlying theory clustered around practical interventions that would ensure previous knowledge could be contextualised within good mental health practice. For us this clearly indicated the need to include reflective practice and clinical supervision as central themes throughout the whole length of the course. In this chapter we will consider the wider context within which this initiative began, the influence of the curriculum, the nature of the supervision, the responses and experiences of those who acted as supervisors and a discussion of the role of supervisor in an educational context.

Supervision in context

Supervision has been present in some form amongst some mental health nurses for decades with many nurses adopting the kinds of practices associated with other professions such as psychologists, counsellors and social workers (UKCC 1996; Faugier and Butterworth 1994). In the early 1990s, the document *A Vision for the Future* (Department of Health 1993) promoted the use of clinical supervision through identified policy targets. Within the profession itself, *Working in Partnership* (Department of Health 1994) and *Pulling Together* (Sainsbury 1997) reinforced the notion of supervision within mental health nursing. Faugier and Butterworth's (1994) report on supervision qualified and quantified the development of supervision within mental health nursing and helped to clarify the models in use.

These developments have occurred at both a macro and micro level. At a macro level, policy initiatives dictate levels of excellence through processes and initiatives that are concerned with promoting quality, for example, clinical governance. At a micro level individual practitioners reflect on their practice through the use of PREP (Post Registration Education and Practice Project (UKCC 1990)) and supervision (UKCC 1996). Nursing no longer utilises a fixed body of knowledge and procedures which is simply delivered to a patient who is a passive recipient of care. Nursing and nurses must constantly reflect on practice and learn from research, theory and new skills gained in practice itself, to develop their knowledge and practice in order to meet the demands of a continually changing health care system.

Part of this learning process is facilitated by supervision with the supervisor enabling the supervisee to reflect on their own practice and explore its knowledge and research rationale thus enabling reflection through insight (Cutcliffe and Burns 1998). The authors believe that group supervision greatly enhances the opportunity for reflection and new learning to occur, it also provides opportunities for support, experiences of group cohesion and enhances opportunities for communication skills training (Markham and Turner 1998). The supervisor facilitates the reflection of both the individual, and the whole group, and focuses this reflection on the clinical issues raised in a session. In addition the supervisor can facilitate examination of the dynamics of the group which may enlighten relationship issues between the supervisee and the client as a parallel of the client–nurse relationship (Playle and Mullarkey 1998).

Supervision of students

The clinical supervision sessions for students were located and sequenced so that the students had sufficient exposure to practice that could be used as a basis for discussions. It was noted in the groups that students often had previous experience of caring in a variety of ways, but mainly as support workers for people who had either a diagnosis of mental illness or learning disability, this proving to be a useful ingredient in addition to their other life experiences. Early sessions with the students were taken up with setting ground rules and checking out and confirming that we all had a clear understanding of what clinical supervision meant to us in the context of this group and relating this closely to the Faugier and Butterworth (1992) approach of seeing clinical supervision as the developing of skills through the medium of sharing and reflecting on experiences (from a work situation).

This approach to the implementation of clinical supervision reflected that of Twinn and Johnson (1998) in that the three stages of normative, formative and restorative practice were followed although each aspect also led into or fed back to each other, so that comfort or competence in one would provide a sound base to move on to the next one. This meant that as the course progressed the level of the sessions moved from focusing on what had happened in their practice to developing some of the aspects identified by Proctor (1986) in the formative part of her model, such as links with ethical and skill enhancement.

In the last six months of the course the students started to take on the lead facilitating role for the groups and the lecturer, as the original facilitator, moved to a type of co-facilitator and providing feedback to the student who had led the session. This in itself was an extension of the clinical supervision, the supported movement from supervisee to supervisor. In undertaking this way of operating the group members experienced a number of positive outcomes. From a content point of view they received opportunities where they could explore caring issues, with the outcome of considering alternative caring strategies, that members should receive opportunities to explore their attitudes in caring situations and that members should be exposed to the ideas and attitudes of others. From a process point of view the students could focus on and model the strategies used initially to enable exploration of caring issues in members, consider how issues were dealt with by the group and quantify the link between work in the group and the impact upon practice outside the group. It is important to note that in this respect the supervision sessions linked with each other as issues were not dealt with in isolation but were seen as ongoing from session to session.

As the sessions progressed the students identified a range of issues that they believed had helped and enhanced their learning within the supervision groups. These included:

- *Establishing boundaries*
  Boundaries are essential to provide an environment where supervisees feel supported in disclosure. Broadcasting (having boundaries written down and distributed) and discussing them is an essential component to enabling work in the group to begin. The boundaries allowed for some initial prescription on the part of the supervisor with greater freedom to explore developing later in the session and through the development of the group. Haddock (1997) highlighted the feelings of anxiety evoked in group where boundaries and structure were not evident and there was little cohesion or support experienced as a result. Supervisees were encouraged to explore and communicate their worries and suggest ways in which they could explore their practice but feel safe. It was not the intention to remove all risks, as risk-taking would be part of developing as a nurse and an aid to disclosure in the group.
- *Confidentiality*
  Initially, through the setting of ground rules, confidentiality and the supervisor's role were explored. For a supervisor who is a registered nurse there were

limits on confidentiality: for example, if a supervisee disclosed serious criminal abuse of clients then action by the supervisor would be inevitable. Generally issues raised in the group would remain in the group. If supervisees needed to raise an issue for themselves with their personal tutor then they would be supported in this, however, it would not be the supervisor's role to report anything of the group to a personal tutor.

Disclosure was also discussed and this was closely aligned to purpose, the purpose being to have a forum where supervisees could reflect on their practice. Disclosure of personal material relevant to practice would be the responsibility of the supervisee. For example, the supervisor may intuit from the supervisee that their caring might be inhibited by a similar experience in their own life which is impacting on their caring. If this were acknowledged by the supervisee it would be up to them whether they wished to disclose and explore this issue. Supervisees were always given the option to opt out.

- *Keeping to focus*
One of the problems for the supervisor was enabling the supervisees to focus on the purpose. Even though the purpose was highlighted in the boundaries, supervisees still drifted away from the purpose. As supervisor it was important to use communication skills to focus supervisees onto a self-reflective cycle rather than an other-reflective cycle. Supervisees tended to confuse reflecting on others' practice with their own, and programme theory or practice issues with their own assessments, judgements or rationales for their caring time. To aid focusing, written explanations as well as verbal examples were given of self-reflection and Mezirow's (1981) critical reflectivity was used as a tool to aid reflection. Enabling supervisees to focus on what was their experience of caring rather than an observation of others, was a fundamental step in the development of their skills.

- *Exploration of issues*
Once supervisees began to bring their own practice issues to the group the supervisor's purpose was to enable as broad an exploration of each issue as possible. Once again Mezirow (1981) was used as a guide along with Hawkins and Shohet's (1989) process model (see Box 21.1).

Box 21.1 Process model of supervision

The focus of the supervision session

- Reflection on the content of the session
- Exploration of the strategies used by the carer
- Exploration of the caring process
- Focus on the carer's blocks to facilitating care.

The focus of the supervisor's session

- Focus on the here-and-now process as a mirror or parallel of the there-and-then process
- Focus on the supervisor's counter-transference

(Adapted from Hawkins and Shohet (1989), *Supervision in the Helping Professions.*)

Actively listening to the supervisee (and encouraging other members to do the same) the supervisor would probe aspects of the issue raised as well as clarify with questions, for example, asking: what do you think about your judgements at the time? What decisions did you make? What was your rationale for your decision? How did the episode make you feel? All these questions enabled exploration of the issue for the supervisee, and in verbalising their thoughts enabled and developed within the supervisee some clarity about the situation. This enabled movement onto the next phase of the process model, exploration of the strategies and interventions used by the carer. The supervisee bringing the issue was encouraged to look at alternative strategies in the situation reflecting on theory and research and their own nursing philosophy. Alternative scenarios were considered and if necessary practice, or plans, initiated by the supervisee were made for practice outside of the supervision session. In this respect outcomes were very important to each session, the supervision not being seen as an isolated bubble but a springboard for change in future practice. Thus work in the supervision group might produce changes in practice reflected in a learner's portfolio of learning or discussed as an issue in theory in one of the Action Learning Groups. Links between supervision and other reflective processes in nursing are well documented (Lowry 1998). Feedback was often expected in the following or subsequent sessions. Lastly in the sessions, exploration of the caring process and relationship as well as focus on the carer's blocks to facilitating care were explored. Was there anything within the supervisee that was hindering their progress with the client? Issues of gender, self-perception, race, discrimination, culture and previous negative experiences were all raised at this point and if the supervisee agreed, gently explored.

- *Credibility*

Throughout the sessions comment was often made to the supervisor's role in relation to that of university lecturer. In the initial sessions there seemed to be an acceptance that lecturers had clinical as well as educational credibility. As the sessions progressed and the students felt more able to challenge and confront it was enormously useful for lecturers as supervisors to be able to relate that they not only worked in the clinical arena for part of their time but also received supervision themselves. *The supervisors were also supervisees and this enabled them, in the views of the students, to play a major role in translating the curriculum into a functioning course at the point of delivery to learners.*

Supervision for supervisors

One of the major criticisms around supervision is that those who supervise are insufficiently equipped for the role of supervision (Fish and Twinn 1997). When setting up the clinical supervision for the students we had to consider the fact that we needed supervision in terms of the course in order to avoid the frequently levelled criticism of lecturers teaching theory without the related practice. In considering the process of setting up supervision for lecturers we had to address a number of issues which highlighted the similarities and differences between health oriented services and educational organisations and the perceived value for those concerned.

- *Occupational stress*

Whilst recognising that all occupations have their own unique pressures, some activities are inherently more stressful than others and therefore it is incumbent on organisations to diligently seek out any measure that will ameliorate the damaging effects stress has on overall well-being. There is literature that identifies the caring professions, including nursing, as being particularly stressful (Parry-Jones *et al.* 1998; Wing 1999; Hardy 1995) either because of the particularly turbulent climate caused by changes in social policy concerning the locus of care or through the primacy of the interpersonal aspects of the role and the essential therapeutic role of self (Peplau 1988; Altschul 1997; Barker 1997; Gallop 1997).

Nursing students, teachers and lecturers engaged in health-focused programmes are also identified as being in particularly stressful situations (Youseff and Goodrich 1996; Sawatzky 1998; Jones and Johnston 1997; Hamill 1995), possibly because the organisational turbulence and personal investment are not dissimilar (Playle 1995; Humphreys 1996). People involved in nurse education can therefore be seen to be doubly at risk as they are constantly exhorted to be active in the clinical as well as the educational domain (Hopton 1996). If, as all the evidence, albeit partially anecdotally, suggests, supervision has a part to play in promoting a person's well-being it is clearly something that should be available to nursing students and nursing lecturers. This may be increasingly important as recent moves into higher education have placed different, if not greater, imperatives on role performance (Rodriguez and Goorapah 1998).

The tendency of those in senior roles to focus on performance and action rather than exploring the subtleties of process, the potential for material offered during supervision to be used in a disciplinary manner, the tendency to focus on management issues as the major agenda, and the confusion caused by the duality of supervisory and managerial roles, all contribute to the difficulties when such people undertake the role of supervisor.

- *Choosing a supervisor*

In seeking supervision, the lecturers concerned elected to ask the head of department to act as their group supervisor based on a number of considerations. Some writers emphasise when choosing a supervisor the primacy of the interpersonal skills of the person such as warmth, trust and understanding (Jones 1996), the possession of relevant knowledge and skills (Sloan 1999a) and the ability to reflect and analyse (Fisher 1996). Undoubtedly many within the university possess this laudable range of skills and attributes but this may not necessarily be sufficient to overcome the inherent dialectic created when heads of department are asked to become supervisors. The tendency of those in senior roles to focus on performance and action rather than exploring the subtleties of process (Morris 1995), the potential for material offered during supervision to be used in a disciplinary manner (Burrow 1995; Wilkin *et al.* 1997), the tendency to focus on management issues as the major agenda (Sloan 1999b) and the confusion caused by the duality of supervisory and managerial roles (Adcock 1999) all contribute to the difficulties when such people undertake the role of supervisor.

Despite these warnings the sessions appeared to go well and feedback from all participants indicated their worthwhileness. This clearly is not wholly congruent with some of the literature and therefore leads to a consideration as to why this may be. Underpinning the above writers' concerns appears, at least in part, to be the potential to misuse the power differential created by hierarchical involvement. Power differentials are created by the extent to which one person is dependent on another in terms of resources and outcomes (Brass and Burkhardt 1992) and therefore is determined not only by the personal approaches of the participants but crucially by the nature and culture of the organisation by whom they are employed (Mullins 1993).

The locus of most literature on clinical supervision is understandably within care delivery arenas. Because of its military origins nursing, and hospitals in general, are often seen as the epitome of bureaucracy. Whilst this term has acquired pejorative overtones and has become synonymous with 'red tape' and 'officialdom', Hoyle (1986) paraphrases Max Weber in describing bureaucracies as organisations containing bureaucracy, specialisation, centralisation, procedural rules and a sense of order, security and predictability.

Many clinicians would look at their current practice and yearn for such order, symmetry and rationality but Hoyle suggests that, whilst seldom seen in its pure form, most organisations approximate it to some degree. The degree to which there is an observable and operational hierarchy within nursing is marked, this being supported by such things as by clinical grading, differing levels of educational qualification, clerical specialists and the various tiers of management either general or clinical.

In contrast higher education, in which most schools of nursing and midwifery now belong, arose from a more monastic, discursive origin which is reflected in their culture and operations. Most positions of apparent authority are roles, not posts, and alternate between people over a set period of time, the main decision making bodies are committees not individual officers and 'academic freedom' is acknowledged as a central facet of operational policy. It is suggested, therefore, that universities as organisations resonate more clearly with the organisational structure known as organised anarchies than with bureaucracies (Enderud 1980). Whilst anarchy is not necessarily less pejorative then bureaucracy it points to organisational characteristics such as ambiguous goals, sub-unit autonomy, less positivistic means-end relationships and a variety of responses to external influences (Cameron 1980) all of which are observable within our own university.

For lecturers working within a less overtly structured culture, issues of power and potential coercion would not be as pervasive and therefore they may not see the hierarchical roles as antagonistic to supervisory roles. It would follow therefore that nurses working within a more hierarchical structure would have a greater concern about the potential abuse of power differentials and that would inform their views and actions regarding the choice of supervisor. For lecturers working within a less overtly structured culture, issues of power and potential coercion would not be as pervasive and therefore they may not see the hierarchical roles as antagonistic to supervisory roles.

It is our view that the differences outlined create a milieu within university departments that is significantly different from the corresponding locus of activity within health care delivery. Therefore when 'managers' are involved in supervision it is significantly less problematic as the power difference is negligible and therefore does not compromise the internal dynamics and processes that are essential to effective supervision. This should not be misinterpreted as suggesting that nurses are more passive and reactive whereas nursing lectures are in some way bolder and more proactive, but is more about the effects of organisational structures and cultures on the perceptions of equally valuable and worthwhile people.

In fact it could be argued that as newer care-oriented developments such as a greater involvement of users and carers, more multidisciplinary working, nurse consultancy, clinical governance, health action zones and primary care groups begin to take effect then current bureaucratic structures will, of necessity, become more anarchic. They will therefore become increasingly reliant on high quality non-power-coercive clinical supervision from people with the appropriate skills irrespective of the position they hold.

- *The value of supervision for educationalists*
  The perceived benefits of supervision have been available to some of the caring professions i.e. midwifery and psychotherapists for some time (Thomas and Reid 1995; Farrington 1995) and it is only relatively recently that, under the guise of clinical supervision, nurses have access to these. Indeed, Fowler (1996) identified the use of supervision by others as being one of the reasons why nurses are now seeking access to such a helpful device. The benefits to nurses appears to outweigh the difficulties associated with supervision and are thought to include developing skills and knowledge that will equip practitioners to meet future health care needs (Barton-Wright 1994), increased feelings of support, well-being, confidence and higher morale (Cutcliffe and Proctor 1998), reduction in staff stress and burnout (Farrington 1995), clarifying status thereby reducing uncertainty and confusion (Lowry 1998) and an increased confidence to tackle work related problems (Bowles and Young 1999).

There is much less published work relating to how supervision can help educationalists, however our own personal experiences would suggest that the benefits listed for nursing can also apply to educationalists. One of the first issues that arose during our sessions resonates with Lowry's (1998) notion that supervision aids role clarity. In supervision it was evident that the course leader felt that he had legitimate power in respect of this role and it was therefore questionable as to how much he had to listen to, consider or take on board the views of the other group participants. Clearly he needed to come to terms with the reality that this was not just an exercise to demonstrate that we practice what we preach but a meaningful attempt at increasing the feelings of support and well-being that Cutcliffe and Proctor (1998) suggested.

Addressing and ultimately resolving this issue arose during a session when one of the lecturers in the group raised the question as to how decisions should be reached and agreed relating to course implementation. Fidelity with the previously agreed ground rules ensured a reasoned and seemly debate ensued with everyone attempting to respect the views and feelings of their peers. By the end of the session a democratic system of reaching agreement through a majority viewpoint had been agreed with the proviso that everyone then accepted and stuck to that decision.

In setting the initial ground rules, it was unanimously agreed that no written record of the meetings would be kept. This was partly to ensure congruency with the approach taken in the student groups but also to ensure total confidentiality within the group setting. Obviously the results of our discussions could be utilised to the benefit of the course as was the case when a better system of disseminating assignment information arose from discussions within the supervision group. Our approach to records did mean, however, that we were in danger of potentially going over the things time after time either through lapses in memory, the identification of further evidence or at times an effort to use prevarication and delaying tactics in order to gain personal advantage. In order to try to avoid an almost farcical situation arising it was decided to ask the supervisor to keep brief notes of the key headings, which were prompted and ratified by the supervisees. This constituted part of the facilitator's summarising function at the end of one session and his introduction at the beginning of the next.

The next challenge came when one supervisee wanted to raise an issue about what had happened in their supervision session with the students. This raised an ethical dilemma in that student supervision groups had an agreement not to raise any matter to others unless it fell into one of the areas where it had to be disclosed e.g. illegal activities. Therefore it was felt not possible to discuss this issue in detail but in an attempt to help it was decided to use hypothetical illustrations. At the end of this particular session there was an agreement that such a course of action had been of great use and had increased the individual's repertoire of skills for helping students in distress.

Perhaps the most meaningful indication that the supervision sessions were of value was the level of attendance. The rules of the sessions stipulated that all members had to be present in order to enhance ownership and commitment. Whilst fully recognising that this rule was incredibly ambitious and could have promoted pressure to attend and therefore resentment in fact attendance was good with only a very small minority of sessions being cancelled, which was particularly noteworthy during a period of increased activity and annual leave.

Conclusion

It is often stated, especially in health arenas, that things appear to be essentially cyclical. Old activities could be seen to reinvent themselves as new and exciting initiatives leading cynics to suggest that things are just the same as they have always been only with a new name. Within higher education it is possible to level this criticism at supervision for nurse lecturers and students. Students have personal tutors whose remit includes a pastoral element, course leaders who often address issues that may affect a student's progress, assessors and mentors during clinical placements who oversee skill development.

Lecturers have annual staff appraisal interviews, peer assessment of teaching and for those new to the organisation a 'probation' period for up to three years that includes regular supervision sessions. A question that arises therefore is that within this milieu is there a niche for the type of supervision described in this chapter or is it merely repetition of other support mechanisms under a different guise? It is the firm belief of the authors that this is not the case and there is something significant and worthwhile about the process we have undertaken. Often other forms of support are task oriented and focused on increasing the person's repertoire of knowledge or how to make something work within the given organisation.

The key thing that emerged from our supervision sessions was the felt sense of well-being and emotional support. These are outcomes that are difficult to empirically quantify and therefore could be questioned in a cost effective, financially driven arena. However perhaps the challenge for those who advocate supervision in either clinical or educational settings is to establish appropriate ways of demonstrating its worth to those who have not experienced the warmth and power of the process.

References

Adcock, L. (1999), Clinical supervision in practice, *Journal of Community Nursing*, 13(5): 4–6.

Altschul, A. (1997), A personal view of psychiatric nursing, in S. Tilley (ed.), *The Mental Health View: Views of Practice and Education*, London: Blackwell Science, pp. 1–14.

Barker, P. (1997), Toward a meta theory of psychiatric nursing practice, *Mental Health Practice*, 1(4): 18–21.

Barton-Wright, P. (1994), Clinical supervision and primary nursing, *British Journal of Nursing*, 3(1): 23–29.

Bowles. N. and Young, C. (1999), An evaluative study of clinical supervision based on Proctor's three function interactive model, *Journal of Advanced Nursing*, 30(4): 958–964.

Brass, D.J. and Burkhardt, M.E. (1992), Centrality and power in organizations, in N. Nohria and R.G. Eccles (eds), *Networks and Organizations: Structure Form, and Action*, Boston, MA: Harvard Business School Press.

Burrow, S. (1995), Supervision: clinical development or management control, *British Journal of Nursing*, 4(15): 879–882.

Butterworth, T. and Faugier, J. (eds) (1992), *Clinical Supervision and Mentorship in Nursing*, London: Chapman & Hall.

Cameron, K. (1980), Critical questions in assessing organizational effectiveness, *Organizational Dynamics*, 9(Autumn): 66–78.

Cutcliffe, J.R. and Burns, J. (1998), Personal, professional and practice development: clinical supervision, *British Journal of Nursing*, 7(21): 1318–1322.

Cutcliffe, J.R. and Proctor, B. (1998), An alternative training approach to clinical supervision, *British Journal of Nursing*, 7(5): 280–285.

Department of Health (1993), *A Vision for the Future*, London: HMSO.

Department of Health (1994), *Working in Partnership: A Collaborative Approach to Care*, London: HMSO.

Enderud, H. (1980), Administrative leadership in organised anarchies, *International Journal of Institutional Management in Higher Education*, 4(3): 235–251.

Farrington, A. (1995), Models of clinical supervision, *British Journal of Nursing*, 4(15): 876–878.

Faugier, J. and Butterworth, T. (1994), *Clinical Supervision: A Position Paper*, Manchester: The Manchester University School of Nursing Studies.

Fish, D. and Twinn, S. (1997), *Quality Clinical Supervision in the Health Care Professions: Principled Approaches to Practice*, London: Butterworth Heinemann.

Fisher, M. (1996), Using reflective practice in clinical supervision, *Professional Nurse*, 11(7): 443–444.

Fowler, J. (1996), The organisation of clinical supervision within the nursing profession: a review of the literature, *Journal of Advanced Nursing* 23(3): 471–478.

Gallop, R. (1997), Caring about the client, in S. Tilley (ed.), *The Mental Health Nurse: Views of Practice and Education*, London: Blackwell Science: pp. 28–42.

Haddock, S. (1997), Reflection in groups: contextual and theoretical considerations within nurse education and practice, *Nurse Education Today*, 17(5): 381–385.

Hamill, C. (1995), The phenomenon of stress as perceived by Project 2000 Student Nurses: a case study, *Journal of Advanced Nursing*, 21(3): 528–536.

Hardy, S. (1995), Promoting a healthy workforce: a clinical case presentation, *British Journal of Nursing*, 4(10): 583–586.

Hawkins, P. and Shohet, R. (1989), *Supervision in the Helping Professions*, Milton Keynes: Open University Press.

Hopton, J. (1996), Reconceptualising the theory practice gap in mental health nursing, *Nurse Education Today*, 16(3): 227–232.

Hoyle, E. (1986), *The Politics of School Management*, London: Hodder & Stoughton.

Humphreys, J. (1996), Educational commissioning by consortia: some theoretical and practical issues relating to qualitative aspects of British nurse education, *Journal of Advanced Nursing*, 24(6): 1288–1299.

Jones, A. (1996), Clinical supervision: a framework for practice, *International Journal of Psychiatric Nursing Research*, 3(1): 290–299.

Jones, M.C. and Johnston, D.W. (1997), Distress, stress and coping in first year student nurses, *Journal of Advanced Nursing*, 26(3): 475–482.

Lowry, M. (1998), Clinical supervision for the development of nursing practice, *British Journal of Nursing*, 4(10): 583–586.

Markham, V. and Turner, P. (1998), Implementing a system of structured clinical supervision with a group of DipHE (Nursing) RMN students, *Nurse Education Today*, 18(1): 32–35.

Mezirow, A. (1981), A critical theory of adult learning and education, *Adult Education*, 32(1): 3–24.

Morris, M. (1995), The role of clinical supervision in mental health practice, *British Journal of Nursing*, 4(15): 886–888.

Mullins, L.J. (1993), *Management and Organisational Behaviour*, 3rd edn, London: Pitman.

Norman, I.J., Redfern, S.J. and Bodley, *et al.* (1996), *The Changing Educational Needs of Mental Health and Learning Disability Nurses*, London: English National Board for Nursing, Midwifery and Health Visiting.

Parry-Jones, B., Grant, G., McGrath, M., Ramcharan, P. and Robinson, C.A. (1998), Stress and job satisfaction among social workers, community nurses and community psychiatric nurses: implications for the care management model, *Health and Social Care in the Community*, 6(4): 271–285.

Peplau, H.E. (1988), *Interpersonal Relations in Nursing*, 2nd edn, London: Macmillan.

Playle, J.F. (1995), Humanism and positivism: contradictions and conflicts in nursing, *Journal of Advanced Nursing*, 22(5): 979–984.

Playle, J.F. and Mullarkey, K. (1998), Parallel process in clinical supervision: enhancing learning and providing support, *Nurse Education Today*, 18(7): 559–556.

Proctor, B. (1986), Supervision: a cooperative exercise in accountability, in M. Marken and M. Payne (eds), *Enabling and Ensuring*, Leicester: Leicester Youth Bureau and Training in Community Work.

Rodriguez, P. and Goorapah, D. (1998), Clinical supervision for nurse teachers: the pertinent issues, *British Journal of Nursing*, 7(11): 663–669.

Sainsbury (1997), *Pulling Together: The Future Roles and Training of Mental Health Staff*, London: Sainbury Centre for Mental Health.

Sloan, G. (1999a), Understanding clinical supervision from a nursing perspective, *British Journal of Nursing*, 8(8): 524–528.

Sloan, G. (1999b), Good characteristics of a clinical supervisor: a community mental health nurse perspective, *Journal of Advanced Nursing*, 30(3): 713–722.

Sawatzky, J.-A.V. (1998), Understanding nursing students' stress: a proposed framework, *Nurse Education Today*, 18(2), 108–115.

Thomas, B. and Reid, J. (1995), Multidisciplinary clinical supervision, *British Journal of Nursing*, 4(15): 883–885.

Twinn, S. and Johnson, C. (1998) The supervision of health visiting practice: a continuing agenda for debate, in T. Butterworth, J. Faugier and P. Burnard (eds), *Clinical Supervision and Mentorship in Nursing*, Cheltenham: Stanley Thornes.

UKCC (1990), *Post Registration Education and Practice Project*, London: United Kingdom Central Council.

UKCC (1996), *Position Statement on Clinical Supervision for Nursing and Health Visiting*, London: United Kingdom Central Council.

Wilkin, P., Bowers, L. and Monk, L. (1997), Clinical supervision: managing the resistance, *Nursing Times*, 93(8): 48–49.

Wing, M. (1999), Nursing makes you sick, *Nursing Times*, 95(7): 24–25.

Youseff, F.A. and Goodrich, N. (1996), Accelerated versus traditional nursing students: a comparison of stress, critical thinking ability and performance, *International Journal of Nursing Studies*, 33(1): 76–82.

Part IV

Contemporary research activity on clinical supervision

22 Nurses' experiences of core phenomena in the supervisor training programme

Ann-Kristin Holm Wiebe, Ingrid Johansson, Ingegerd Lindquist and Elisabeth Severinsson

There is a long tradition of nursing supervision at the Institute for Caring Sciences and Health at Göteborg University, Sweden. Its pedagogic development began in 1989 when process oriented supervision was provided to assist nursing students at different educational levels. Since 2008, students have received three terms of supervision, which is compulsory in nursing education. The students are supervised by nurse teachers as well as by professionally active clinical nurses, all of whom hold the postgraduate degree for Nurse Supervisors. In this chapter, the authors identify, describe and synthesise the core phenomena in nursing supervision based on their work with students. The three emerging dimensions regarding the core phenomena were: (1) value-based phenomena; (2) upholding and nurturing relationship, and (3) the meaning of supervision space.

We believe that this chapter is very interesting for clinical supervisors, educators and researchers. The authors highlight important core phenomena that deepen our understanding of the process of nursing supervision and the supervisor-supervisee relationships. The reported findings also provide an interesting starting point for the development of the theoretical concept of nursing supervision.

We respectfully acknowledge that three of the authors – Ann-Kristin, Ingrid, and Ingegerd – are teachers at the Institute for Caring Sciences and Health and received the 2008 Göteborg University Pedagogical team prize for this work.

Background

This chapter is intended for clinical nurses, especially those involved in supervision and the education of student nurses in the clinical field. The goal of nursing supervision is to ensure and enhance quality of care (Holm *et al.* 1998, 2003; Halvarsson and Johansson 2000). An additional goal is to integrate practice and theory, promote the development of the student nurse's professional identity and preparedness to act as well as to provide an opportunity for reflection (Holm *et al.* 1998; Severinsson 2001, 2005).

A prerequisite for nursing supervision is educated professional supervisors who can influence the development of the prospective nurses' professional identity. First we will briefly describe the education, and thereafter, the applied part, with a focus on the phenomena inherent in the supervision process.

Process-oriented nursing supervision

The nurse supervisors' academic education is both theoretical and applied. The curriculum states (1995, revised 2004): *The aim of the course 'Supervision as a process in nursing practice – training programme for supervisors' is to develop the student's competence to supervise in on-going process-oriented nursing supervision. An additional aim is to develop the students' ability to increase their professionalism and critically analyse their supervisory skills.*

The education is divided into different modules corresponding to 30 higher education credits (15 for theoretical and 15 for applied supervision) and takes place on an on-going basis over four semesters (part-time, 25 per cent). The mode of working in the applied part includes systematic reflection on one's own experiences of theoretical as well as practical learning situations. Therefore the applied module involves 80 hours of supervision on professional identity and 40 hours on working in a group, in addition to acting as a supervisor for 40 hours (total 160 hours). The supervisors are nurse teachers trained in process-oriented group supervision. Specific examination areas include a literature review of core phenomena in supervision, which takes the form of a written report and an oral presentation at a seminar.

Over the years, the curriculum has become more academic and scientific, with evidence-based criteria for the selection of published articles. *Little is known about the phenomena inherent in the supervision process.* The choice of phenomena is related to the student nurses' interest in knowledge development, their identification of phenomena and their supervisor paradigm. Overall, when gathering and analysing the data it was interesting to note that although the criteria changed, the phenomena remained the same. Several of the examination reports were based on the caring sciences, while the theoretical understanding of the phenomenon was guided by two nursing theorists, Professor Katie Eriksson and Professor Elisabeth Severinsson.

What are the most common phenomena in nursing supervision?

To answer this question we identified the phenomena described by the nurses attending the supervisor programme. The data were based on self-reports and covered a period of ten years (1998–2008). All the documents were read through with focus on the students' own thoughts and reasoning. The aim was to analyse the students' reflections on the phenomena they had chosen to describe. In total, 32 self-reported documents were analysed. All the students consented to the analysis of their texts.

Thereafter, we applied thematic content analysis (see Graneheim and Lundman 2004) and sorted the topics into three groups: value-based phenomena; upholding and nurturing relationships; and the meaning of supervision space. The third part of the analysis involved interpreting the three groups in relation to each other in order to reach a deeper understanding of core phenomena in the context of nursing supervision. The following research questions were applied: 'How do the selected phenomena become visible in nursing supervision?' and 'How do the most common phenomena relate to each other?' The fourth part of the analysis comprised a synthesis of the three groups in relation to each other aimed at contributing to a deeper understanding of core phenomena in the context of nursing supervision.

Value-based phenomena

We assumed that the value-based phenomena inherent in nursing supervision include: *guilt, shame and inadequacy; forgiveness and reconciliation; suffering and relief; power and responsibility; and courage.*

Guilt, shame and inadequacy

In the context of nursing supervision, guilt and shame are two strongly related phenomena, although the guilt is more common than the others. Human beings feel guilty about negative things that they have done i.e. guilt is related to 'doing'. The nurse supervisee constructs an image of him/herself as the perfect and ideal nurse. We speculated: could it be that the idealism in caring leads to feelings of guilt among staff and that when the self-image cracks it results in feelings of inadequacy and failure? Reflecting on his/her professional situation for the first time makes the nurse aware of his/her shortcomings and leaves him/her standing 'naked' in his/her own eyes and in front of others. *Nursing supervision can alleviate feelings of guilt and inadequacy.* Sharing experiences with colleagues and reflecting on the work may lead to changes related to improved working routines and result in a positive feeling of deriving more benefit from one's working conditions. It is of great importance to be able to view, present, articulate and share feelings of guilt in nursing supervision. Another way to help the supervisee to reflect is by allowing him/her to assume responsibility for his/her situation. On the other hand, shame concerns the individual's self-value, which can be difficult to address in supervision as it may require a more therapeutic intervention. *Daring to face feelings of shame and inadequacy and sharing them in supervision requires courage.* If someone judges him/herself too harshly during supervision it will become a central part of the session, thus supervision could have a negative impact on that person and it might be advisable for him/her not to attend the supervision group for a while.

Difficult caring situations that give rise to feelings of powerlessness and meaninglessness can result in a sense of inadequacy, abandonment and exclusion. Powerlessness and feelings of inadequacy often exist in parallel processes. One explanation may be that the person's own standpoint is not articulated and therefore subordinated. Experiences of inadequacy are common in caring situations. The phenomena that constitute inadequacy are closely related to the moral aspect of caring. Burnout is also associated with feelings of inadequacy.

Forgiveness and reconciliation

Forgiveness is present in the relationship between and reciprocal actions of the supervisee and supervisor. Reconciliation is defined as a process that takes place within a person. Both forgiveness and reconciliation have a deep religious meaning but are present in everyday situations. They can also imply healing, since reconciliation concerns wholeness, integration and acceptance. It is essential to address feelings of discouragement and dissatisfaction in supervision in order to be able to integrate the goodness and evil within each individual. In the context of nursing supervision, it is important that the supervisees' experiences of weakness are not concealed, but accepted and given space to exist, since it must be possible to be weak and at the same time strong and competent.

Suffering and relief

Feelings of suffering can occur when the nurse experiences shortcomings due to his/her inability to encounter patients or team members in an appropriate fashion. Feelings of anger, injustice, degradation, self-pity and powerlessness can make the supervisee disheartened and unsure in her/his professional role. This can damage his/her self-confidence and trust in other people, thereby leading to a lack of joy and difficulty developing a professional identity. In what way can the supervisor encounter suffering and create the necessary conditions for professional growth and change? *In encounters with the supervisee the supervisor must respect him/her by being accepting, nurturing, assuming a forgiving stance and eschewing contempt, as it is essential to confirm the supervisee.* The supervisor has an obligation not to abandon the supervisee and leave him/her feeling isolated.

Another way of supporting the supervisee is to reflect on his/her responsibility. Experiences of guilt may make it more difficult for the supervisee to face and understand him/herself. While the supervisor assumes responsibility for the supervisee he/she does not take over the latter's responsibility. The supervisee must be willing to take responsibility, choose between different ways of acting and have the courage to adhere to what he/she considers right and good.

The organisation and structure of continual supervision provide the health care professional with support, time to reflect and allow him/her to narrate his/her experiences. The supervisor is responsible for allowing the supervisee space in which to express his/her stress and suffering. It is often difficult to admit one's weakness and therefore it can be helpful to use metaphors to express such experiences.

Power and responsibility

Power is a central phenomenon in nursing supervision and the supervisor's power influences the group process in various ways. *Power requires the supervisor to reflect on his/her way of leading the group.* The supervisee may have different experiences of people in authority, which can be a challenge for the supervisor.

Exercising power in the group can have both negative and positive consequences depending on whether the supervisor assumes responsibility for his/her power. Positive consequences are the supervisor's strength and ability to be patient as well as to inspire hope and courage. Inability to exercise power can mean that the supervisor lacks structure in his/her leadership, has difficulty setting boundaries, summarising the supervision session and motivating the supervisees.

Insight into power and responsibility constitutes an ethical challenge. A dominant group member may take up so much space that it damages the group process. This implies that the supervisor must have the courage to confront him/her. It is important to be aware that fear of exercising power may hinder one's leadership. *In the supervision process, the supervisees are trained to reflect on their actions and values in a deeper way.* Nurses and student nurses often narrate stories related to powerlessness, which concern situations where they had no opportunity to influence the care. It takes courage to choose new ways of thinking and acting. Nurses may have difficulties handling conflicts between what they are supposed to do when caring for patients and the subordinate role they are expected to maintain. Supervision is a space in which questions of gender and social order can be illuminated, expressed in words, reflected upon and discussed, thus leading to change.

Courage

Courage is a virtue. In order to change and develop identity, one needs a model that allows virtues to exist. *When the supervisor is courageous, he/she can serve as a model that may help the supervisees to develop courage.* In supervision, courage can concern daring to share a story with others in the group and reflecting together on the individual's role as a nurse and a person. Describing negative issues requires courage. The supervisee must be aware of his/her fear in order to understand and overcome it, thus allowing courage to emerge. Moreover, willingness to share the growth and experiences of other human beings requires courage. *The supervision process broadens self-awareness and allows the supervisee to take responsibility for his/her own weakness without blaming others.* Supervision can provide courage to be the person one wants to be. Having courage means acting and reacting in a more autonomic way.

Upholding and nurturing relationships

The following phenomena: *confirmation; understanding and empathy; being present in an encounter; creating trust and security*, are fundamental for relationships.

Confirmation

In supervision, confirmation is the most valuable component for achieving professional growth. The deepest wish of all human beings is to be loved and confirmed. *Being confirmed leads to a process of growth in terms of professional identity and increases the supervisees' self-confidence and self-knowledge.* Confirmation influences professional identity, professional stance and caring relationships. The goal of confirmation is to eliminate doubt and achieve a professional identity. Confirming interventions demand active listening, the ability to put oneself in the other person's situation, turn to the other person and verbally confirm him/her. Thus, confirmation is a stance. We are all dependent on each other's confirmation. If one is unable to accept confirmation from the other person, it may undermine one's identity development. In supervision, confirmation occurs at the beginning of the session when the supervisor invites and welcomes everyone into the group and also when the person focused upon is given space to tell his/her story. *Receiving supervision is a confirmation that one is needed as a human being and nurse.* Being seen, emotionally touched and listened to, being good enough, daring and having courage enable one to experience confirmation. Self-affirmation and confirmation are necessary in order to feel whole. It is also important that confirmation is received from colleagues other than the leader of the department. It is in the dialogue between the supervisor and the supervisee that the latter experiences confirmation and learns how to confirm others. In supervision, the source of confirmation, i.e. the view of oneself and external confirmation, is important. Experiencing support in an open working climate does not mean always agreeing with each other. The feeling of being able to discuss different perceptions is also an important aspect.

Understanding and empathy

Achieving an intellectual understanding of the situation focused upon in supervision can relieve the supervisee's anxiety. It is therefore important that the supervisor has the theoretical knowledge to comprehend what the supervisee expressed about his/her situation. *Theoretical knowledge provides the supervisor with security and the potential to act.* It is possible to guide the supervisee by means of intellectual understanding and the ability to put oneself in his/her position. Emotional understanding implies sensitivity towards the other person, as well as sympathy for his/her experiences and emotional reactions. Working as a nurse can mean balancing on a tightrope with the risk of falling off at any moment. Supervision is a lifeline, as shortcomings and imperfections may be expressed without the fear of being judged and/or considered incompetent.

Being present in an encounter

Good supervision is a pedagogical process grounded in the encounter. The first meeting sets the tone for the following sessions, where acceptance of the supervision contract, i.e. time, place and group members' expectations of the supervision process, is an important element. Each session starts with the 'round' where everyone relates something about themselves. The time is 'here and now' and the starting point is who meets who and what they plan to do together. *The most important aspect is that the supervisor encounters the supervisees at their emotional level using his/her skills, knowledge and warmth.* Communication is the foundation of the encounter with other people and can take different forms, including body language, words, facial expression, tone of voice, environment and context. The art of listening requires knowledge, sensitivity and emotional involvement, but above all the ability to listen with an open mind. It means not only silence but the ability to be present in the here and now and the courage to allow oneself to be emotionally touched, which is one of the most difficult things to achieve. Insight based on one's emotions may be the only way to trust one's inner guide. Each time the supervisee attends supervision together with others he/she learns about him/herself and the subject of the dialogue. The supervisee can learn from both the inner and external world.

Creating trust and security

The feeling of being able to trust the other members of the supervision group means that one dares to narrate experiences, even those related to inadequacy. This statement highlights the importance of trust, which is a beautiful concept that concerns being able to rely on another human being. *In supervision, a trusting relationship means that the supervisee has the courage to tell about his/her shortcomings and failures without losing control of the situation.* Trust is a central concept in supervision and is facilitated by the supervisor's structure, knowledge and ability to create a positive environment. It is important for the supervisor to understand that it takes time to create a climate of trust in supervision, which is a prerequisite for daring to describe experiences, thoughts and feelings. Trust influences the supervisees' learning ability and is necessary for personal growth. As the supervisor might not be aware of the self-image of the different people in the group, he/she must exercise caution.

The meaning of the supervision space

The supervision space is characterised by the creation of mental space. The space and existential becoming are created by means of *storytelling*, *sharing* and *reflection*. *Playing* and *acting* are considered to have a healing function for the human being and are thus an important part of caring. Finally, there is a space for *challenges* that create meaning and can provide an insight into gifts that were never noticed or experienced before.

Storytelling

The nurse puts words to his/her innermost thoughts and reflects over the situations experienced by means of storytelling. The supervisee is invited by the other group members to analyse and examine the story. He/she can formulate a problem, discover what happened and what he/she needs help with. Together with the other supervisees, he/she can identify the underlying idea and learn from it. Inviting 'the other' and creating trust are of the utmost importance.

It is essential to listen to one's own stories as well as those of the other members of the group. No one can have an authentic dialogue with another human being without being authentic with him/herself. As a supervisor it is important to be aware of one's own ethical stance – a part of one's life story. When encountering the supervisee, the supervisor can stimulate both an inner and external dialogue. Supervisees who are not very talkative may need help to start the inner dialogue in order to be able to express thoughts and feelings in words. The stories are ever present and linked to each other, thus creating a chain. Every story is unique. Some stories may have similarities that one can recognise, but they can never replace one's own story. It is important to confirm both the storyteller and the story. Moreover, it is not easy to tell a story and one needs help to learn how to articulate in a colourful way so that others can feel involved, reflect and find their own points of reference.

Sharing and reflection

Sharing means being open and revealing aspects of oneself that are not visible to other people. Some supervisees recognise their own experiences when listening to the stories of other group members, which can be considered a form of healing. Sharing something one does not fully understand can encourage others to share their experiences and may strengthen the persons involved. *Communicating and sharing experiences lead to new knowledge and help the supervisees to get to know each other well so that they can develop a deeper and more trusting relationship with each other.* Reflection flourishes in the supervision space. When the supervisee reflects on his/her own and others' stories he/she becomes aware of his/her reactions as well as consequences of his/her actions. A more reflective stance increases maturity and facilitates the development of a professional identity. It is also important to reflect on the story.

'Playing'

'Playing' in supervision facilitates creativity, learning, courage and professional growth. The supervisor's role is to create a climate characterised by trust, closeness, openness and eagerness. Preparedness and structure are of fundamental importance for the creation of space for 'playing'. *When the supervisor creates a structure for 'playing' it becomes possible to use different forms of communication, language, thoughts and feelings.* One of the supervisor's roles is to support the supervisee to find his/her own solutions, thereby enabling professional growth.

Challenges

The concept of challenge, which concerns inspiring, inviting, encouraging, defying and/or provoking someone to assume responsibility, has both a positive and a negative aspect. *While it is easy to adopt the positive part, one may question whether it is wrong to provoke in supervision.* And is it wrong to increase the level of tolerance with regard to anxiety? That which is different challenges the 'normal' as well as norms and values. The 'different-ness' affects the individual when someone narrates about an event that is so unusual that it might be difficult to reflect on. Accepting different-ness and being able to say: 'I cannot understand this, what does it mean?' and 'What can I learn from it?' can be a part of the inner and external dialogue if we are open and willing to learn from other people. This is important for those who work with other human beings. Challenges are necessary for personal growth. Learning to challenge as a part of the supervisory role requires openness and sensitivity. The supervisor has a responsibility to encounter the supervisee in a spirit of trust and confidence. This is necessary for growth, as is confirmation, being asked about and invited to describe what one is unsure of and allowing the group to react to the supervisor's challenges. Such challenges can be seen as a struggle for the supervisees. It is therefore not surprising that they prefer to be confirmed. It may be difficult to find a balance between challenges and confirmation in relation to professional growth.

Comprehensive understanding

Three dimensions of nursing supervision emerged in our study: (1) value-based phenomena; (2) upholding and nurturing relationships; and (3) the meaning of supervision space, all of which are important, more or less common phenomena inherent in and dependent on each other in the supervision process. All three dimensions also relate to individual growth and thus offer potential for developing nurses' professional ethical stance and consciousness of their own value base. Personal growth and the development of professional identity are dependent on upholding and nurturing the relationship between the supervisor and the supervisee. This specific relationship can be viewed as a parallel process to that between the nurse and patient. It seems that if a nurse is encountered in a confirming manner, it makes it possible for him/her to encounter and confirm others as well as develop the courage and strength to relate to the patient in deeper way. Moreover, the relationship in the supervision process includes understanding of others, the need for empathy as well as the importance of trust and security. This also applies to the supervision space developed by means of storytelling, sharing and reflection in the form of 'playing' and being challenged. In the supervision space the supervisee can share his/her worries about not being a good enough nurse, how to act and how to maintain the ethical stance taught in the education. The desire to develop moral responsibility and cope with the demands of others in nursing practice is of the utmost importance. Understanding and feeling empathy as well as being seen and confirmed by others enhance the development of a professional identity.

This study provides evidence for the development of the theoretical concept of nursing supervision and adds a new and deeper understanding of the process of supervision i.e. its substance and most common phenomena. In this way it provides evidence for nursing practice and the nurse supervisees' relationship with colleagues and patients. This finding is in accordance with research by Johansson *et al.* (2006) on the value of caring in nursing supervision. Caring is inherent in all aspects of nursing supervision; in the narratives pertaining to the patients' situations; the professional role; and the benefits of participating in supervision.

References

Curriculum (1995, revised 2004), *Sahlgrenska akademien vid Göteborgs universitet, Institutionen för vårdvetenskap och hälsa. Curriculum. Kontinuerlig processhandledning i omvårdnad- handledarutbildning*, 20 p [*The Sahlgrenska Academy University of Gothenburg Institute of Health and Care Sciences Curriculum Supervision as a Process in Nursing Practice – Training Program for Supervisors*, 20 credit], 6 June 1995, revised 4 May 2004.

Graneheim, U.H. and Lundman, B. (2004), Qualitative content analysis in nursing research: concepts, procedures and measures to achieve trustworthiness, *Nurse Education Today*, 24(2): 105–112.

Halvarsson, M. and Johansson, I. (2000), Att ge och ta emot bekräftelse. En studie av bekräftelse i processorienterad handledning i vårdarbete [Giving and Receiving Confirmation in Process-Oriented Supervision within Nursing], *Vård i Norden*, 20(1): 9–14.

Holm, A.K., Lantz, I. and Severinsson, E. (1998), Nursing students' experiences of continual process-oriented group supervision, *Journal of Nursing Management*, 6(2): 105–113.

Holm, A.K., Lantz, I. and Severinsson, E. (2003), A theoretical perspective of the core concepts of nursing supervision, *Norsk tidskrift for sykepleieforskning [Norwegian Journal of Nursing Research]*, 5(2): 71–82.

Johansson, I., Holm, A.K., Lindqvist, I. and Severinsson, E. (2006), The value of caring in clinical nursing supervision, *Journal of Nursing Management*, 14(8): 644–651.

Severinsson, E. (1995), *Clinical Nursing Supervision in Health Care*, doctoral dissertation at the Nordic School of Public Health, Göteborg.

Severinsson, E. (2001), Confirmation, meaning and self-awareness as core concepts of the nursing supervision model, *Nursing Ethics*, 8(1): 36–44.

23 Efficacy of clinical supervision

Influence on job satisfaction, burnout and quality of care

Kristiina Hyrkäs, Kaija Appelqvist-Schmidlechner and Riina Lemponen

This chapter introduces findings of a nationwide clinical supervision (CS) evaluation study conducted in Finland. The authors first review earlier effectiveness studies and the different types of evaluation methods. The chapter introduces key results of the evaluation study and focuses on discussing: (1) how the supervisees' background variables and infrastructure of CS relate to evaluations of the effectiveness of CS; and (2) how evaluations of CS effectiveness predict supervisee job satisfaction, burnout and assessments of quality of nursing care.

We believe that this chapter demonstrates important developments in the area of clinical supervision. First, it shows that progress has been made in the field of evaluation research due to the availability and use of validated and reliable instruments. The importance of evaluation is also evident in that the study shows that there are significant differences among supervisees regarding their experiences and evaluations of CS. In order to develop CS further in the twenty-first century, the results of evaluations are crucial. Second, this chapter confirms the results from earlier studies regarding the significance of the infrastructure and practical arrangements for clinical supervision and that these are strongly associated with the supervisees' evaluations. This is an important chapter for supervisors, supervisees, managers and researchers who are part of the planning, implementation and evaluation of clinical supervision in their organisations. This study was originally published in the *Journal of Advanced Nursing* (Hyrkäs *et al.* 2006) and interested readers can find a thorough discussion of the results and statistical analyses in that original research paper.

Introduction

Research-based understanding of clinical supervision (CS) is quite extensive in Scandinavian countries, the United Kingdom and Australia (Hyrkäs *et al.* 1999; Hyrkäs and Munnukka 2002). During the past decades, empirical research has focused on the effects of CS and has been critiqued on the basis of weak scientific rigor (Hyrkäs *et al.* 1999; Teasdale *et al.* 2001). However the current research challenge is not about CS effectiveness or analysis of the concept (Lyth 2000), but the CS intervention itself. It is possible to claim, based on the literature (e.g. Fowler and Chevannes 1998) that evaluation is an inseparable part of CS process. However, most evaluation has been based on supervisees' own subjective criteria and these have been impossible to compare or study empirically (Herrmann 1996).

Literature review and theoretical background

Clinical supervision in Finland and Scandinavian countries

The Finnish history of CS in helping professions is long. The literature indicates that CS started gradually in health care organizations in the 1950s, first carried out by psychoanalysts in psychiatric units (Paunonen 1991). Towards the end of the 1980s, CS expanded and slowly moved into the different specialties in health care organizations (Paunonen and Hyrkäs 2001). The numbers of empirical studies focused on the effects of CS and published in Finnish have increased since the early 1980s reflecting the growth of CS in practice (Paunonen and Hyrkäs 2001). The first national level survey exploring the prevailing state of CS was completed and reported by the Ministry of Social and Health Affairs in the beginning of the 1980s (Sosiaali- ja terveysministeriö 1983).

The research-based knowledge of the effects of CS has clearly increased during the 1990s (Hyrkäs *et al.* 1999). The empirical studies have tried to demonstrate for example the effects of CS on professional (Hallberg *et al.* 1994) and personal growth (Arvidsson *et al.* 2000), knowledge base and competencies (Hallberg 1994; Arvidsson *et al.* 2000), professional independence (Paunonen 1991), tedium (Berg *et al.* 1994, Hallberg 1994) and strain (Berg and Hallberg 1999), quality of care (Hallberg 1994; Edberg *et al.* 1996; Edberg 1999; Hyrkäs and Paunonen-Ilmonen 2001) and documentation (Hallberg *et al.* 1994), increased creativity (Berg *et al.* 1994; Berg and Hallberg 1999) and job satisfaction (Hallberg *et al.* 1994; Arvidsson *et al.* 2000). An interesting finding is that both positive and negative evidence concerning the effects of CS have been reported, and these have focused for example on professional identity (Segesten 1993), burnout (Berg *et al.* 1994; Pålsson *et al.* 1996; Butterworth *et al.* 1997), sense of coherence (Pålsson *et al.* 1996; Berg and Hallberg 1999) and empathy (Pålsson *et al.* 1996). The relatively high number of papers reporting non-desired or even negative effects gives a strong rationale to examine and evaluate the intervention itself more closely (Hyrkäs *et al.* 1999; see also Teasdale *et al.* 2001).

CS evaluation research: earlier studies and methods of evaluation

The utility and usefulness of CS has not been questioned in the literature, but instead the notion that CS has an inherent value in health care and that it is 'equally good' for every nurse became generalized in the 1990s along with the reported positive experiences (Bowles and Young 1999). However, supervisees' subjective 'feel-good' evaluation reports or multi-focused effectiveness studies provide an inadequate rationale for decision making in health care management. The expanded use of CS among nursing and other health care staff increased pressure in the late 1990s to develop systematically CS evaluation methods utilizing research. Development of such methods was also required to justify the investment of resources in CS (Dudley and Butterworth 1994; Hyrkäs *et al.* 2001b). The ability to assess objectively the impact of CS on organizations, individuals in the workforce and patient outcomes was therefore essential (Winstanley 2000).

There were few CS evaluation studies reported in the literature in the late 1990s (Bowles and Young 1999; Butterworth *et al.* 1999; Lees 1999; Stanton *et al.* 2000; Cheater and Hale 2001). The focus of these studies and the methods used to make the evaluations varied considerably. For example, Sloan (1998) used focus group techniques and thematic content analysis to define what made a good supervisor. This pioneering study was without doubt interesting, but the findings, like in many other studies, were not directly associated with the evaluation of the efficacy of the CS intervention. White *et al.* (1998) reported 'lived experiences of CS' based on in-depth interviews. The findings of this study indicated positive and valuable outcomes, but similar to Scanlon and Weir's (1997) study of mental health nurses' perceptions and experiences of CS, these studies did not quite focus on evaluation of the efficacy of CS. Rather, they only mapped out some of the substantive domains. Only a few evaluation studies reported successful use of reliable and valid self-completion questionnaires focusing on evaluation of the efficacy of CS in the late 1990s (Nicklin 1997a, 1997b; Mahood *et al.* 1998; Winstanley 2001).

Instruments

In our study, the supervisees were asked to complete the following questionnaires:

1 Background questionnaire.
2 Manchester Clinical Supervision Scale (MCSS) (Winstanley 2000).
3 The Maslach Burnout Inventory (MBI) (Maslach and Jackson 1986; see also Schaufeli *et al.* 1993).
4 The Minnesota Job Satisfaction Scale (short form) (MJSS) (Weiss 1967; see also Koelbel *et al.* 1991).
5 Good Nursing Care – questionnaire (Leino-Kilpi 1990).

All the instruments are well-established research scales, with extensive data on their reliability and validity. They have also been used in earlier CS studies reported by Butterworth *et al.* (1997, 1999) and Winstanley (2000). Permission to use the instruments was obtained. The study design is presented in Figure 23.1.

Results

Demographic

Data collection took place between October 2000 and February 2001 and involved 12 regional, central and university hospitals across Finland. Approval for the study was obtained from each participating organization. Responses were received from 799 respondents (i.e. supervisees), an overall response rate of 62 per cent. Most of the respondents were female and the mean age was 42 years. The majority reported that their supervisor was a woman with an average age of 42 years. Most had prior experience of CS. Only one in five was receiving CS for the first time. Most frequently, the ongoing supervision had lasted less than two years. The sample had nearly equal numbers of those receiving one-to-one and group supervision.

Respondents' backgrounds and evaluations of CS

Female supervisees gave more positive evaluations of CS than their male colleagues with the best evaluations given by respondents who: worked on day shifts, had

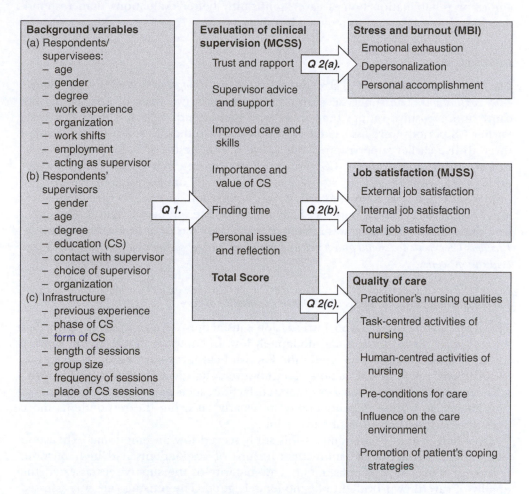

Figure 23.1 Study design and theoretical framework of the study.

tenured positions in psychiatric organizations; and were specialized nurses. Respondents who were supervisors themselves gave better evaluations than non-supervising respondents. Supervisees' specialty, gender and supervising experience were predictors for the highest CS evaluation scores. The best evaluation scores were given to female supervisors who had an academic degree other than psychology. *Supervisors who had been educated in CS were evaluated statistically significantly better than their colleagues without CS education. The best evaluation scores were given when supervisors were selected by supervisees, there was contact at least once a month, and the supervisor was from the same organization as the respondent.* The ability to choose a supervisor and the supervisor's occupation were background variables that predicted the highest evaluation scores.

The most critical evaluations were given by physiotherapists, non-tenured staff, night shift workers and respondents in somatic organizations. The supervisees who worked in other organizations such as psychiatric outpatient clinics, mental health clinics or rehabilitation homes gave significantly better evaluations than respondents in university, central or regional hospitals.

Infrastructure details

The infrastructure and practical arrangements of CS were strongly associated with the respondents' evaluations. The supervisees who had more than two years of CS gave significantly more positive ratings than those who had attended CS less than one year. Earlier CS periods were associated with the ratings so that those who had attended three to five earlier supervision periods gave the highest scores. Respondents who had no prior experience of CS gave the lowest scores. When CS occurred every other week with 45 minute sessions in the form of one-to-one supervision, the ratings were better as compared with group supervision, with a lower frequency and longer duration. As for group CS, smaller groups received better ratings. CS organized outside the work place was rated better in all aspects than CS in the workplace. *Previous CS experience, small group size and high frequency of sessions all predicted the highest evaluation scores.*

Job satisfaction, burnout and evaluations of the quality of care

The respondents' overall and intrinsic job satisfaction were moderately high, but the extrinsic job satisfaction was moderately low. In comparison with the normative scores of MJSS (Koelbel *et al.* 1991) the Finnish health care professionals, extrinsic, intrinsic and total job satisfaction were, however, slightly above the average normative scores. The intrinsic factors of job satisfaction, such as 'steady employment' or 'the chance to work independently' were clearly satisfying the respondents more than the extrinsic factors of job satisfaction.

Over half of the respondents of this study scored low on emotional exhaustion and depersonalization, but more than a third of respondents had high burnout scores for personal accomplishment. The majority of the supervisees assessed the quality of care they provided to be moderately good. The nursing care was assessed as good especially in the subscale of 'Human Centred Activities' of nursing.

Respondents' backgrounds as predictors for job satisfaction, burnout and quality of care

Age predicted the supervisees' extrinsic job satisfaction and burnout levels related to 'Personal Accomplishment'. In comparison to the youngest respondent group (under 30 years) the other age groups had lower extrinsic job satisfaction. Personal accomplishment was, however, lower in the next age group indicating a higher burnout level. Among the 41–50-year-old respondents, burnout in the form of distracted personal accomplishment was more likely than for younger respondents. The respondents' education predicted also 'Personal Accomplishment'. The polytechnic level education (i.e. BNSc) was the best predictor for lower level of burnout compared to the Nursing School level (i.e. Diploma) education. The respondent's gender predicted only the evaluations related to the quality of care. The female supervisees were more likely to evaluate the 'Preconditions of Care' with higher than median scores.

Employment status was related to job satisfaction, strain and assessment of quality. This background variable predicted non-tenured respondents' lower 'Intrinsic Job Satisfaction', and part time workers' higher 'Depersonalization' and low evaluations related to the 'Preconditions of Care'. The non-tenured respondents were more likely to indicate intrinsic job dissatisfaction.

The respondents' speciality was a predictor for 'Depersonalization' and evaluations of quality related to 'Practitioner's Nursing Qualities' and 'Human Centred Activities of Nursing'. The supervisees working in somatic specialities of nursing were more likely to get high scores of depersonalization in comparison to their colleagues representing psychiatric specialities. The respondents working in somatic units had, however, a tendency to evaluate practitioners' nursing qualities and human-centred activities higher compared to colleagues in psychiatric units.

The full rotation working hours predicted respondents' 'Intrinsic-' and 'Total Job Satisfaction' and 'Emotional Exhaustion'. The supervisees working on all shifts were more likely to experience 'Intrinsic Job Dissatisfaction' and 'Total Job Dissatisfaction'. Emotional exhaustion was also more likely among respondents who worked on all shifts in comparison for example to the respondents who were working only on day shifts.

The respondents' work experience was related to levels of burnout and predicted 'Emotional Exhaustion', 'Depersonalization' and evaluations of quality related to 'Practitioner's Nursing Qualities'. The supervisees who had over ten years' work experience were likely to be less exhausted, but likely to get higher than median scores of depersonalization in comparison to less experienced supervisees. The supervisees with long work experience (ten years or more) were quite critical in their evaluations concerning practitioners' nursing qualities. These respondents were more likely to give lower evaluations than the median in comparison to their less experienced colleagues.

Having supervising experience was a significant predictor for 'Extrinsic-', 'Intrinsic-' and 'Total Job Satisfaction' The respondents who did not act as supervisors were more likely to be dissatisfied on extrinsic, intrinsic and some selected overall factors related to work.

Evaluations of CS as predictors for job satisfaction, burnout and quality of care

Supervisees' evaluations of 'Trust and Rapport' towards their supervisors were related to respondents' job satisfaction and quality of care. The respondents who had given high evaluations for trust and rapport in their CS relationship were more likely to score higher than median 'Intrinsic Job Satisfaction', but also likely to give higher than median evaluations concerning the 'Task-Centred Activities of Nursing', more likely to give higher evaluations related to the 'Preconditions of Care' and more likely to assess 'Care Environment' with higher scores than the median.

The evaluations concerning 'Supervisor Advice and Support' were significant predictors for job satisfaction, burnout and quality of care. The respondents who had assessed their supervisors' advice and support as effective were more likely to get higher than median scores for 'Extrinsic Job Satisfaction' and more likely to score higher than median for 'Total Job Satisfaction'. On the other hand, the supervisees who assessed their supervisor's advice and support as effective were also more likely to get higher than median scores for 'Emotional Exhaustion'. The evaluations of 'Supervisor Advice and Support' predicted also such qualities of good nursing care as 'Task-Centred Activities of Nursing' and 'Human-Centred Activities of Nursing'. The supervisees whose supervisor was assessed as effective with advice and support were more likely to evaluate the 'Task-Centred' and 'Human-Centred Activities of Nursing' higher than the median.

The supervisees' evaluations concerning the 'Improved Care and Skills' due to CS predicted respondents' extrinsic job satisfaction. The respondents who evaluated that CS had highly improved care and their skills were, however, more likely to score lower than median for 'Extrinsic Job Satisfaction'.

The assessments concerning 'Importance and Value of CS' focused on predicting the evaluations of quality care. The supervisees who assessed that CS was a very important and valuable part of their work were also more likely to evaluate the 'Pre-conditions of Care' and 'Care Environment' with high scores, and likely to give high scores for 'Promotion of Patient's Coping Strategies'.

The supervisees' evaluations of 'Finding Time for CS' were the predictors for job satisfaction and burnout. The respondents who had had time for CS were more likely to score positively for 'Extrinsic-', 'Intrinsic-' and 'Total Job Satisfaction' and these supervisees were also more likely to get lower scores than the median for 'Depersonalization'.

The 'Total Score for CS' was a significant predictor for the respondents' burnout and assessments related to the quality of care. The total CS evaluation score predicted the respondents' 'Emotional Exhaustion' and 'Personal Accomplishment'. The supervisees who had evaluated their CS as effective were more likely to have higher scores than the median for emotional exhaustion, but more likely to score well for 'Personal Accomplishment'. The high total evaluation score for CS predicted respondents' high evaluations for 'Practitioner's Nursing Qualities', 'Human-Centred Activities of Nursing' and 'Promotion of Patient's Coping Strategies'. The supervisees who evaluated their CS as effective were also more likely to evaluate 'Practitioner's Nursing Qualities', 'Human-Centred Nursing Activities' and 'Promotion of Patient's Coping Strategies' with higher than median scores.

Discussion

Our findings show that there were statistically significant differences among supervisees regarding their experiences and evaluation of CS. These differences support the argument that CS has been naively accepted 'as being good for every nurse and likely to be equally good for every nurse' (see also Bowles and Young 1999).

The most positive CS evaluations were given by specialist nurses working day shifts in tenured positions. In organizations such as psychiatric outpatient clinics, mental health clinics or rehabilitation homes, supervisees gave statistically significantly better evaluations than respondents in university, central or regional hospitals. This may be explained by the history of CS in Finland where psychiatric care has the longest history and most advanced understanding of CS.

Several earlier studies have identified and described the characteristics of a good supervisor (Scanlon and Weir 1997; Spence *et al.* 2002). Characteristics described prior to this study have been mainly personal attributes with no evaluation context or examination from a wider CS intervention perspective (Sloan 1998). Previous research by Butterworth *et al.* (1997) and Cutcliffe and Proctor (1998a, 1998b) emphasized the importance of training for supervisors and supervisees as education and training influence the quality of CS that supervisees receive. In our study, we found characteristics in a supervisor's background, including education and training, and showed that these were statistically significant variables which were related to the best evaluation scores.

Although we have shown that supervisor education and training are related to the efficacy of CS, there also seem to be benefits to combining supervisee and supervisor training (see also Spence *et al.* 2002), including establishing a non-administrative/non-hierarchical relationship. Furthermore, the findings reflect the importance of a supervisee choosing their own supervisor and having regular sessions at least once a month that are not held at the supervisees' workplace. These background variables and infrastructure were statistically significantly related to high evaluation scores indicating the efficacy of CS. Interestingly, these main findings reflect directly the policy of CS recommended by the Finnish Ministry of Social Affairs and Health (Sosiaali- ja terveysministeriö 1983) in the early 1980s (see also Nicklin 1997a, 1997b).

Earlier studies have demonstrated that a variety of approaches and forms of CS are used in hospital organizations (Sosiaali- ja terveysministeriö 1983; Stanton *et al.* 2000). At the time of this study, CS was most commonly provided on a one-to-one basis (Kelly *et al.* 2001; Winstanley 2001). *We found that small group size was associated with more positive evaluations of the efficacy of CS.* Several researchers have considered this as the most effective way to organize CS (Butterworth *et al.* 1997; Nicklin 1997a, 1997b), but contradictory findings have been reported as well. For example, Winstanley (2001) reported that group supervision can be more effective than one-to-one CS because other members of the CS group can offer collective advice and support.

Our study showed that supervisors from other disciplines can be successful supervisors for nursing staff. For example, supervisors who were occupational therapists, physicians and social workers were given high evaluation scores in comparison to the RN supervisors' evaluation scores. However, studies published in international journals have reported differing results concerning supervisors' disciplines. For example, Kelly *et al.* (2001) conducted a survey in Northern Ireland demonstrating that under 50 per cent of respondents agreed with the idea of having supervisors from different disciplines.

We also found that supervisees have quite different experiences, and evaluations vary depending on previous experiences of CS, form and group size, frequency, duration and place of sessions (see also Edwards *et al.* 2005). In our survey, the most critical evaluations were given when supervisees' CS experience was less than one year, and sessions were infrequent and long in duration. Our findings seem to suggest that supervisees learn to use CS best after three to five periods of CS, or after attending sessions for two years (see also Bowles and Young 1999; Hyrkäs *et al.* 2001a). In this study, supervisees' years of work experience were not related to the evaluations. However, Bowles and Young (1999) have reported an inverse correlation between length of service and benefits of CS. Therefore, the findings of this and earlier studies were somewhat contradictory. Such contradictions show that the efficacy of different modes, forms or approaches to CS have not been studied sufficiently (see also Bartle 2000; Edwards *et al.* 2005) and thus more research and systematic evaluation are required.

The aim of the study was to determine if CS evaluations predicted levels of burnout, job satisfaction and perceptions of the quality of care. *The findings did demonstrate that evaluations of CS were predictors for job satisfaction, burnout and assessments of care.* However, this was the first time these questions had been explored, and thus more research is required to better understand the factors that influence the efficacy of clinical supervision.

Conclusions and recommendations

This study showed that the supervisees' evaluations of CS varied significantly in Finland. The scores varied in association with the respondents', and their supervisors', background and also with the infrastructure. These findings demonstrate the importance of systematically evaluating CS in its different forms, modes and organization for different healthcare professionals' groups. This will help to build the knowledge to develop effective CS.

The findings give support to recommendations that it is beneficial to invest resources in CS and offer it to nursing professionals in older age groups with more than ten years of work experience, who work in somatic care, have a diploma type of degree, in non-tenured positions, with part-time work and who work on three shifts. The study showed that effective CS improved these supervisees' levels of job satisfaction, reduced their burnout and stress, and initiated fresh new perceptions related to quality of services and good nursing care. The findings also support the recommendation to make greater investments in supervisor education, and to encourage nursing professionals to start working actively in the supervisor/supervisee roles. This is not merely a function of offering CS, but it is also a factor with positive effects on job satisfaction.

References

Arvidsson, B., Löfgren, H. and Frilund, B. (2000), Psychiatric nurses' conceptions of how group supervision in nursing care influences their professional competencies, *Journal of Nursing Management*, 8(3): 175–185.

Bartle, J. (2000), Clinical supervision: its place within quality agenda, *Nursing Management*, 7(5): 30–33.

Berg, A. and Hallberg, I. (1999), Effects of systematic clinical supervision on psychiatric nurses' sense of coherence, creativity, work related strain, job satisfaction and view of the effects from clinical supervision: a pre-post design, *Journal of Psychiatric and Mental Health Nursing*, 6(5): 317–381.

Berg, A., Welander-Hansson, U. and Hallberg, I. (1994), Nurses' creativity, tedium and burnout during 1 year of clinical supervision and implementation of individually planned nursing care: comparison between a ward for severely demented patients and a similar control ward, *Journal of Advanced Nursing*, 20(4): 742–749.

Bowles, N. and Young, C. (1999), An evaluative study of clinical supervision based on Proctor's three function interactive model, *Journal of Advanced Nursing*, 30(4): 958–964.

Butterworth, T., Carson, J., Jeacock, J., White, E. and Clements, A. (1999), Stress, coping, burnout and job satisfaction in British nurses: findings from the clinical supervision evaluation project, *Stress Medicine*, 15(1): 27–33.

Butterworth, T., Carson, J., White, E., Jeacock, J., Bishop, V. and Clements, A. (1997) *It is Good to Talk: An Evaluation of Clinical Supervision and Mentorship in England and Scotland*, Manchester: University of Manchester.

Cheater, F. and Hale, C. (2001), An evaluation of a local clinical supervision scheme for practice nurses, *Journal of Clinical Nursing*, 10(1): 119–131.

Cutcliffe, J.R. and Proctor, B. (1998a), An alternative training approach to clinical supervision: Part One, *British Journal of Nursing*, 7(5): 280–285.

Cutcliffe, J.R. and Proctor, B. (1998b), An alternative training approach to clinical supervision: Part Two, *British Journal of Nursing*, 7(5): 344–350.

Dudley, M. and Butterworth, T. (1994), The costs and some benefits of clinical supervision: an initial exploration, *International Journal of Psychiatric Nursing Research*, 1(2): 34–40.

Edberg, A-K. (1999), *The nurse-patient encounter and the patient state*, doctoral thesis, Lund, Sweden: The Medical Faculty, University of Lund.

Edberg, A-K., Hallberg, I. and Gustafson, L. (1996), Effects of clinical supervision on the nurse patient co-operation quality, *Clinical Nursing Research*, 5(2): 127–149.

Edwards, D., Cooper, L., Burnard, P., Hannigan, B., Adams, J., Fothergill, A. and Coyle, D. (2005), Factors influencing the effectiveness of clinical supervision, *Journal of Psychiatric and Mental Health Nursing*, 12(4): 405–414.

Fowler, J. and Chevannes, M. (1998), Evaluating the efficacy of reflective practice in the context of clinical supervision, *Journal of Advanced Nursing*, 27(2): 379–382.

Hallberg, I. (1994), Systematic clinical supervision in a child psychiatric ward: satisfaction within nursing care, tedium, burnout and the nurses' own reports on the effects of it, *Archives of Psychiatric Nursing*, 8(1): 44–52.

Hallberg, I., Welander-Hansson, U. and Axelsson, K. (1994), Satisfaction with nursing care and work during a year of clinical supervision and individualized care: comparison between two wards for the care of severely demented patients, *Journal of Nursing Management*, 1(6): 297–307.

Herrmann, N. (1996), Supervisor evaluation: from theory to implementation, *Academic Psychiatry*, 20: 205–211.

Hyrkäs, K. and Munnukka, T. (2002), Kansainvälisen työnohjaustutkimuksen kehityslinjat [Development of clinical supervision research from international perspective], in K. Hyrkäs, T. Munnukka and M. Sorsa (eds), *Työnohjaus hoitotyössä: pysyvä perusta vai turha taakka? [Clinical Supervision in nursing: a solid foundation or an unnecessary burden?]*, Tampere, Finland: Perhekeskeisen hoidon tutkimus- ja opetuskeskus, Julkaisuja 4. Tampereen Yliopistopaino Oy Juvenes Print, pp. 26–41.

Hyrkäs, K. and Paunonen-Ilmonen, M. (2001), The effects of clinical supervision on the quality of care. Examining the results of team supervision and the conceptions of multiprofessional teams, *Journal of Advanced Nursing*, 33(4): 492–502.

Hyrkäs, K., Appelqvist-Schmidlechner, K. and Metsänoja, R. (2006), Efficacy of clinical supervision: influence on job satisfaction, burnout and quality of care, *Journal of Advanced Nursing*, 55(4): 521–532.

Hyrkäs, K., Appleqvist-Schmidlechner, K. and Paunonen-Ilmonen, M. (2001a), Hoitotyöntekijöiden työnohjaus: miten järjestelykäytännöt ovat yhteydessä työnohjauksen onnistumiseen? [Clinical supervision for health care professionals: how are the arrangements associated with its success?], *Hoitotiede [Nursing Science]*, 1: 43–51.

Hyrkäs, K., Koivula, M. and Paunonen, M (1999), Clinical supervision in nursing in the 1990s – current state of concepts, theory and research, *Journal of Nursing Management*, 7(3): 177–187.

Hyrkäs, K., Lehti, K. and Paunonen-Ilmonen, M. (2001b), Cost-benefit analysis of team supervision: the development of an innovative model and its application as a case study, *Journal of Nursing Management*, 9(5): 1–15.

Kelly, B., Long, A. and McKenna, H. (2001), A survey of community mental health nurses' perceptions of clinical supervision in Northern Ireland, *Journal of Psychiatric and Mental Health Nursing*, 8(1): 33–44.

Koelbel, P.W., Fuller, S.G. and Misener, T.R. (1991), Job satisfaction of nurse practitioners: an analysis using Herzberg's theory, *Nurse Practitioner*, 16(4): 43–56.

Lees, C. (1999), Clinical supervision: an initial evaluation, *Journal of Community Nursing*, 13(6): 14–16.

Leino-Kilpi, H. (1990), *Hyvän hoitamisen arviointiperusteet [Assessment basics for good nursing care]*, Lääkintöhallituksen julkaisuja 163, Helsinki: Valtion Paintauskeskus.

Lyth, G. (2000), Clinical supervision: a concept analysis, *Journal of Advanced Nursing*, 31(3): 722–729.

Mahood, N., McFadden, K., Colgan, L. and Gadd, P. (1998), Clinical supervision: the Cartmel NDU experience, *Nursing Standard*, 12(26): 44–47.

Maslach, C. and Jackson, S. (1986), *The Maslach Burnout Inventory*, Palo Alto, CA: Consulting Psychologists Press.

Nicklin, P. (1997a) *Clinical Supervision – Efficient and Effective?* Unpublished final report to research steering group, Hexham General Hospital.

Nicklin, P. (1997b), A practice-centred model of clinical supervision, *Nursing Times* 93(46), 52–54.

Pålsson, M-B., Hallberg, I., Norberg, A. and Björvell, H. (1996), Burnout, empathy and sense of coherence among Swedish district nurses before and after systematic clinical supervision, *Scandinavian Journal of Caring Sciences*, 10(1): 19–26.

Paunonen, M. (1991), Testing a model for counselor supervision in three public health care organizations, *Nurse Education Today*, 11(4): 270–277.

Paunonen, M. and Hyrkäs, K. (2001), Clinical supervision in Finland – history, education, research and theory, in J.R. Cutcliffe, T. Butterworth and B. Proctor (eds), *Fundamental Themes in Clinical Supervision*, London: Routledge, pp. 284–302.

Scanlon, C. and Weir, W. (1997), Learning from practice? Mental health nurses' perceptions and experiences of clinical supervision, *Journal of Advanced Nursing*, 26(2): 295–303.

Schaufeli, W., Enzman, D. and Girault, N. (1993), Measurement of burnout: a review, in W. Schaufeli, C. Maslach and C. Mareck (eds), *Professional Burnout: Recent Developments in Theory and Practice*, Washington, DC: Taylor and Francis.

Segesten, K. (1993), The effects of professional group supervision of nurses: utilizing the nurse self-description form, *Scandinavian Journal of Caring Sciences*, 7(2): 101–104.

Sloan, G. (1998), Focus group interviews: defining clinical supervision, *Nursing Standard*, 12(42): 40–43.

Sosiaali- ja terveysministeriö (1983), *Työnohjaustyöryhmän muistio [Ministry of Social Affairs and Health. Report of the working group of clinical supervision]* Helsinki.

Spence, C., Cantrell, J., Christie, I. and Samet, W. (2002), A collaborative approach to implementation of clinical supervision, *Journal of Nursing Management* 10(2): 65–74.

Stanton, A., Strupish, L., Seaton, A. and Fawcett, K. (2000), Effective clinical supervision, *Nursing Management* 7(2): 12–15.

Teasdale, K., Brocklehurst, N. and Thom, N. (2001), Clinical supervision and support for nurses: an evaluation study, *Journal of Advance Nursing*, 33(2): 216–224.

Weiss, D.J., Davis, R.W., England, G.W. and Lofquist, L.H. (1967), *Manual for the Minnesota Satisfaction Questionnaire*, Minneapolis, MN: University of Minnesota, Industrial Relations Center.

White, E., Butterworth, T., Bishop, V., Carson, J., Jeacock, J. and Clements, A. (1998), Clinical supervision: insider reports of a private world, *Journal of Advanced Nursing*, 28(1): 85–192.

Winstanley, J. (2000), Manchester clinical supervision scale, *Nursing Standard*, 14(19): 31–32.

Winstanley, J. (2001), Developing methods for evaluating clinical supervision, in J.R. Cutcliffe, T. Butterworth and B. Proctor (eds), *Fundamental Themes in Clinical Supervision*, London: Routledge, pp. 210–224.

24 Multidisciplinary attitudinal positions regarding clinical supervision

A cross-sectional study

John R. Cutcliffe and Kristiina Hyrkäs

An issue that remains underexamined is that of multidisciplinary attitudes towards/ about clinical supervision (CS); as a result this chapter focuses on a study that attempted to bridge some of this knowledge gap. After describing the research design, sample composition and the approach used to analyse the statistical data, the chapter includes detailed results. Following this, the authors discuss the findings and focus in particular on the two most conspicuous findings: the respondents' agreement concerning the importance of confidentiality in clinical supervision and the almost total agreement amongst the respondents concerning the clear separation between clinical supervision and managerial supervision.

The apparent importance of having a clinical supervisory relationship that remains separate from administrative/managerial supervision and one where confidentiality is assured has once more been highlighted by empirical study. Furthermore, these attitudes are not restricted to one professional or disciplinary group. In times which have been described as being epitomised by uncertainty, low morale, high stress, high rates of burnout (and the ever closer pending mass exodus of much of the nursing workforce as the 'baby-boom' demographic starts to retire), one could even make the case that the need for CS is greater. It is the editors' strongly held view, then, that the effective support system of CS should therefore not be 'watered-down' by awkward and unnecessary amalgamations with administrative/managerial supervision (AM/S).

Introduction

While attention to clinical supervision (CS) within academic nursing literature may have passed beyond its zenith[1] examination of the extant literature reveals that CS is very much still a matter of high interest for nurses, nurse researchers, nurse educationalists and nurse managers. The visible decline in the number of papers notwithstanding, a closer inspection of the extant literature shows a number of interesting things. First, the papers that continue to be published appear to add something new, meaningful and/or significant to the literature.[2] Second, while it might be said that some of the earlier published work could have delved a little deeper into the substantive issues, the more recent published work appears to do just that.

As with any longitudinal, evolutionary, cumulative approach to knowledge generation, the existence of earlier work by no means serves to suggest that there is nothing new worth saying; what this actually means is that we have more questions now than perhaps we did before (Toulmin 1967; Popper 1972). A further outcome of interrogating the extant literature is that of the discovery of gaps in our knowledge base. Accordingly, it is perhaps worthy of note that some existing questions do not appear to have been fully debated or resolved and others have yet to be asked. As a result, this chapter hopes to make a small contribution to the extant CS literature by focusing on one issue that remains underexamined – that of clinical supervision within a multidisciplinary context.

Literature review: studying attitudes towards clinical supervision

The extant social psychology literature is replete with studies purporting to examine attitudes, to the extent that authors describe attitudes as social psychology's most central concept (see, for example, Atkinson *et al.* 2002). Not surprisingly given the theoretical and conceptual congruence with social psychology and nursing, studies of attitude in nurses and nursing are common (Alfredson and Annerstedt 1994; Anderson 1997; Samuelsson *et al.* 1997). This is despite that fact that attitude remains an elusive and ill-defined concept and the study of attitude is methodologically problematic. A number of authors, researchers and theoreticians have drawn attention to problems in measuring attitude and highlight three confounding variables: context, variability and constitution. Context can easily be lost in typical attitudinal scales where brief unitary responses to predetermined questions are required (Potter and Wetherell 1988). Variability is manifest wherein people will say different things at different times; and the constitution of attitudes is itself a matter of debate (McGuire 1985; Potter 2005). There is consensus that attitudes clearly involve some form of internal evaluation; though how additional factors such as moral obligation, personal choice, mood, emotion and personality affect these evaluations is unclear. Despite methodological difficulties, potentially illuminating findings can still be obtained by attempting to determine some aspect(s) of attitude towards certain phenomena, though it would be prudent to view these findings with a degree of caution. Accordingly, though beset with epistemological and methodological problems, studies of attitudes towards CS (or aspects of CS) would still appear to have the potential to expand or deepen our understanding. There may be particular utility in undertaking such endeavours before one attempts to introduce CS into practice and as a means to further our understanding of any associated resistance to CS. Indeed for some, such is the importance of attitudes in the context of CS that any attempt to introduce it into practice is prefaced by the need to examine prevailing attitudes (Hancox *et al.* 2004). The same authors continue:

> unless nurses were receptive to the idea of receiving supervision and viewed the (introduction) strategy positively, it would be unlikely that the widespread introduction of supervision would take place.
>
> (Hancox *et al.* 2004: 199)

Accordingly, a review of the recent literature that focuses on CS and attitudes in nurses(ing) is in order.

In a small scale qualitative study that followed the introduction of CS nine months previously, Malin (2000) used direct observation of supervision sessions, critical incident questionnaires and semi-structured interviews in order to evaluate CS in practitioners working in community homes with adults with learning disabilities. The findings that speak to attitudes indicated that practitioners felt CS was a positive experience overall, but one that perhaps was accompanied by a sense of confusion; particularly around the formative/restorative and normative confluence. It is maybe noteworthy that the research participants also highlighted the need for CS to be non-hierarchical. Landmark *et al.* (2003) attempted to determine the factors (including attitudes), thought by nurses to be influential upon the development of competence and skill in CS. Using a qualitative method[3] they collected data by means of three focus groups consisting of nurses from two local hospitals. Data were analysed according to Kvale's (1996) approach to qualitative data analysis. Three principal themes (factors) were described, namely: didactics, role functions and organisational framework. Interestingly, and in keeping with previous published work (see Earnshaw 1995; Wilson-Barnett *et al.* 1995; Andrews and Wallis 1999) their findings suggest that the success (or otherwise) of CS is dependent upon the organisational framework used and, moreover, the particular organisation's ability to create a supportive framework or infrastructure for CS. Hyrkäs and colleagues (2005) reported findings from a study of front-line managers' views of the long term effects of CS. Data were collected in the form of narrative responses or 'empathy-based stories' (Hyrkäs *et al.* 2005: 213). These data were then subjected to a qualitative, thematic analysis and this produced seven 'themes' where the respondents felt unequivocally that CS had a long-term positive effect on their practice and self-development. It may be worthy of note that all the respondents in this student engaged in 'peer-CS' not hierarchical CS.

Teasdale *et al.* (2001) describe a mixed methods study which attempted to evaluate (or assess the effects) of CS within a region of the United Kingdom. The authors claim they accessed a sample of 211 registered nurse participants, who completed two instruments/questionnaires and 146 completed critical incident forms, which appear to have served as the qualitative data and indicate the sample size. The paper appears to contain evidence of methodological slippage, e.g. there is no theory induced from what claims to be, at least in part, a grounded theory study; neither is there any evidence of the constant comparative approach to data collection/analysis (see Glaser 1992, 1998). It is interesting to note that where the respondents could choose their own supervisor, the majority (78 per cent) elected not to have a line manager act as a supervisor; whereas where the supervisees were afforded no choice, then 63 per cent of line managers predominated also as supervisors. However, the authors report some quantitative data that suggested supervisees reported higher (more positive) factor scores when their supervisor was also their manager. The authors, quite rightly, include a cautionary caveat noting that these findings were produced using a hitherto untested instrument.

In summary, as with many other aspects of CS literature, there exist only a small number of studies that focus on attitudes towards CS and even fewer that have examined attitudes towards certain forms or aspects of CS. Significant gaps remain in the extant literature. There is a noticeable absence of quantitative studies and according to the search undertaken by the authors of this paper, nothing at all that has examined attitudes towards CS from a multidisciplinary perspective. As a result, the following study was undertaken in an attempt to begin to bridge that gap.

Methods and research design

Data was collected using a questionnaire-type form (see Box 24.1). The form was composed of seventeen (17) statements. The respondents were asked to rank-order the statements starting from one for the most important statement, two for the next most important up to 17. In order to do so, the respondents were asked to consider the characteristics of a CS group that represented the type of CS they would wish to engage in. In ranking these elements, particular attitudes towards CS would become more apparent. The respondents were informed that there were no 'right or wrong' answers; that they should answer according to what they felt/thought/believed was important for the organisation/delivery of CS and what was not.

The total number of respondents was 74 (see Figure 24.1). The sample was composed of eight different professional groups:

1. Registered Nurses – hospital-based (RNs) (n=12)
2. Chiropodists (n=7)
3. Occupational Therapists (n=7)
4. Learning Disability Nurses (n=10)
5. Registered General Nurses – community-based (n=15)
6. Registered Psychiatric/Mental Health Nurses (n=14)
7. Health Visitors (n=4)
8. Physiotherapists (n=5).

Box 24.1 Group Supervision Ranking Form

Your task is to rank the following statements that you believe should describe the characteristics of a supervision group. To do this place a (1) alongside the most important statement and a (2) along the next most important until all the statements are ranked in order of importance from (1) to (17). There are no right or wrong answers; you should answer according to what you feel/think/believe is important for the organisation/delivery of CS and what is not.

1. Time should be allowed to facilitate personal issues if they emerge.   ....
2. Supervisor and supervisees should share the same theoretical orientation.   ....
3. Supervision groups should be of a closed membership.   ....
4. Each member has the opportunity to facilitate supervision.   ....
5. Members freely express negative feelings.   ....
6. The facilitator directs the focus of the group.   ....
7. Members feelings are considered during supervision.   ....
8. Time is allocated for each member by the supervisor.   ....
9. Members provide support for each other.   ....
10. Members should challenge each other's practice.   ....
11. Confidentiality is assured and agreed.   ....
12. A written contract for supervision is completed.   ....
13. The goals of supervision are explicitly formulated.   ....
14. Supervisees should be of roughly equal experience and status.   ....
15. The supervisor should be an expert practitioner.   ....
16. Supervision notes should be maintained by the supervisor.   ....
17. The supervisor should be a manager.   ....

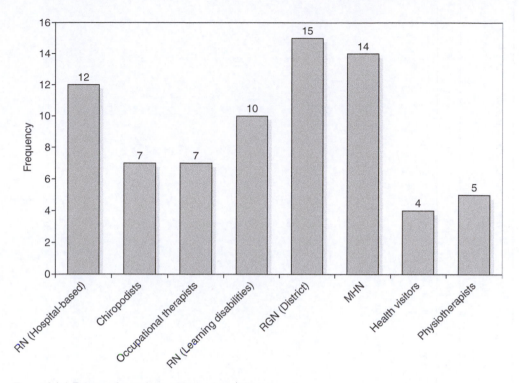

Figure 24.1 Respondents/supervisees (n = 74).

The data was collected in different occasions during the years 1999–2001. Each of the study participants had undertaken a four-day CS training/education course over eight weeks that was offered under the auspices of Sheffield University. Participation in the research was entirely voluntary and the data collected was anonymous as no names were used. The only identifying information was the particular discipline of the participant. As the data collection occurred after the conclusion of the course, no participant would have experienced a sense of coercion: a sense of fear of not answering the way the course instructor expected them to.

Data were analysed by descriptive and non-parametric statistics. The statistical package used for data analysis was SPSS (Windows Release 14.0, SPSS Inc. Chicago IL, USA). Data were entered in the database coding the highest ranked item as one, the second highest ranked item as two up to 17 as the lowest ranked item. Some respondents had given the same rankings for a few items/characteristics and these rankings were entered unaltered in the database. The material was presented as counts, modes, and percentages. The data were analysed first at group level and after that differenced between the groups were studied using non-parametric tests.

Findings

The respondents' agreement was high concerning the rankings of the item (11) *'Confidentiality is assured and agreed'*. Almost all respondents ranked this item as the most important characteristic for group CS (mode = 1). An interesting finding, on

Table 24.1 Mode values of the ranks concerning the characteristics of clinical supervision

Mode-values	RNs hospital-based	Chiropodists	Occupational therapists	RN learning disabilities	RGN district community-based	MHN community	Health visitors	Physiotherapist	Mode all respondents
	Mo	Mo	Mo	Mo	Mo	Mo	Mo	Mo	Mo
1. Time should be allowed to facilitate personal issues if they emerge.	6 [a]	8	8	3 [a]	12	12	3 [a]	10	8
2. Supervisor and supervisees should share the same theoretical orientation.	14	14	12 [a]	13	11 [a]	11	13	9 [a]	14
3. Supervision groups should be of a closed membership.	7 [a]	7 [a]	7 [a]	8 [a]	13	7 [a]	13	1 [a]	13
4. Each member has the opportunity to facilitate supervision.	8	10	8	8 [a]	6	8 [a]	4 [a]	4 [a]	10
5. Members freely express negative feelings.	6	6	6	5 [a]	7	6	3 [a]	4 [a]	6
6. The facilitator directs the focus of the group.	7	9 [a]	11	10	6	9	12	6 [a]	6
7. Members' feelings are considered during supervision.	5	4	9	4	8	4	2 [a]	2 [a]	4
8. Time is allocated for each member by the supervisor.	3	5 [a]	3	2	4	3	6	8	3

9. Members provide support for each other.	4	4	4	3	4[a]	4[a]	4[a]	5	4
10. Members should challenge each other's practice.	11[a]	15	13	5[a]	14	12	4[a]	5[a]	15
11. Confidentiality is assured and agreed.	1	1	1	1	1	1	1[a]	1	1
12. A written contract for supervision is completed.	12	2	2[a]	1	2	2	2	2	2
13. The goals of supervision are explicitly formulated.	2[a]	3	2[a]	7[a]	3	2[a]	1[a]	3	3
14. Supervisees should be of roughly equal experience and status.	8[a]	11	13[a]	11	15	14	15	16	11[a]
15. The supervisor should be an expert practitioner.	15	13	15[a]	15[a]	16	16	16	14	16
16. Supervision notes should be maintained by the supervisor.	16	16	16	16	16	16	11	15	16
17. The supervisor should be a manager.	17	17	17	17	17	17	16[a]	17	17
Number of respondents	12	7	7	10	15	14	4	5	74

Note

a Multiple modes exist. The smallest value is shown.

the other hand, was that the respondents shared almost a total agreement concerning the item (17) *'The supervisor should be a manager'.* This was ranked as the least important characteristic for group CS (mode = 17). The variation of modes between the respondents' rankings was also quite low in the item of (7) *'Members feelings are considered during supervision'.* The respondents shared quite high agreement concerning this item and among all respondents the item was ranked the fourth important (mode = 4) characteristic of group CS (Table 24.1).

We also calculated the agreement percentages concerning the rankings of the items within the groups and among all supervisees who participated in the study. We considered that the agreement of the rankings was excellent if there was a total 100 per cent or greater than or equal to 80 per cent, good for 60–79 per cent, moderate for 40–59 per cent, fair for 20–39 per cent, and poor if the agreement was 19 per cent or under. In this study, the agreement percentage was excellent for the majority of the items among all respondents and good for items (6) *'The facilitator directs the focus of the group'* (74.64 per cent), (10) *'Members should challenge each other's practice'* (73.84 per cent), (12) *'A written contract for supervision is completed'* (74.32 per cent), and (13) *'The goals of supervision are explicitly formulated'* (76.95 per cent). We found a moderate agreement only in the group of health visitors concerning the item (10) *'Members should challenge each other's practice'* (42.64 per cent). See Table 24.2.

Significant differences were found between the groups concerning the respondents' rankings of (14) *'Supervisees should be roughly equal experience and status'* and (17) *'The supervisor should be a manager'.* The group of hospital-based nurses ranked the supervisee's experience and status of highest importance compared to the other group of the study (p = .021). The health visitors, on the other hand ranked this characteristic lowest among the eight professional groups, but manager's role as supervisor highest compared to all other groups (p = .001). See Table 24.3.

Discussion

Examination of the findings shows two immediately clear and significant findings: 1) the vast majority of participants in this study (always more than 90 per cent), and across all the various disciplines and specialties, held the attitude that *their supervisor should not also be their manager.* 2) Similarly, the vast majority of participants in this study (always more than 90 per cent), and across all the various disciplines and specialties, held the attitude that *confidentiality is assured and agreed.* It may be significant to note that the health visitors' highest ranking of the manager's role as a possible supervisor (when compared to the other disciplinary groups) is likely to be related to their different conceptualization of CS; one that encapsulates direct responses to child protection laws. Even so, the health visitors still ranked the statement relating to supervisors as managers as the least important for them, perhaps indicating that their highly important normative function vis-à-vis child protection can still be carried out if their supervisor is not also their manager. Far from being detached or incongruous with one another, these issues of the requirement for confidentiality and not having one's manager as one's supervisor are inextricably linked together. These issues will thus form the basis for our discussion.

For those readers who are familiar with the extant CS literature, the issue of managers also acting as supervisors and the resultant conflicts and confusion that this

Table 24.2 Agreement percentages concerning the rankings of the items within the groups and among all supervisees

	RNs hospital-based	Chiropodists	Occupational therapists	RN learning disabilities	RGN District Community-based	MHN community	Health visitors	Physiotherapist	All respondents
Agreement percentage									
1. Time should be allowed to facilitate personal issues if they emerge.	78.43	98.00	89.92	70.00	76.47	76.05	67.64	95.29	84.58
2. Supervisor and supervisees should share the same theoretical orientation.	89.71	97.50	90.76	80.59	83.53	85.29	95.59	77.65	85.61
3. Supervision groups should be of a closed membership.	88.23	89.90	68.90	84.12	88.63	74.79	85.29	52.94	82.11
4. Each member has the opportunity to facilitate supervision.	93.12	94.95	85.71	85.29	79.61	84.87	75.00	75.29	86.65
5. Members freely express negative feelings.	85.29	92.44	94.12	86.47	93.33	93.28	86.76	75.29	89.59
6. The facilitator directs the focus of the group.	81.86	90.77	90.76	83.53	74.12	82.35	85.29	67.06	74.64
7. Members' feelings are considered during supervision.	88.24	95.80	87.39	91.76	71.76	91.18	79.41	80.00	89.11
8. Time is allocated for each member by the supervisor.	78.90	82.35	80.67	86.47	86.67	86.55	95.59&	87.06	82.75
9. Members provide support for each other.	91.18	96.60	94.12	92.35	94.12	91.60	80.89	88.23	91.81
10. Members should challenge each other's practice.	81.37	78.99	87.39	70.59	77.65	85.71	42.64	67.06	73.84
11. Confidentiality is assured and agreed.	92.60	97.48	95.80	92.94	97.65	93.70	76.47	92.94	93.64
12. A written contract for supervision is completed.	76.96	77.31	88.23	71.18	72.55	75.63	82.35	74.12	74.32
13. The goals of supervision are explicitly formulated.	73.00	81.51	89.92	77.06	73.73	77.73	71.43	87.06	76.95
14. Supervisees should be of roughly equal experience and status.	82.35	94.96	89.08	82.35	90.20	90.34	95.59	78.82	84.82
15. The supervisor should be an expert practitioner.	85.78	95.80	94.96	91.76	79.22	86.97	83.82	81.18	84.18
16. Supervision notes should be maintained by the supervisor.	80.89	99.16	84.03	91.18	80.78	88.66	94.12	75.29	84.26
17. The supervisor should be a manager.	100.0	100.0	100.0	99.41	100.0	100.0	97.06	95.29	99.44

Table 24.3 Comparison of the mean ranks concerning the characteristics of clinical supervision

	RNs hospital-based	Chiropodists	Occupational therapists	RN learning Disabilities	RGN district community-based	MHN community	Health visitors	Physiotherapist	Kruskall-Wallis	df	p-value
	Mean Rank	Mean Rank	Mean Rank	Mean Rank	Mean Rank	Mean Rank	Mean Rank	Mean Rank			
1. Time should be allowed to facilitate personal issues if they emerge.	39.00	32.86	39.43	34.50	35.57	37.29	41.13	47.20	1.916	7	.964
2. Supervisor and supervisees should share the same theoretical orientation.	42.54	57.21	38.71	27.15	30.37	38.14	32.25	40.60	11.120	7	.133
3. Supervision groups should be of a closed membership.	38.75	22.14	46.68	33.90	43.30	39.21	34.38	30.40	7.141	7	.414
4. Each member has the opportunity to facilitate supervision.	37.29	40.29	32.79	38.65	39.30	38.89	33.00	32.70	1.096	7	.993
5. Members freely express negative feelings.	45.00	36.57	25.79	36.00	42.33	36.21	19.13	44.00	8.034	7	.303
6. The facilitator directs the focus of the group.	32.75	34.14	36.64	44.80	39.33	33.64	34.38	48.00	3.798	7	.803
7. Members' feelings are considered during supervision.	28.79	29.57	55.71	33.90	39.47	37.29	43.75	40.90	9.029	7	.251
8. Time is allocated for each member by the supervisor.	35.96	36.21	45.29	34.70	36.50	34.54	46.00	42.20	2.375	7	.936
9. Members provide support for each other.	31.46	39.43	30.21	33.20	40.27	35.54	38.63	64.40	10.788	7	.148
10. Members should challenge each other's practice.	31.85	45.07	42.39	33.85	35.30	40.54	38.88	38.70	2.916	7	.893
11. Confidentiality is assured and agreed.	43.46	30.43	35.00	38.50	31.60	36.11	50.88	45.50	7.204	7	.408
12. A written contract for supervision is completed.	50.04	36.00	26.14	35.50	37.83	37.43	25.88	37.90	7.546	7	.374
13. The goals of supervision are explicitly formulated.	37.38	35.71	21.86	53.35	41.23	35.43	32.75	28.90	10.935	7	.141
14. Supervisees should be of roughly equal experience and status.	25.46	29.07	42.00	26.95	46.43	38.89	63.13	41.80	16.431	7	.021
15. The supervisor should be an expert practitioner.	32.25	28.21	49.86	47.20	32.70	39.61	44.50	29.50	8.677	7	.277
16. Supervision notes should be maintained by the supervisor.	33.96	55.64	35.29	42.60	36.37	38.86	14.13	31.80	11.694	7	.102
17. The supervisor should be a manager.	40.00	40.00	40.00	36.40	40.00	40.00	22.00	24.60	24.549	7	.001

can (and does) create, will be neither new nor surprising. This confusion is well documented in the literature (see White 1996; Butterworth *et al.* 1997; Cutcliffe and Proctor 1998a, 1998b; Deery 1999; Yegdich 1999; Cutcliffe 2003; Hyrkäs *et al.* 2005, 2006). Yet, no such confusion or conflation with administrative/managerial supervision (AM/S) was ever intended in the original conceptualizations and justifications for CS. Such conceptualizations are clearly evident if one examines the historical inception of CS in the United States, or during more contemporary history in the United Kingdom, or indeed, in Scandinavian countries during the 1960s. In the United States in the 1920 and 1930s, CS was predicated as being a democratic process concerned with professional growth, was to occur in a wholesome atmosphere of partnership, permissiveness and support, had no authoritarian overtures or undercurrents and was in no way conflated with, or wrapped up by, AM/S (see Yegdich 1999 for a comprehensive review on this matter.) In the United Kingdom, along with other pioneers, Butterworth and Faugier (1992) were clear in asserting that CS was principally concerned with supporting the nurse–patient relationship. More vehemently, when introducing CS, the Scandinavian countries stated unequivocally that having line managers also acting as clinical supervisors was considered complex and difficult due to possible role conflicts and thus was not introduced this way (Paunonen and Hyrkäs 2001).

In addition to these conceptualizations that were prevalent during the introduction of CS into nursing, contemporary policy, at least in parts of Europe, echoes these views. The United Kingdom Central Council's position (2006) could not be clearer about the delineation between CS and AM/S. In response to the rhetorical question, 'What is clinical supervision?' it states,

1. Clinical supervision is not a managerial control system. It is not, therefore:
12.1 the exercise of overt managerial responsibility or managerial supervision;
12.2 a system of formal individual performance review; or
12.3 hierarchical in nature.

Similarly, in Finland, having managers, first-line managers or head nurses acting as clinical supervisors with their subordinates would be in direct contradiction of the recommendations of the Ministry of Health and Social Services. In light of these original conceptualizations and recent policy statements, in some ways, then, the two principle significant findings from this study should have been expected. What was somewhat surprising to the researchers however, was the degree of consensus across very different disciplines in addition to the depth or strength of feeling regarding having managers also acting as one's clinical supervisor. Yet the authors of this paper confess to experiencing some surprise because, despite the very well documented case for ensuring CS does not become conflated with AM/S, it is our experience, and there are examples in the literature, that often CS *is* arranged in a hierarchical, top-down or pyramidal way with managers also acting as CS for the staff they manage, resulting in the most obvious conflation of CS and AM/S (see Wolsey and Leach 1997; Teasdale *et al.* 2000; Kelly *et al.* 2001; Barriball *et al.* 2004). Even the most cursory examination of the current literature will show that there are examples of conflation of CS with AM/S and there are those who advocate for such a model within nursing (see Teasdale *et al.* 2001). As Malin (2000) eloquently points out, CS now (somehow) inevitably includes activities to, and to phrase this simplistically, serve the needs of the organization (and the managers) and activities to serve the needs/desires of the nursing workforce. It is unclear exactly how this conflation of CS with AM/S became so, but there appears to be little doubt in the extant literature that such developments were/are linked to:

a   an increased concern in health care policy and subsequent practice around the notions of safeguarding the patient (and public), quality of care, professional accountability (i.e. *normative issues)* and furthermore,

b   (not least) as a means to 'prevent' further nursing 'disasters' such as those indicated in the Allitt inquiry (Clothier *et al.* 1994; Yegdich 1999).

Now, the authors need to be clear about this point and that is that there are obvious links between CS and AM/S; and that these links exist on a number of levels. The UKCC's (now NMC's) position (2006) statement also makes this point stating:

> Links between clinical supervision and management are important. These links are best described in the local policy and ground rules. Management will wish to evaluate the impact of clinical supervision and its service benefits. Development and establishment of clinical supervision should, therefore, involve managers and practitioners with the emphasis on a 'light touch' management influence.

Thus managers are involved in supporting, evaluating, and facilitating CS. There are also links around the desired increase in professional accountability. So there is clear utility in maintaining a close link between CS and AM/S. Captivatingly, advocating for the continued separation of CS from AM/S supervision does not mean and has never meant the demise of AM/S and with it the various processes for assuring professional accountability. Nowhere, to the best of our knowledge, has any CS advocate suggested that such processes of accountability are not necessary. To the best of our knowledge no CS advocate has ever argued for the abandonment of AM/S. Yegdich (1999) constructs a similar argument when she points out that CS neither substitutes nor supersedes the need for nursing to continue to develop and produce normative standards. However, as the findings in this study appear to indicate, as indeed the body of existing literature does (see for example Yegdich 1999; Kelly *et al.* 2001; Epling and Cassedy 2001) combining CS with AM/S inevitably severely diminishes the more democratic, emancipatory, supportive and developmental aspects of CS. The first author summarized the documented and anecdotal difficulties that arise from conflating CS and AM/S into the same process and when provided by the same person. Cutcliffe (2003: 140) highlighted that:

- [T]here is a tendency for those in senior roles to focus on performance and action rather than exploring the subtleties of process;
- There is the potential for material offered during supervision to be used in a disciplinary manner;
- There is the tendency to focus on management (normative) issues as the major agenda;
- And there is a confusion caused by the duality of supervisory and managerial roles.

Accordingly, these arguments need to be considered in the context of the fact that there already exist mechanisms for surveillance and professional accountability in nursing, yet there are few enough existing opportunities for personal/practice development in an entirely safe, yet challenging and supportive, yet stimulating interpersonal environment.

What may be worthy of particular note is that, to the best of the knowledge of the authors, no one has yet produced a robust argument for why this should be the case, why CS *should* be amalgamated with AM/S? There have been theoretically based arguments, such as Wolsey and Leach's (1997) view that CS should adopt 'business in health care' as a means to improve the normative outcomes. Some audit literature speaks to how having a manager/clinical supervisor would be mean that this person serving in the dual role would be well placed to deal with some of the issues that might arise in clinical supervision and/or would have an increased understanding of the roles and responsibilities of the supervisee (see Barriball *et al.* 2004). For example, a supervisee discovers through reflection in CS that he/she would benefit from in-service training regarding a specific practice, or that he/she would like to gain more experience of a certain clinical practice. Thus the manager could theoretically help facilitate such activities. This argument has a certain degree of intuitive logic to it but, in and of itself, cannot be seen to represent a robust argument. Indeed, there is nothing to prevent a clinical supervisee from gaining a new awareness of an issue in CS and then taking this to the manager. There is also the (we believe mistaken) argument that a manager would wish to know about any errors that are occurring on his/her unit and that such errors might become known through supervisee disclosures in CS. Interestingly, there is a dearth of empirical evidence to support this position, and an argument can be made that opposite is more accurate, namely that supervisees are less willing to share information during CS on any errors they have made if they know that the manager is duty bound to report such incidents. This dynamic was evident in the findings in this study whereby the vast majority wished to have a supervisory situation where confidentiality is guaranteed.

Lastly, the findings in this study perhaps contribute to the evidence base for CS and this in turn casts further doubt on blending CS with AM/S. If the accumulating evidence continues to show that the significant majority (in this study over 90 per cent) of supervisees do not want their managers to act as their supervisors, in part because of fears around confidentiality, then would managers as supervisors be an evidenced-based practice? In face of the extant evidence, in all its various forms, it would be a difficult argument to make.

Limitations of the study

In this study 74 supervisees returned the completed form and the respondents represented eight different professional groups. It is possible to assume that the sample represents well the multi-professional supervisee population attending the CS training in UK. The respondents registered for this course on a voluntary basis; they were interested in learning more about CS, and their attitudes were probably positive concerning CS. Since the findings of this study are based on a convenience sample, what remains unknown are the attitudes of those professionals in health care organizations who did not enroll and attend the CS courses.

The data for this study was collected by the first author and instructor of the CS course, and thus it is important to assess whether this has affected the supervisees' attitudes and responses. Specific efforts were taken to minimize the influence of the instructor. The respondents were informed of the voluntary nature of the study and no demographic or respondent specific identifiers were collected. Earlier studies have shown that CS seems to increase supervisees' critical thinking and reflection (Paunonen-Ilmonen 2001), and thus it is possible to claim that it is difficult to influence supervisees' attitudes, rather, they create their own opinions.

The problem of studies trying to describe attitudes is that opinions as well as attitudes change over time. This was cross-sectional study by its design and the data was collected at the end of CS course. It would have been interesting to complete a follow-up survey after the supervisees had returned to their organizations and study how strong and sustainable the attitudes are. Longitudinal study design, on the other hand, would have been difficult to arrange and impossible without registration and identification of the respondents (see also Arvidsson *et al.* 2000, 2001).

Conclusion

The apparent importance of having a clinical supervisory relationship that remains separate from AM/S and one where confidentiality is assured has once more been highlighted by empirical study. Furthermore, these attitudes are not restricted to one professional or disciplinary group. While the authors of this paper have no wish to contradict their own previously documented views pertaining to the value in not forcing one model or approach of CS upon all practitioners, we wish to add a caveat to these earlier statements and that concerns the parameters of CS. CS is a discrete form of practice and, as such, has its own conceptual boundaries. Even allowing for the fluidity of such boundaries (and the fluid nature of concepts themselves notwithstanding – see Wittgenstein 1968; Rodgers 1989) historical and current conceptualizations and policy statements clearly indicate that CS is not AM/S; neither should these two similarly valuable concepts be conflated.

The need for a process and/or mechanism of support and development for the variety of disciplines involved in providing twenty-first century health care is as evident today as it was when CS was first touted as an idea. In times which, according to Yegdich (1999) are epitomized by uncertainty, low morale, high stress, high rates of burnout (and the ever-closer pending mass exodus of much of the nursing workforce as the 'baby-boom' demographic starts to retire), one could even make the case that the need for CS is greater. The effective support system of CS should therefore not be watered-down by awkward and unnecessary amalgamations with AM/S.

Notes

1 Arguably this occurred during the 1990s.
2 And it would be inaccurate to assert this of the papers produced during the 1990s when there was a great deal of repetition.
3 Though the authors do not state which type of qualitative method.

References

Alfredson, B.B. and Annerstedt, L. (1994), Staff attitudes and job satisfaction in the care of demented elderly people: group living compared to long term care, *Journal of Advanced Nursing*, 20(5): 964–974.

Anderson, M. (1997), Nurses' attitudes towards suicidal behaviour: a comparative study of community mental health nurses and nurses working in accident and emergency departments, *Journal of Advanced Nursing*, 25(6): 1283–1291.

Andrews, M. and Wallis, M. (1999), Mentorship in nursing: a literature review, *Journal of Advanced Nursing*, 29(1): 2001–2007.

Arvidsson, B., Löfgren, H. and Fridlund, B. (2000), Psychiatric nurses' conceptions of how group supervision in nursing care influences their professional competence, *Journal of Nursing Management*, 8(3): 175–185.

Arvidsson, B., Löfgren, H. and Fridlund, B. (2001), Psychiatric nurses' conceptions of how group supervision program in nursing care influences their professional competence: a four year follow-up study, *Journal of Nursing Management*, 9(3): 161–171.

Atkinson, R.L., Atkinson, R.C., Smith, E. and Hilgard, E. (2002), *Introduction to Psychology*, New York: HBJ.

Barriball, L., While, A. and Much, U. (2004), An audit of clinical supervision in primary care, *British Journal of Community Nursing*, 9(9): 390–396.

Butterworth, T. and Faugier, J. (1992), *Clinical Supervision and Mentoring in Nursing*, London: Chapman & Hall.

Butterworth, T., Carson, J., White, E. *et al.* (1997), *It is Good to Talk. An Evaluation of Clinical Supervision and Mentorship in England and Scotland*, Manchester: The School of Nursing Studies, University of Manchester.

Clothier, C., MacDonald, C.A. and Shaw, D.A. (1994), *The Allitt Inquiry: independent inquiry relating to the deaths and injuries on the children's ward at Grantham and Kevestan General Hospital during the period February to April 1991*, London: HMSO.

Cutcliffe, J.R. (2003), Clinical supervision and reflective practice: symbient and integral aspects of the role of community psychiatric nurses, in B. Hannigan, M. Coffey and P. Burnard (eds), *A Handbook of Community Mental Health Nursing*, London: Routledge, pp. 132–144.

Cutcliffe, J.R. and Proctor, B. (1998a), An alternative training approach in clinical supervision: Part One, *British Journal of Nursing*, 7(5): 280–285.

Cutcliffe, J.R. and Proctor, B. (1998b), An alternative training approach in clinical supervision: Part Two, *British Journal of Nursing*, 7(6): 344–350.

Deery, R. (1999), Professional issues: improving relationships through clinical supervision: Part Two, *British Journal of Midwifery*, 7(4): 251–254.

Earnshaw, G.J. (1995), Mentorship: the students' views, *Nursing Education Today*, 15(4): 274–279.

Epling, M. and Cassedy, P. (2001), Visions from the classroom, in J.R. Cutcliffe, T. Butterworth and B. Proctor (eds), *Fundamental Themes in Clinical Supervision*, London: Routledge, pp. 64–83.

Glaser, B.G. (1992), *Basics of Grounded Theory Analysis: Emerging versus Forcing*, Mill Valley, CA: Sociology Press.

Glaser, B.G. (1998), *Doing Grounded Theory: Issues and Discussions*, Mill Valley, CA: Sociology Press.

Hancox, K., Lynch, L., Happel, B. and Biondo, S. (2004), An evaluation of an educational program for clinical supervision, *International Journal of Mental Health Nursing*, 13(3): 198–203.

Hyrkäs, K., Appleqvist-Schmidlechner, K. and Kivimäki, K. (2005), First-line managers' views of the long-term effects of clinical supervision: how does clinical supervision support and develop leadership in health care? *Journal of Nursing Management*, 13(3): 209–220.

Hyrkäs, K., Appelqvist-Schmidlechner, K. and Metsänoja, R. (2006), Efficacy of clinical supervision: influence on job satisfaction, burnout and quality of care, *Journal of Advanced Nursing*, 55(4): 521–535.

Kelly, B., Long, A. and McKenna, H.P. (2001), A survey of community mental health nurses' perceptions of clinical supervision in Northern Ireland, *Journal of Psychiatric and Mental Health Nursing*, 8(1): 33–44.

Kvale, S. (1996), *Interviews – An Introduction to Qualitative Research Interviewing*, Thousand Oaks, CA: Sage.

Landmark, B.T.H., Hansen, G.S., Bjones, I. and Bohler, A. (2003), Clinical supervision – factors defined by nurses as influential upon the development of competence and skills in supervision, *Journal of Clinical Nursing*, 12(6): 834–841.

McGuire, W.J. (1985), Attitudes and attitude change, in G. Lindzay and E. Aronson (eds), *Handbook of Social Psychology*, 3rd edn, New York: Random House.

Malin, N.A. (2000), Evaluating clinical supervision in community homes and teams serving adults with learning disabilities, *Journal of Clinical Nursing*, 31(3): 548–557.

Paunonen-Ilmonen, M. (2001), *Työnohjaus toiminnan laadunhallinnan varmistaja [The Appropriateness of Supervising the Activities of Quality Management]*, Helsinki, Finland: WSOY.

Paunonen, M. and Hyrkäs, K. (2001), Clinical supervision in Finland: history, education, research and theory, in J.R. Cutcliffe, T. Butterworth, and B. Proctor (eds), *Fundamental Themes in Clinical Supervision*, London: Routledge, pp. 284–302.

Popper, K.R. (1972), *Objective Knowledge: An Evolutionary Approach*, Oxford: Clarendon Press.

Potter, J. (2005), Making psychology relevant, *Discourse and Society*, 16(5): 739–747.

Potter, J, and Wetherell, M. (1988), Accomplishing attitudes: fact and evaluation in racist discourse, *Text*, 8(1–2): 51–68.

Rodgers, B. (1989), Concepts, analysis and the development of nursing knowledge: the evolutionary cycle, *Journal of Advanced Nursing*, 14(4): 330–335.

Samuelsson, M., Sunbring, Y., Winell, I. and Asberg, M. (1997), Nurses' attitudes to attempted suicide patients, *Scandinavian Journal of Caring Science*, 11(4): 232–237.

Teasdale, K., Brocklehurst, N. and Thom, N. (2001), Clinical supervision and support for nurses: an evaluation study, *Journal of Advanced Nursing*, 33(2): 216–224.

Toulmin, S.E. (1967), The evolutionary development of natural science, *American* Scientist, 55(4): 456–471.

UKCC (2006), *Position Statement on Clinical Supervision for Nursing and Health Visiting*, London: UKCC.

White, E. (1996), Clinical supervision and Project 2000: the identification of some substantive issues, *NTResearch*, 1(2): 102–111.

Wilson-Barnett, J., Butterworth, T., White, E., Twinn, S., Davies, S. and Riley, L. (1995), Clinical support and the Project 2000 nursing student: factors influencing the process, *Journal of Advanced Nursing*, 21(6): 1152–1158.

Wittgenstein, L. (1968), *Philosophical Investigations*, 3rd edn, trans. G.E.M. Anscombe, New York: Macmillan.

Wolsey, P. and Leach, L. (1997), Clinical supervision: a hornet's nest? *Nursing Times*, 93(44): 24–27.

Yegdich, T. (1999), Clinical supervision and managerial supervision: some historical and conceptual considerations, *Journal of Advanced Nursing*, 30(5): 1195–1204.

25 Clinical supervision in multidisciplinary groups

Qualitative evaluation using a focus group technique

James Dooher and John Fowler

This chapter reports on the findings from a qualitative study that used multidisciplinary focus groups to evaluate the experience of receiving clinical supervision. It provides findings from each of the multidisciplinary groups who participated in the research and it contains a summary of the actions, outputs, and outcomes of clinical supervision. It concludes with a summary of the key findings and draws a very insightful analogy of clinical supervision as a campfire.

It is interesting to note that the findings in this chapter lend support to the editors' position that there is no one 'best way' of conducting clinical supervision. Models and formats of supervision, that fitted within the parameters identified in Chapter 1, were developed to meet the needs of the different situations and individual members. As a consequence, practitioners gained a sense of ownership of the supervision and were thus perhaps more committed to ensuring it worked for them. It is also worth noting that across the wide variety of health care disciplines who participated in this research, the benefits of clinical supervision was unanimously recognised.

The philosophy underpinning this evaluation of clinical supervision

Traditional evaluation of health care practice has relied largely on professional judgement and the subjective experience of those either directly involved, or in positions of authority. The relatively recent demand for 'evidence-based practice' has stimulated managers and researchers to review this customary approach to evaluation. The factors that have triggered this move towards more rigorous evaluation are, according to Jenkinson (1997), twofold. First, there is the fear that many health care procedures are of no benefit and may even be harmful, second is the acknowledgement that health care resources are finite, and that provision must be effective in terms of both cost and health gain. Thus the providers of health care look to research and other forms of enquiry to provide evidence of successful practices, and the resources they consume.

The often stated 'gold standard' of evaluative research is the randomised controlled study (RCT) (McGee and Notter 1995; Greene and D'Oliveira 1998). This method is frequently used for evaluating specific physical and chemical treatments and, if applied with scientific rigour, can allow the researcher to make statements regarding the effectiveness of a particular treatment. Arguably the strength of the

RCT lies in the ability of the researcher to identify and isolate a single variable and measure its effect against a control group. This requires three things: first, the isolation of the variable; second, a tool which can accurately measure its effect; and third, two groups which are the same in every respect, one to be the experimental group and the other to be the control. Whilst these criteria can be met in laboratory conditions there are many health care practices which cannot be isolated into single variables, accurately measured or manipulated onto an experimental group.

Caring aspects of nursing practice and the interpersonal interactions associated with clinical supervision are difficult to isolate. This may lead to the false assumption that this lack of measurability indicates that they are of no use. Conversely, the blind acceptance of practices that are somehow on a higher intellectual or aesthetic plain, because they are difficult to isolate or measure, is equally misplaced.

Where does this leave evaluation of clinical supervision? Although it is unlikely that clinical supervision will do harm, it does have the potential to consume and divert both human and financial resources from direct clinical contact. Although there are some published examples of evaluative studies (Dudley and Butterworth 1994; Edberg *et al.* 1996; Butterworth *et al.* 1997; Fowler and Chevannes 1998) they form the minority of published work regarding clinical supervision. If we accept that we should evaluate clinical supervision, the next question must be what are we going to evaluate? And how should we do it? Jenkinson (1997) postulates that evaluative research should be as critical and objective as possible and may use a variety of research methods to achieve this. In the evaluation of clinical supervision the strength and weaknesses of different research methods need to be examined against the problems to be investigated, and the questions of which answers are sought. In this regard, no one method should be assumed to be appropriate to every investigation but rather considered in relation to the identified problem or efficacy of the intervention.

The study

In Leicestershire, an NHS Trust developed a strategy regarding clinical supervision, and this study considers its implementation. Some areas and clinical teams within the Trust had previously established a form of clinical supervision; others underwent a training day to prepare them for its introduction. This study represents the independent evaluation of ten pilot sites. The aim of the study was to evaluate from the staff's perspective:

- the general structure of clinical supervision;
- the outcomes of clinical supervision for staff;
- the outcomes of clinical supervision for patient/client care.

Method: The Trust commissioning the study had already implemented clinical supervision making any form of pre- and post-evaluation (Bowling 1997) difficult, and we agreed to produce an objective evaluation based upon reflective discussions with staff who had been involved with clinical supervision.

An adapted focus group (Wright and Baker 2005; Ruff *et al.* 2005) was considered the most appropriate method of collecting data. Evaluation using focus groups would allow open questions to be posed to approximately 70 people. The disadvantages of this method were explored in that some staff might not be able to express dissatisfactions with other group members present, and more vocal members may dominate the discussions. To overcome these potential disadvantages it was planned that the group members would be given the opportunity to talk to the researchers on an individual basis either following the focus group or at a suitable time. A structured interview based upon the Trust's original objectives was developed, and presented to the local ethics committee.

Notes were taken and an audiotape of each focus group helped gather data. The analysis was carried out thematically based upon the objectives set by the Trust but including any emerging themes.

Procedure: The facilitators of the ten pilot sites were written to informing them of the evaluation study. They were then contacted by phone and a convenient date, time and venue arranged for the focus group meeting, which usually commenced with informal 'chat', then the formal focus group took approximately 60 minutes. All of the ten pilot sites were visited as part of the evaluation, and of a potential 78 staff in the official membership list, 78 per cent (N = 61) attended focus groups.

Set questions were posed to eight of the ten groups although for two groups it became apparent that these questions were not appropriate as the groups' clinical supervision sessions had either never really started off, or discontinued after only one or two sessions. For these groups the evaluation was focused on the reason for the groups not developing.

The ten pilot sites

Group 1: health visitors

This group consisted of seven health visitors meeting for 90 minutes every two months. They appreciated the clinical supervision meetings as a time when they could mix with their peers in a way that other professional meetings did not allow. The health visitors felt that the clinical supervision sessions provided an arena where they could spend a little time discussing difficult clients, brainstorming ideas and gaining support from their peers. Initially the first three meetings had been about setting up the group, discussing ground rules and generally getting to know each other. The subsequent last three meetings were seen to be very useful although some members found the setting aside of time for the meeting and then protecting it, a stressful process.

Comment: This system allowed staff to review difficult clinical situations and discuss issues of professional concern. It served as a valuable professional support forum and had the potential to become even more supportive as the group continued to meet and relationships developed.

Group 2: physiotherapists

This was a group of community physiotherapists and was the only group to structure clinical supervision on a purely individual basis.

Junior physiotherapists: Junior physiotherapists on a rotational placement to the community met up once a week individually with a senior physiotherapist. The main focus of this meeting was to review the caseloads. Each patient was reviewed, with any immediate problems identified and discussed. The junior physiotherapists felt that these clinical supervision meetings were a useful and supportive system. Being new to community work they appreciated the opportunity to have a regular meeting with an experienced supportive senior physiotherapist.

Senior physiotherapists: The senior physiotherapists met approximately monthly for an hour to review the workloads and the organisation of the department. The content of the meeting tended to be rather ad hoc with the demands of the department dictating the discussions.

Comment: This was a system that supported and monitored the work of junior staff working in a new and very different environment, allowing individual patient treatments to be reviewed and unusual conditions, treatments or family relationships to be discussed in detail. The supervision meetings for the senior staff were useful but with a little more structure and focus have greater potential than was currently being realised.

Group 3: community hospital nursing staff

This was the only ward-based hospital group to be part of the clinical supervision pilot study. It was set up with the ward manager and five staff nurses. After the first couple of meetings that focused on discussing the ground rules, however, the ward manager and one of the staff nurses left the hospital for alternative jobs. This posed two main problems for the remaining members of the group. First, the person who led and motivated the group had gone, and none of the remaining group took on that motivating role. Second, neither the staff nurse nor the ward manager was replaced, leading to the remaining staff covering the shifts on the ward. After the ward manager left the group no longer met. They admitted that their morale was low and that they 'just couldn't raise themselves any more'. They said that it would have been 'really nice if the group had advanced enough so that we stayed as a peer group'.

Comment: The absence of a key motivator, lack of managerial interest and disempowered staff resulted in the failure of this group. Paradoxically the area where the benefits of clinical supervision would be extremely valuable was the area least able to implement it. It was felt that this group would need resources and expert support to engender motivation and the basic ability to develop a useful system.

Group 4: community nurses

This consisted of two groups, qualified nursing staff and health care assistants (HCA), the structure of which was planned to accommodate both group and individual supervision. Group meetings were held once a month for two months and then in the third month, individual clinical supervision. The person taking the supervisor role was decided upon by the department manager who did not participate in either of the groups. The HCA group continued for a further two or three meetings, but the qualified group never really started. The reasons why clinical supervision was not adopted were complex. The department was relatively new and as such was developing its role, function and structure. At the time that clinical supervision was introduced, the lines of professional and personal management appeared unclear to the staff within this team. There appeared to be no formal or informal leader responsible for the direction of the team, indeed the concept of 'team' did not appear to be a dominant feature of these workers. Into this structure a number of the group felt that clinical supervision was 'thrown in by the management' and in their own way they 'threw it out'. Choice of supervisors was said to have been imposed on both supervisors and supervisees. Both groups expressed feelings that demonstrated that they felt no ownership of the process citing, 'The way it was done put your back up'. In discussion as to why clinical supervision did not take off with either group the following factors were identified by the group:

Qualified group

- *role of supervisor imposed upon us;*
- *did not know what to expect and the training did not help;*
- *meetings took on the same format as others;*
- *senior managers did not appear motivated;*
- *no one was clear about roles and which hat to put on;*
- *there was a lack of enthusiasm;*
- *we were not getting anything out of it;*
- *covering 24 hours of patient care makes meetings difficult.*

HCA group

- *the supervisor was from the team, someone from outside would have been better – not the facilitator herself but just someone from outside the team;*
- *they would be able to ventilate more;*
- *how can a manager who bullies you one minute, be your friendly supervisor the next?*
- *covering 24 hours of patient care made meetings difficult;*
- *false hierarchical registered/HCA divide.*

Comment: A lack of managerial commitment, team restructuring and the interpersonal difficulties caused by role ambiguity created a dysfunctional group of workers who made a conscious decision to abdicate from clinical supervision. This factor may indicate the decision to retake some of the power and control which was felt to be absent from the team which, according to Dooher and Byrt (2003), could be considered an empowered action. They felt that the role of supervisor should be less formal.

Group 5: community nursing staff

All twelve people at the focus group were community nurses and included health care assistants and qualified nurses of various grades. The groups met for approximately 60–90 minutes every four to six weeks. The groups identified a number of examples in which clinical supervision had impacted upon their clinical practice. These included diabetic care, management of incontinence, accountability issues, development of critical thinking and feeling happier at work.

Comment: Clinical supervision was a useful and professionally supportive system. It provided a forum in which staff could discuss professional issues, clinical conditions and explore difficult areas of communication or relationships. Staff felt supported and valued by being part of the group.

Group 6: health visitors and school nurses

This group consisted of six health visitors and three school nurses. They meet together for one hour every month during their lunch hour. They decided that they did not want a 'chatty or poor me group', it should be focused on clinical situations. Clinical supervision sessions tended to focus on clinical situations looking at 'what happened?' and 'could it have gone better?'

This group felt that it was not appropriate for their sessions to be used for 'burdening others with personal stress' although issues of professional concern were discussed. The opportunity to discuss difficult client scenarios with peers was seen to be extremely valuable in that it gave reassurance that what was being proposed was appropriate, and this increased clinical confidence, and 'it gave power to move forward having discussed it with other professionals'. This reduced the potential stress of professional practice.

Although clinical supervision was seen as a positive experience and they 'got a lot out of it'. The group commented that they were fed up with yet more lunchtime meetings, and felt clinical supervision survives because staff donate their own lunchtimes.

Comment: This was a motivated and assertive group. It focused on professional work but in a way that was outside of the standard management structure, and utilised a reflective cycle to review incidents. 'I wouldn't have attended if it was more management-type meetings.'

Group 7: school nurses

This group consisted of six school nurses who met for one hour a month over lunch, spending five to ten minutes in general chat, and the remaining 50 minutes on the 'business'. All the group were experienced school nurses and as such said that they tended not to talk about 'hands on clinical issues' but concentrated on issues of policy, time management or general management situations. All the staff worked in isolation and talked about the benefits of clinical supervision as being one of mutual support and the opportunity to discuss issues with colleagues.

Clinical supervision sessions were used to discuss difficult situations and a comment, 'it was good to share and gain support, we are all in the same boat' highlighted the usefulness.

Comment: This system provided a valuable time for staff to meet together and discuss issues that were pertinent to their specialty. It allowed difficult or unusual clinical situations to be discussed with peers working in similar situations.

Group 8: occupational therapists

The staff present at this focus group represented two separate clinical supervision groups of occupational therapy (OT) staff. Initial allocation to either of the groups appeared fairly random. Both groups met for two hours once a month. The department's work was either adjusted or covered by the remaining staff of the department. The groups developed differently.

First group: gelled immediately and began focusing on clinical issues via presentations of patient studies. All participants found the group a 'pleasure to be a part of' and saw it as valuable time out. Discussions used a reflective format with a patient case study being presented for general discussion. A number of specific clinical issues were discussed usually via a case study presentation.

Second group: Initially the group did not gel and for the first six months they seem to be working through a number of role and personality issues. Attendance tended to be poor, 50–60 per cent attending each group and about five groups being cancelled in the first year. Following a six month review the group began to progress, attendance was improved and people began to share clinical situations and clinical problems. At the time of the evaluation, trust and respect were beginning to develop and staff were beginning to work together.

Comment: Both groups contained a mixture of OTs specialising in physical and mental health: this proved to be very beneficial particularly in the exchange of experience regarding dealing with patients with disruptive behaviour and mental health problems. Staff commented that their confidence in dealing with clinical situations had increased resulting from the reassurance they had received about clinical outcomes.

Group 9: health visitors

This group consisted of eight health visitors meeting every two months for 90 minutes over a lunchtime period. The meetings covered areas such as topics of interest, cases of interest and the possibility of guest speakers. An agenda was set for each meeting.

Although this group felt able to discuss difficult clients it had currently not done so. Issues such as UKCC policies, hormone replacement therapy, measurement of head circumference and dealing with the police were covered. This has led to a general questioning of some traditional health visiting practices. There was a general feeling that these were more than just professional discussions: 'at other meetings I tend not to be listened to or no action is taken, but here we can do something'.

Comment: Staff were using the clinical supervision sessions to discuss issues of professional interest and concern. They felt that their contributions were valued and that they were able to act upon some of the issues discussed.

Group 10: clinic staff

This group consisted of four nurses and a consultant doctor. The group met once a month for one hour over lunchtime and had been meeting for approximately 15 months. Sociological and ethical issues relating to their specialty were discussed and the boundaries and extent of their role debated. The group felt that they had gained a lot of reassurance from finding out that they all faced similar anxieties and had explored different ways of dealing and coping with the professional problems. This had resulted in increased personal confidence, clinical ability and recognition of the nature and limitations of their role.

Comment: This was the only group to contain a consultant doctor and nurses. The mixing of disciplines proved useful and served to build relationships and helped both disciplines appreciate each other's role and routine functions. Specific clinical situations were discussed and support was gained in difficult areas. Despite being experienced staff, the group felt that clinical supervision had increased their clinical confidence.

An overview of the pilot site responses

In eight of the ten pilot sites clinical supervision could be said to be up and running. In the other two groups clinical supervision had either never commenced or floundered after two meetings. The reasons why clinical supervision did not take off in these two groups were complex but tended to focus on organisational and staffing issues.

As a general observation it appeared that the more frequently a group met the more likely it was to discuss and reflect upon specific patient/client care.

Groups that met on average once a month tended to review one client in depth for part of the meeting and then discuss pertinent issues during the rest of the meeting. It could be concluded from this that if a group wishes to focus in greater detail on individual patients/clients they will need to meet quite frequently.

The general view was that clinical supervision was a genuinely supportive system in terms of dealing with difficult or new clinical situations. Reassurance, confidence-building and empowering were three terms that were frequently mentioned. Those staff that worked predominately on their own or were the only member of their specialty working in a team felt that simply meeting with and discussing 'specialist' issues very supporting. In a number of the groups there was a very definite, yet difficult to quantify, 'warmth of atmosphere', and what was evident in the majority of groups was the willingness to discuss such issues in a positive and problem solving way.

Actions, outputs and outcomes of clinical supervision

Structure of the sessions

- Most of the sites had implemented group clinical supervision with only two examples of individual supervision. Both models were effective in the situations in which they were introduced.
- Group supervision was particularly useful for staff who worked predominately on their own.
- Some sites had staff of mixed grades and disciplines. Others were segregated according to grade and discipline. As a general finding it appeared that a mixture of disciplines and grades was useful in giving staff insight and understanding of other people's ways of working. At times, however, these groups would be restricted in focus in terms of the professional interest and the potential depth of their discussions.
- Clinical supervision needs time for a relationship of mutual trust and respect to be developed between the staff. Depending on the frequency of the meetings this seems to take between three and six months. The 'productivity' or qualitative outcomes of clinical supervision sessions seems to be significantly greater once the relationships have gelled.
- Clinical supervision sessions ranged from weekly meetings to those occurring once every two months. Sessions lasted between 60–90 minutes. Where used to review patient caseload, weekly clinical supervision is appropriate. Where clini-

cal supervision is used to review longer-term patient situations and general professional issues then monthly meetings seem to be appropriate. Groups that met every two months found it harder to focus on specific clinical issues and discuss individual problems.

- Staff who cover 24 hour patient care by working shifts have considerable difficulty in organising and safeguarding a set time for a clinical supervision meeting.
- Staff who are in charge of their own diary and are experienced in managing their own time were most effective in organising and safeguarding clinical supervision sessions.

Process of clinical supervision

- Different clinical supervision groups developed different focuses, functions and 'personalities'.
- Those groups where *all* members feel that they have ownership and control of clinical supervision appear to be the most productive.
- Those sites where clinical supervision became established and productive had mature leadership. The style of leadership varies within each site and there does not seem to be one style that is more favourable than another. With experienced staff groups a 'low key' leader that encouraged equality and joint responsibility between all members seemed particularly effective. With groups that had less experienced staff a slightly more dominant leader who took responsibility for direction and focus appeared productive. There is a delicate balance between leadership that encourages, organises, motivates and empowers without appearing to dominate and take over.
- Mutual trust and comfortable working relationships appeared to be a feature of groups that met regularly and formed the basis for a number of beneficial outcomes.

Outcomes of clinical supervision

The following outcomes are based upon a general summary of the eight groups where clinical supervision had become established.

- Feedback to individuals that clinical actions and professional practices undertaken were appropriate and reassurance that these actions were 'good/best practice'.
- Discussion of alternative ways of dealing with unusual clinical problems and identification of creative solutions.
- Acted as stimulus to reflect upon one's own practice and helped prevent complacency developing.
- The safeguard and sanction of time to focus in depth on a specific client problem.
- Support from clinically knowledgeable peers regarding difficult relationships concerned with clients, relatives or colleagues.
- A formalised, structured system for staff to seek advice and gain support relating to professional work situations.

- A valuable support system for all staff but particularly effective for new staff and those changing roles.
- Provision of a platform from which individuals felt able to influence their practice and, at times, the organisation's policy and practices.
- Provided a safe environment where one's areas of weakness could be disclosed, reviewed and positively managed.

Conclusions

1   No single model of clinical supervision emerged as better than any of the others. Each developed to meet the needs of different situations and individual members.
2   Sufficient autonomy should be given to each group to allow them to develop and tailor a model that is seen to be useful to themselves.
3   When new groups are being established they should be encouraged to explore different approaches and established good practices but given the authority to develop and build upon these models so that they can develop a system specific to their needs.
4   Implementation of clinical supervision required the support, permission and encouragement of the organisation and immediate managers but it is essential that the ownership should be taken and maintained by the individual practitioners.
5   Where the working environment is in a state of considerable organisational change, or staffing levels are significantly below the norm, then the introduction of clinical supervision is probably not appropriate at that time.
6   Clinical supervision has to be seen as a long-term investment from both the organisation's and practitioners' perspectives. The benefits appear to be related to the cumulative effect of regular, planned meetings and the building up of trust and friendship between the health care practitioners.
7   The actual and potential benefit of clinical supervision to staff was unanimously recognised and praised as a legitimate and professionally acceptable process by all participants. The wholly positive perception of benefits was illustrated by a range of clinical examples and anecdotal accounts, citing improved performance, increased confidence, a reduction in the use of both professional and personal support mechanisms, and a greater understanding of colleagues' clinical work.
8   The benefits to clients were less tangible, with secondary gains being acquired from new knowledge of contemporary treatment methods, previously shared during clinical supervision. The professionals' increased self-assurance in their own practice was said to have been projected onto clients, who were on the whole more confident and relaxed about the care they received.
9   Where clinical supervision had been successfully established, the benefits to the organisation seemed to have their basis in an increased level of job satisfaction and morale. Staff felt clinical supervision had created an opportunity to consider the method and style of their clinical interventions which in turn made them more effective professionals.

The final picture: clinical supervision as a campfire!

All of the groups where clinical supervision was up and running felt that the sessions had been worthwhile. People tended to feel that individually and professionally they gained from clinical supervision. For all staff it meant committing the time to attending, being prepared to talk honestly and having genuine respect for others. In both of the areas where clinical supervision did not take off, staff were noticeably demotivated, lacked energy and appeared to have no professional leadership. These individuals did not feel in control of their daily working environment and poor staffing seemed to be a significant factor in one of the areas. Both areas were undergoing considerable organisational change, which appeared to be poorly planned and poorly implemented. The introduction of clinical supervision appeared to be something else that was being imposed upon them and in which they had little say. Somewhat ironically, the support and direction that clinical supervision has the potential to offer, was exactly what these two areas needed. However, the motivation and leadership required to introduce and develop such a system were not there.

An analogy of clinical supervision could be that of a group of people sitting around a campfire. If a group had dry wood they could with relative ease get a fire going and enjoy its warmth. Once the fire was established it would be relatively easy to keep it going. Even if it began to rain and their wood got damp the fire would keep going because the warmth of the existing fire would dry out the damp wood. However, another group is already wet and their wood is damp. They are sitting in a field where it is raining and the wood they bring to the fire is damp. This group will find it very difficult to get a fire started. People who are particularly skilled may be able to start the fire, but it will probably require some outside input, such as a carefully controlled dose of petrol.

In this analogy the wood is likened to people's motivation and energy, those who have an excess of energy, enthusiasm and motivation can throw it into the fire where it generates warmth, support and encouragement for others in that group. Once the group is established and positive relationships forged, then they will be able to 'keep the fire going' even when people are going through a hard, demotivating time. Those groups in which people do not have any spare motivation or energy – and this can occur due to a variety of reasons – will not be able to get the fire going. Ironically it is these 'damp' groups that need the warmth and support of the 'fire'.

The moral of this analogy is to establish clinical supervision when the team is strong. When the team is weak and feels disempowered, outside motivation will need to be injected and maintained until the group is established and self-supporting.

References

Bowling, A. (1997), *Research Methods in Health*, Buckingham: Open University Press.

Butterworth, T., Carson, J., White, E., Jeacock, J., Clements, A. and Bishop, V. (1997), *It is Good to Talk. An Evaluation Study in England and Scotland*, Manchester: University of Manchester.

Dooher, J. and Byrt, R. (2003), *Empowerment and Participation: Power Influence and Control in Contemporary Healthcare*, Salisbury: Quay Books.

Dudley, M. and Butterworth, T. (1994), The cost and some benefits of clinical supervision, *The International Journal of Psychiatric Nursing Research*, 1(2): 34–40.

Edberg, A., Hallberg, I. and Gustafson, L. (1996), Effects of clinical supervision on nurse patient cooperation quality: a controlled study in dementia care, *Clinical Nursing Research*, 5(2): 127–149.

Fowler, J. and Chevannes, M. (1998), Evaluating the efficacy of reflective practice within the context of clinical supervision, *Journal of Advanced Nursing*, 27(2): 379–382.

Greene, J. and D'Oliveira, M. (1998), *Learning to use statistical tests in psychology*, Milton Keynes: Open University Press.

Jenkinson, C. (1997), *Assessment and Evaluation of Health and Medical Care*, London: Open University Press.

McGee, P. and Notter, J. (1995), *Research Appreciation*, Salisbury: Mark Allen Publishing.

Ruff, C.C., Alexander, I.M. and McKie, C. (2005), The use of focus group methodology in health disparities research, *Nursing Outlook*, 53(3): 134–140.

Wright, M. and Baker, A. (2005), The effects of appreciative inquiry interviews on staff in the UK National Health Service, *International Journal of Health Care Quality Assurance*, 18(1): 41–51.

26 Clinical supervision for nurses in administrative and leadership positions

A review of the studies focusing on administrative clinical supervision

Pirjo Sirola-Karvinen and Kristiina Hyrkäs

This chapter focuses on reviewing and discussing the literature regarding clinical supervision for nurses in administrative and leadership positions. Many papers regarding the topic have been published in Finland, but international literature has also been included in this systematic literature review. The authors conducted an extensive, systematic literature search and utilised Proctor's model for the analysis of the selected literature. The chapter discusses the challenges for conducting a literature review due to discrepancies regarding the concept and the use of keywords in the electronic databases.

It is obvious to us that the nurses in administrative and leadership positions need and benefit from administrative clinical supervision and that it has a positive impact on the quality of the services at the organisational level. We believe that this is an important chapter for managers and administrators pursuing excellence of leadership and outcomes of nursing.

Acknowledgment

The original article was published in the *Journal of Nursing Management*, 14(8): 601–609, and has been reproduced here with the kind permission of Blackwell Science.

Background

The future challenges of health care are to provide high quality services, to respond to the changing needs of the population and to provide for the well-being of the health care personnel. Projections of scarce financial resources and the lack of personnel have to be considered when planning different scenarios in order to provide high quality health services. (Hätönen and Rintala 2002.) The managers and administrators are facing high demands when it comes to developing the content and quality of nursing care. The leadership role is central for giving directions when organizations are pressured by continuous changes and learning requirements. Administrative clinical supervision (ACS) is a unique form of clinical supervision in the Finnish clinical supervision culture. ACS is organized, among others, for nursing managers, ward sisters, and head nurses in health care organizations. The goal of ACS emphasizes quality management based on the organization's mission and vision statements in addition to the supervisee's learning in order to support career development. The aim of ACS is to support manager and/or administrator supervisees to find their own personal and natural style as a leader. ACS is a process-like intervention that empowers managers and administrators, increasing their trust and confidence in successfully managing their leadership role, related tasks, and challenges regarding change. ACS is a strategic method of support for management and at the same time a part of a manager's well-being (Ollila 2008). At its best it is part of the structure of the organization and the management system. It is also a way to ensure sustainable development in health care organizations.

ACS is a timely and important topic since organizational structures in health care and nursing leadership are changing in addition to the increasing number of complex challenges present in health care. Notable to international developments in recent years is the rise of the "Magnet Recognition Program" for hospitals recognizing nursing excellence. There is increasing interest in Finland regarding this program. Some of the criteria for achieving Magnet Status include: transformational leadership; structural empowerment; exemplary professional practice; new knowledge, innovations and improvement; and empirical quality outcomes (Magnet Model Components and Sources of Evidence 2008). ACS could be one of the tools to aim at these goals.

Administrative clinical supervision

ACS or clinical supervision for managers and administrators has been scantily studied because of its unique perspective. The number of effectiveness studies in clinical supervision is also quite low (Hyrkäs et al. 1999). However, the most recent literature has significantly increased understanding of the nature of ACS, its potential, and capacity to develop.

The excellence of leadership is often seen to include abilities to create a vision of one's own as well as skills and abilities to make independent decisions. Even though democracy and teamwork are increasingly emphasized today in organizations, managers still often make the final decisions and ultimately carry the responsibility alone. There is not much support or help available in leadership work. Managers do not necessarily always get enough honest feedback from employees or supervisors in regards to their activities in everyday work. It is thus possible to assume that the benefits of ACS are emphasized for nurses in leadership positions because of the nature of their work (Lohiniva and Purola 2004). Because strategic competence-based management in health care organizations is a very demanding and multidimensional function, it needs a great deal of support. Therefore, the significance of ACS should be emphasized more in the management of health services (Ollila 2008).

In the international literature, clinical supervision for nursing managers and administrators is not widely acknowledged and the concept is not well known. However, the idea of clinical supervision throughout the career has been discussed briefly by some authors, and it is possible to interpret this as ACS since it is organized for nurses at the higher/highest levels of their career (Butterworth et al. 1997). However, it is important to clarify the difference between the concepts in order to avoid confusion among supervision, clinical supervision, and ACS. In the international literature, these three terms have quite often been used interchangeably, and thus misunderstandings have emerged concerning the role of managers and administrators as supervisors/clinical supervisors for their employees. As a result, another misunderstanding is that the role of managers and administrators as clinical supervisors has been described as a means of administration. Furthermore, it is thought of as a wider concept than the conventional definition of clinical supervision.

ACS is defined as clinical supervision for nursing managers, administrators, head nurses, and respective superiors in the organization. The focus of the ACS is to discuss and process nursing leadership issues aligned towards achieving set goals. ACS concerns issues and topics of nursing leadership and development challenges of nursing (Lohiniva and Purola 2004). In this literature review, *ACS is defined as clinical supervision targeted at nursing managers, administrators, and leaders.*

The aim of the literature review

The aim of this literature review was to describe the empirical evidence concerning ACS based on empirical studies. The focus of interest was the intervention and its effects on the nursing leadership. This review was narrowed down to scrutinize only ACS for nursing managers and administrators. The framework utilized in the literature review was the commonly accepted model of three main elements and functions of clinical supervision: normative, formative and restorative (see Figure 26.1 and Proctor 1988).

Approach

The purpose of reviewing the literature was to systematically and critically collect and review a pre-defined, selected set of literature and/or studies utilizing well-justified questions (Vuorinen *et al.* 2005: 271; Kääriäinen and Lahtinen 2006). The systematic literature review proceeded in stages, starting with the research question and defining the focus for the literature search comprehensively covering all elements of the research topic (see Figure 26.2).

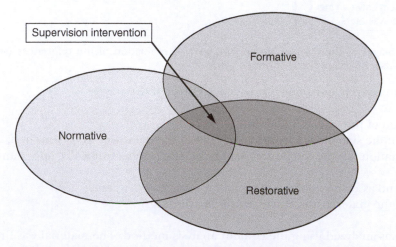

Figure 26.1 Three main elements and functions of clinical supervision (see also: Proctor 1988).

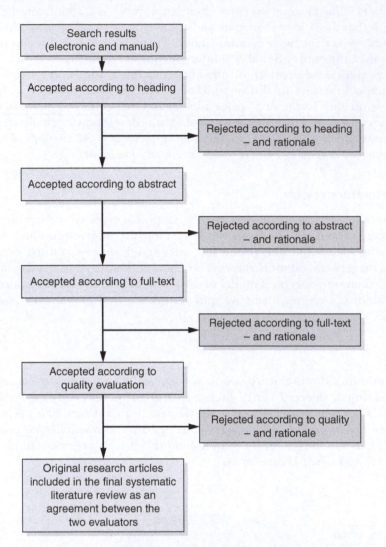

Figure 26.2 Stages of the original search strategy and evaluation of the references (see also: Kääriäinen and Lahtinen (2006)).

The literature search and analysis proceeded through five stages:

1   specification of the research question;
2   planning of the systematic literature search and the databases to be searched;
3   implementation of the literature search in stages: electronically and hand-search;
4   selection and assessment of the material for critical review; and
5   analysis of the material and summarizing the findings.

The material was analyzed using the content analysis method. The material was first classified into three main categories using Proctor's model of (1) normative, (2) formative, and (3) restorative functions of clinical supervision. The next step was to

---

Box 26.1 The databases and selected journals used in this literature review

Databases
- CINAHL (Cumulative Index to Nursing and Allied Health)
- MEDLINE (The United States National Library of Medicine)
- The British Nursing Index (BNI) is a database of nursing, midwifery and community health care.
- MEDIC (Database of the Finnish Health Sciences)
- LINDA (Common Database of the Finnish University Libraries)

Selected journals
- *Journal of Nursing Management*
- *Health Care Manager*
- *Journal of Advanced Nursing*

---

analyze and describe each category with more specific subcategories for each of the main categories.

The material for this literature search was found mainly in electronic databases. Specific journals were selected in order to make certain that the search was thorough (Box 26.1).

The inclusion criteria were:
- research studies published in years 1996–2006 in the electronic databases, and older research studies if these were repeatedly referred to in the more recent studies;
- two main concepts were used to evaluate the content of the study (administrative clinical supervision; clinical supervision and leadership);
- the focus of the study was ACS as an intervention for leadership;
- scientific publications that had been approved through a review process based on established criteria of the scientific journal (and the criteria listed above);
- doctoral dissertations (and the criteria listed above);
- university level theses that have a specific value or importance due to the focus of the study, its findings and publication year (and the criteria listed above).

The exclusion criteria were:
- research studies published more than ten years ago, without specific significance;
- research studies with doubtful research methods, such as telephone interviews;
- only one, or none, of the key concepts was used in the study;
- the intervention in the study was something other than what was defined above and the target group was other than nurse managers, directors or leaders;
- research was not available or accessible through library services;
- overlapping research reports.

The material of this review included three national doctoral dissertations, ten articles published in international journals, three national studies, and three merited university level theses that have been cited in the Finnish national scientific journal of nursing. Nearly all were empirical studies, except one that was based on the researcher's field notes. The doctoral dissertations were published in 1989–2006, the articles in 1994–2005 and the university level theses during the years 1995–2005. The countries of origin were Finland (n=9), Sweden (n=1) and the UK (n=8).

The total number of studies included in this review was 18. The methods applied were action research, follow-up, questionnaire, and interview surveys. Research data were mainly collected from individual respondents, but diaries and observation were used as additional data collection methods. The data were analyzed using both qualitative and quantitative methods. The number of respondents varied from seven to 586. The literature review was updated in November–December 2009, which yielded two (n=2) Finnish research articles on ACS.

What did we learn from the literature?

Normative function and managerial element of clinical supervision

In this literature review, ACS was found to have beneficial effects especially on the quality of care. (Butterworth *et al.* 1997; Hyrkäs 2002; Hyrkäs *et al.* 2002; Lohiniva and Purola 2004). Apparently, the changes in the quality of care were also directly, or indirectly, associated with nursing managers' clarified actions, values (Paunonen 1989; McCormack and Hopkins 1995; Swanljung 1995; Ayer *et al.* 1997; Freshwater *et al.* 2002; Ashburner *et al.* 2004; Hyrkäs *et al.* 2005), and intensified leadership activities (Ayer *et al.* 1997; Bowles and Young 1999; Freshwater *et al.* 2002; Hyrkäs 2002; Lohiniva and Purola 2004).

ACS was seen to be a means of leadership beneficial to practice (Ollila 2006) since it increased work motivation and commitment to the organization (Hyrkäs 2002). It was also found that ACS provided, in the long run, a wider perspective on leadership activities (Hyrkäs *et al.* 2005) since it helped to illuminate the managers'/administrators' work in a different way (Ashburner *et al.* 2004).

In the reviewed literature, the effects on quality assurance were found in developed work processes (Hyrkäs 2002), improved management of human resources and activities, clarified principles and value-based directing activities in practice (Lohiniva and Purola 2004), and development of collective shared knowledge (Hyrkäs 2002). It was also possible to conclude that ACS helped to clarify goals (McCormack and Hopkins 1995), reference values and ethical issues (Swanljung 1995), and adoption of norms (Ayer *et al.* 1997). The intensification of activities was seen especially in everyday leadership work, strategic planning, and change management (Lohiniva and Purola 2004). The described organizational developments resembled organizational learning (Ayer *et al.* 1997) as well as intensification of team work (Hyrkäs 2002). According to Ollila's recent study, ACS includes dialogue and reflective thinking as features of competence-based management and its development. It seems to be a strategic method of support for management and at the same time an element in a manager's well-being. ACS as one support system clarifies strategic competence-based management, provides support to leadership know-how, and helps a manager to feel better at work (Ollila 2008).

Formative function and educative element of clinical supervision

The formative function of ACS seemed to have positive improving effects on leadership skills (Paunonen 1989; Johns and Graham 1994; McCormack and Hopkins 1995; Swanljung 1995; Severinsson and Hallberg 1996; Ayer *et al.* 1997; Bowles and Young 1999; Laaksonen 1999; Freshwater *et al.* 2002; Hyrkäs 2002, Hyrkäs *et al.* 2002; Johns 2003; Lohiniva and Purola 2004; Hyrkäs *et al.* 2005, Toivakka 2005). This was described as professional growth and development. In ACS, the managers/administrators learned problem solving skills (McCormack and Hopkins 1995; Swanljung 1995; Laaksonen 1999; Lohiniva and Purola 2004). It was also possible to conclude that this type of clinical supervision had a positive influence on the development of the working community's activities (Johns and Graham 1994; McCormack and Hopkins 1995).

The literature demonstrated that new communication and leadership methods were used among the supervisees (Ayer *et al.* 1997; Hyrkäs 2002). The adoption and development of reflection skills were reported (Johns and Graham 1994), including increased individual and personal growth (Hyrkäs *et al.* 2002), and development of interaction skills (Laaksonen 1999). The self-piloting (Swanljung 1995) and utilization of one's own strengths increased among the supervisees (McCormack and Hopkins 1995).

The increased leadership skills manifest themselves, for example, in the form of new innovative solutions (Laaksonen 1999). The literature reports the development of supervisees' self-evaluations to be more positive and clearer in direction (Hyrkäs 2002), with improved motivation in performance and leadership (Laaksonen 1999). By reviewing one's own working patterns, the manager was also able to measure his/her own knowledge and presence in the working team and strengthen the direction of leadership (Freshwater *et al.* 2002). ACS was also seen as a means of leadership (Ollila 2006) and development of the manager's own work (Freshwater *et al.* 2002).

Sirola-Karvinen and Hyrkäs's (2008) recent study showed that overall the supervision for nurse managers and directors was very successful. The contents of the supervision sessions differed depending on the nurse leader's position. Significant differences were found in the evaluations between specialties and within years of work experience. Clinical supervision was utilized best in psychiatric and mental health nursing. The respondents with long work experience rated the importance and value of clinical supervision highest. The study demonstrated that clinical supervision is beneficial for nursing leaders. The experiences were positive and the nursing leaders appreciated the importance and value of clinical supervision.

Restorative function and supportive element of clinical supervision

The literature review demonstrated that it was possible to link the development of leadership skills to the normative, as well as restorative, functions of clinical supervision (Swanljung 1995; Ayer *et al.* 1997; Butterworth *et al.* 1997; Bowles and Young 1999; Hyrkäs *et al.* 2002; Lohiniva and Purola 2004; Ollila 2006). It was found that when leadership skills developed, self-awareness increased (Paunonen 1989; Laaksonen 1999; Hyrkäs 2002; Lohiniva and Purola 2004; Hyrkäs *et al.* 2005), and interaction and cooperation skills improved (Paunonen 1989; Swanljung 1995; Hyrkäs 2002; Hyrkäs *et al.* 2002; Johns 2003; Lohiniva and Purola 2004; Toivakka

2005). As a result, coping at work, including with its challenges, increased (Paunonen 1989; Butterworth *et al.* 1997; Bowles and Young 1999; Ashburner *et al.* 2004).

ACS appeared to enhance interdisciplinary cooperation by fostering a more open approach to issues, resulting in a more effective team (Johns and Graham 1994; see also Hyrkäs 2002). The literature also demonstrated that interaction increased perceptions of support regardless of supervisory position (Lohiniva and Purola 2004; Ollila 2006).

ACS facilitated dealing with problematic situations (Ashburner *et al.* 2004) and providing support to teams, thus increasing team members' well-being (Toivakka 2005). The intervention emphasized accountability, interaction, and independence. In staff administration, human relations and interaction skills were accentuated (Ollila 2006). Improved leadership skills were evidently based on an increase in self-knowledge, confidence, consideration, and collaboration (Lohiniva and Purola 2004).

Improved interaction and cooperation skills were demonstrated by teamwork and streamlining the flow of information (Lohiniva and Purola 2004). The team's cohesion intensified and practices developed and grew stronger. As a result, the team's functionality improved (Hyrkäs 2002). Through interaction, a more positive work environment emerged (Paunonen 1989; Swanljung 1995). The focus in human relations was on attitudinal changes (Hyrkäs 2002). By becoming more flexible, colleagues and staff were able to listen to and hear each other in a new way (Johns and Graham 1994).

Increased self-knowledge helped to clarify one's own work, individual working methods, recognition of different sources of knowledge (Hyrkäs 2002), clarification of leadership skills, awareness of one's own actions, and understanding of one's own personality (Lohiniva and Purola 2004).

Coping at work was demonstrated as improved stress management (Bowles and Young 1999), decreased burnout (Butterworth *et al.* 1997), morbidity (Ashburner *et al.* 2004), and exhaustion (Paunonen 1989) among supervisees. According to Ollila (2008) ACS should be seen as a preventive function of burnout and thus it should also contribute to the well-being of a manager.

Discussion

Due to the wide range of definitions within the concept, the main challenge of the literature review was to narrow the search without losing important research studies. Reading the abstracts and following the steps of the literature review process helped to clarify the focus of the study. These also helped to determine and specify inclusion and exclusion criteria for the literature search. Another challenge was the variation of the use of keywords in different databases. In this study, the hand-search was completed in order to overcome the discrepancies of the use of certain keywords and to ensure that all the relevant material was collected for the literature review.

In this literature review, Proctor's model proved useful. It helped to focus the analysis, answer research questions, and synthesize findings. It is possible to argue that different types of confounding factors may or may not have influenced (biased) the findings of effectiveness studies. It could be possible to try to control the confounding factors during the study, or at least speculate on the effects on the intervention and its outcomes when reporting the findings. Interestingly, the findings of many studies were often considered to be suggestive (Laakso 2004: 10).

The method of content analysis applied in the literature review required interpretation of the findings to some extent, and the interpretation was based on the researcher's judgment and understanding of the phenomenon under study. This means that the objectivity of the study is not the same as in conventional quantitative studies, but the interpretation may have influenced and biased the reported findings.

During the early stages of the systematic literature review, non-scientific publications were excluded from consideration. The material under review was composed of research studies applying quantitative and qualitative methods with varying sample sizes and varying quality of research designs. Overall, the papers and studies were of moderately high quality.

Multi-professional collaboration will play an increasingly important role in health care since there will be an increase in competition and requirements. *The findings of this review confirmed that ACS promotes collaboration, team functionality, and cohesiveness.* It is thus possible to claim that ACS is an effective, but underutilized, intervention to respond to increasing competition and requirements. Today, it is required that administrators and managers are qualified professionals when working in a health care organization. *The findings of this literature review confirmed that ACS strengthened, developed, and clarified leadership skills as well as managers'/administrators' professional identity.* Thus, ACS could be an efficient intervention and solution to the current and future challenges related to leadership skills.

The findings of this literature review demonstrated that ACS seems to be well known among psychiatric nurses in comparison to nurses representing other specialties. It is possible to claim that there are still prejudices in Finland preventing nurses and other health care professionals from actively seeking and attending clinical supervision, especially among physicians who are members of multi-professional teams as well as in administrative positions (Toivakka 2005). These problems are slowing down the optimal utilization of ACS and therefore benefits to health care.

ACS includes dialogue and reflective thinking as features of competence-based management and its development. It is a strategic method of support for management and at the same time an element in a manager's well-being. ACS as one support system clarifies strategic competence-based management, supports leadership know-how, and helps a manager to feel better at work (Ollila 2008). ACS can increase the capacity of the organization, well-being at work, and targeted operations. *It enables sustainable development and good care of clients in health care organizations also in the future.*

The future challenge is to increase nursing managers' and administrators' awareness of ACS. The challenges of future research from the ACS perspective is to explore the profitability of this intervention as an investment and its financial benefits to an organization in the form of more efficient practices, decreased incidence of malpractice and complaints, and increased retention of staff. *It also seems that there is a distinct need to redefine the concept of ACS.* Furthermore it is important to plan and coordinate a longitudinal evaluation so that clinical supervision for nursing leaders is systematically implemented and continuously developed.

References

Ashburner, C., Meyer, J., Cotter, A., Young, G., and Ansell, R. (2004), Seeing things differently: evaluating psychodynamically informed group clinical supervision for general hospital nurses, including commentary by V. Bishop, *Nursing Times Research*, 9(1): 38–49.

Ayer, S., Knight, S., Joyce, L., and Nightingale, V. (1997), Practice-led education and development project: developing styles in clinical supervision, *Nurse Education Today*, 17(5): 347–358.

Bowles, N. and Young, C. (1999), An evaluative study of clinical supervision based on Proctor's three function interactive model, *Journal of Advanced Nursing*, 30(4): 958–964.

Butterworth, T., Carson, J., White, E., Jeacock, J., and Bishop, V. (1997), *It is Good to Talk: An Evaluation of Clinical Supervision and Mentorship in England and Scotland*, Manchester: University of Manchester.

Freshwater, D., Walsh, L., and Storey, L. (2002), Prison health care. Part 2: developing leadership through clinical supervision, *Nursing Management*, 8(9): 16–20.

Hätönen, H. and Rintala, A. (2002), Hallinnollinen työnohjaus ja johtajuuden haasteet [Administrative supervision and leadership challenges], in K. Hyrkäs, T. Munnukka, and M. Sorsa (eds.), *Supervision in nursing: Permanent foundation or useless burden? [Työnohjaus hoitotyössä: pysyvä perusta vai turha taakka?]*, Department of Nursing Science, Perhekeskeisen hoidon tutkimus- ja opetuskeskus [Family-centered care research and education center], Tampere, Finland: University of Tampere, Publications 4: 85–92.

Hyrkäs, K. (2002), *Clinical Supervision and Quality Care*, doctoral dissertation, Acta Universitatis Tamperensis 869, Tampere, Finland: Tampere University Press.

Hyrkäs, K., Appelqvist-Schmidlechner, K., and Kivimäki, K. (2005), First-line managers' views of the long-term effects of clinical supervision: how does clinical supervision support and develop leadership in health care? *Journal of Nursing Management*, 13(3): 209–220.

Hyrkäs, K., Koivula, M., and Paunonen, M. (1999), Clinical supervision in nursing in the 1990s – current state of concepts, theory and research, *Journal of Nursing Management*, 7(3): 177–187.

Hyrkäs, K., Koivula, M., Lehti, K., and Paunonen-Ilmonen, M. (2002), Nurse managers' conceptions of quality management as promoted by peer supervision, *Journal of Nursing Management*, 11(1): 48–58.

Johns, C. (2003), Clinical supervision as a model for clinical leadership, *Journal of Nursing Management*, 11(1): 25–34.

Johns, C. and Graham, J. (1994), The growth of management connoisseurship through reflective practice, *Journal of Nursing Management*, 2(6): 253–260.

Kääriäinen, M. and Lahtinen, M. (2006), Systemaattinen kirjallisuuskatsaus tutkimustiedon jäsentäjänä [Systematic review as a method of analyzing previous scientific knowledge], *Hoitotiede [Nursing Science]*, 18(1): 37–45.

Laakso, H. (2004), Työnohjaus ja mentorointi johtamisen tukena [Supervision and mentoring as support for leadership], *Ylihoitajalehti*, 32(4): 9–12.

Laaksonen, M. (1999), *Vuoden kestäneen hallinnollisen työnohjauksen vaikutukset osastonhoitajien työhön – Työnohjauskuvaukset osastonhoitajien itsearvioimana* [The Effects of a Year of Regular Systematic Administrative Supervision on Clinical Nurse Manager Work – assessed by the Clinical Nurse Managers], Master's thesis, Tampere, Finland: University of Tampere, Faculty of Nursing.

Lohiniva, V. and Purola, H. (2004), Hallinnollinen työnohjaus johtamistehtävän tukena hoitotyössä [Administrative clinical supervision as a support of leadership in nursing], *Hoitotiede [Nursing Science]*, 16(1): 2–13.

Magnet Model Components and Sources of Evidence (2008), *The Magnet Recognition Program*, Silver Spring, MD: American Nurses Credentialing Center

McCormack, B. and Hopkins, E. (1995), The development of clinical leadership through supported reflective practice, *Journal of Clinical Nursing*, 4(3): 161–168.

Ollila, S. (2006), *Osaamisen strategisen johtamisen hallinta sosiaali- ja terveysalan julkisissa ja yksityisissä palveluorganisaatioissa: Johtamisosaamisen ulottuvuudet työnohjauksellisena näkökulmana* [The Mastery of Strategic Competence-based Management in Public and Private Social and Health Service Organizations: The Dimensions of Managerial Competence from the Viewpoint of Management Supervision], doctoral dissertation, Acta Wasaensia No 156. Department of Public Management, Vaasa, Finland: University of Vaasa.

Ollila, S. (2008), Strategic support for managers by management supervision, *Leadership in Health Services*, 21(1): 16–27.

Paunonen, M. (1989), *Hoitotyön työnohjaus. Empiirinen tutkimus työnohjauksen kehittämisohjelman käynnistämistä muutoksista* [Supervision in nursing. An empirical study of the changes initiated by a supervision development program], doctoral dissertation, Helsinki, Finland: Nurses' Education Foundation.

Proctor, B. (1988), A co-operative exercise in accountability, in M. Marken and M. Payne (eds.), *Enabling and Ensuring: Supervision in Practice*, Leicester: National Youth Bureau and Council for Education and Training in Youth and Community Work.

Severinsson, E. and Hallberg, I. (1996), Clinical supervisors' views of their leadership role in the clinical supervision process within nursing care, *Journal of Advanced Nursing*, 24(1): 151–61.

Sirola-Karvinen, P. and Hyrkäs, K. (2008), Administrative clinical supervision as evaluated by the first-line managers in one health care organization district, *Journal of Nursing Management*, 16(5): 588–600.

Swanljung, S. (1995), *Hoitotyön työnohjaus työnohjaajina toimivien sairaanhoitajien kokemana* [Clinical supervision in nursing as experienced by RN supervisors], Master's thesis, Tampere, Finland: University of Tampere, Department of Nursing Science.

Toivakka, I. (2005), *Työnohjaus johtamisen ja työyhteisön kehittämisen välineenä sosiaali- ja terveydenhuollossa* [Clinical supervision as a tool for management and developing work communities in social work and public health care], Master's thesis, Kuopio, Finland: University of Kuopio, Faculty of Health Care Administration and Finances.

Vuorinen, R., Meretoja, R. and Eriksson, E. (2005), Hoitotyön ohjatun harjoittelun sisältö, edellytykset ja vaikutukset–systemoitu kirjallisuuskatsaus [The contents, preconditions and influences of guided clinical practice – a systematic review], *Hoitotiede [Nursing Science]*, 17(5): 270–281.

27 Personal, professional and practice development

Case studies from clinical supervision practice in psychiatric/mental health nursing

John R. Cutcliffe

This chapter focuses on efforts to contribute to the evidence-base for clinical supervision (CS) and attempts to advance the extant qualitative evidence. The chapter contains a brief review of the evidence-based practice phenomena: the well-documented movement towards 'methodological pluralism', and the value of qualitative findings, specifically the utility of case study evidence, is put forward. Following this, three cases of CS are included, followed by phenomenological analysis of the cases and discussion of these findings. The findings indicate how clinical practice can be influenced (indirectly) by engaging in CS; the lived experiences can be seen to offer a deeper insight into, and evidence of, specific areas of growth and development. They indicate how the supervisee (and supervisor) can experience change as a direct result of CS and how real clinical problems can be overcome.

The editors are mindful of the long-standing dispute often phrased as the 'great quantitative-qualitative debate'. Perhaps because each of us belongs to a discipline that arguably straddles medical and social science, the editors can see the merits and limitations of studies that use either research paradigm. There is clearly a contribution to be made to the knowledge base of clinical supervision by means of qualitative inquiry; similarly in order to have the deepest, most comprehensive understanding of clinical supervision, clearly quantitative studies are necessary. A logical methodological step forward is to conduct studies that can be characterised as 'mixed methods'. It is the hope of the editors that the academe of clinicians, scholars, educationalists who are interested in forwarding the knowledge base of clinical supervision might set aside any limiting philosophical and socio-political agendas that they may have (as these agendas slowed the advance of knowledge in so many areas during the 1970s and 1980s – see Greene 2007). In a methodological pluralist stance, there remains room for retaining an allegiance to one methodological tradition (paradigm) while simultaneously accepting the legitimacy of plurality.

Acknowledgement

This chapter is based on a paper that was originally published as: Cutcliffe J.R. and Burns, J. (1998), Personal professional and practice development: clinical supervision in the *British Journal of Nursing*, 7(21): 1319–1322, and has been reproduced here with the kind permission of Mark Allen Publishing.

Introduction: evidence-based (informed) practice and clinical supervision

Health care and, with that, nursing, currently exist within the epoch of the evidence-based (or evidence-informed) practice movement. Rightly or wrongly this means that all nursing practice ought to be examined within this overarching framework.[1] Given that, in many parts of the world, clinical supervision (CS) is firmly ensconced as a key element of nursing practice, CS should therefore be subjected to the same degree of scrutiny and critique as any other element of nursing practice. To this end, this chapter focuses on efforts to contribute to the evidence base for CS in nursing and concentrates on the need for qualitative as well as quantitative evidence. It begins with a brief review of the evidence-based practice movement and the shift towards methodological pluralism. Following this the need for qualitative findings is made; more specifically the value and utility of case study evidence. Three cases of CS being provided to psychiatric/mental health (P/MH) nurses are included, followed by a phenomenological analysis of the case and discussion of these findings.

Brief overview of the movement towards methodological pluralism in the evidence-based (informed) practice movement

Though it is epistemologically inaccurate to speak of one single, unified view as to the nature and composition of evidence-based (informed) practice, these divergent views often included so-called 'hierarchies of evidence' (see, for example, Evidence-Based Medicine Working Group 1992; Sackett *et al.* 1996; Sackett *et al.* 1997). An example of such a hierarchy is provided in Box 27.1.

Such hierarchies inevitably attempt to place the different forms of evidence in some linear and taxonomic list. Furthermore, such hierarchies inescapably tend to give precedence and hegemonic positions to evidence produced from quantitative studies, or more accurately, systematic reviews of the findings from multiple quantitative studies. However, it needs to be acknowledged that such hierarchies of evidence are by no means universally accepted, particularly within health science. An alternative and well-accepted view posits that research methods within quantitative and qualitative paradigms can be regarded as a toolkit; a collection of methods that are purposefully designed to answer specific questions and discover particular types of knowledge. To attempt to place these designs (and the evidence they produce) into some artificial and linear hierarchy only serves to confuse and obfuscate. If what is needed to answer a particular problem (e.g. the comparison of the therapeutic effects of two drugs) is a meta-analysis of the current studies in one particular area, then for

---

Box 27.1   Hierarchy of evidence

Level 1: meta-analysis of a series of randomised controlled trials
Level 2: at least one well-designed randomised control trial
Level 3: at least one controlled study without randomisation
Level 4: non-experimental descriptive studies
Level 5: reports or opinions from respected authorities

Based on Muir Gray (1997)

that particular problem, that is clearly the best form of evidence. Concomitantly, if what is required to answer a particular problem (e.g. what is the lived experience of experiencing violent incidents) is rich, thorough, sophisticated understanding, then for that particular problem, that is clearly the best form of evidence.

Indeed, some definitions of evidence-based (informed) practice clearly allude to this position of multiple forms of non-hierarchical evidence. In their often quoted work, Sackett *et al.* (1996) state that evidence-based practice is:

> the conscientious, explicit and judicious use of current best evidence in making decisions about the care of individual patients.

Similarly, McKibbon and Walker (1994) offer an even less rigid definition of evidence-based practice, representing it as:

> an approach to health care that promotes the collection, interpretation and integration of valid, important and applicable patient reported, clinician observed, and research derived evidence.

Literature emanating from key evidence-based centres and institutes shows that there has been a gradual (and still growing) acceptance amongst the scientific community within health care that there is a definite role for both methodological forms (see, for example, Mueser *et al.* 1998; Fenton 2000; Florence *et al.* 2005; Roen *et al.* 2004; Pluye *et al.* 2004). Greenhalgh (1999) described this as the dissonance between the 'science' of objective measurement and the 'art' of clinical proficiency and judgement.

Pressure for the inclusion of qualitative research studies and other forms of evidence to be included within the scope of evidence-based practice came from several sources including professional academia, the social sciences, clinical psychology, nursing and medicine (particularly psychiatry). There are known phenomena that in themselves are not susceptible to quantitative processes, e.g. belief structures, feelings, interactions etc. (and an argument has been suggested which purports that much of health care may be invisible or immeasurable and, thus, not accessible using quantitative methods). Thus qualitative methods are required in order to understand the nature and complexity of these phenomena. Health care and CS, it can be argued, are inextricably bound up with human interactions, cultural contexts, existential issues, lived-experiences, and psycho-social processes. Qualitative researchers argue that these phenomena are precisely those that require qualitative methods in order to deepen our understanding of them.

Literature emanating from key evidence-based centres and institutes, and perhaps more significantly, the systematic review literature, also shows that methodological pluralism is becoming the latest orthodoxy. Inextricably linked to this development is the growing recognition and valuing of findings from qualitative studies. Moreover, the criticisms that qualitative studies can sometimes be 'isolated' and parochial in nature is being addressed by means of a number of processes, not least the development of methods for systematic review of qualitative studies and the increasing attention given to qualitative meta-synthesis (see, for example, the work emerging from the various international Cochrane Centres, such as Florence *et al.* 2005; Roen *et al.* 2004; Pluye *et al.* 2004).

Qualitative researchers do not seek to generalise their findings in the same way that a quantitative researcher might. That is, they do not seek *nomothetic* generalisations relating to universal laws and absolute 'truths'. They do seek, however, to produce *idiographic or naturalistic* generalisations. That is, generalisations about and drawn from case (Denzin and Lincoln 1994), generalisations drawn from purposeful samples who have experience of the 'case' and thus applicable to similar 'cases', questions, and problems, irrespective of the similarity between the demographic group. In clinical supervision, focused studies for example, each 'case' of nursing will bear a clear resemblance to CS as a 'whole' and any related, similar 'cases'. Denzin and Lincoln (1994: 201) make this point most cogently when they state: 'Every instance of a case or process bears the general class of phenomena it belongs to.' Thus, a process that is identified in one setting, group or population (i.e. one case), can be similarly experienced by another related setting, group or population. Thus a grounded theory concerned with how P/MH nurses are supported (as supervisees) through receiving CS, is likely to be generalisable to, and bear similarity with, any population that shares the process of engaging in CS as a supervisee.

Work on the systematic review of qualitative studies using the Joanna Briggs Institute Qualitative Assessment and Review instrument (Florence *et al.* 2005) perhaps illustrates the nature of idiographic generalisable findings. Individual researchers from UK, Spain, the US, Canada, Thailand, Hong Kong, China and Australia independently produced a meta-synthesis of qualitative studies; with 18 pairs of reviewers from diverse cultures and contexts. The results of the meta-synthesis exercise were analysed to identify the degree to which inter-reviewer agreement was achieved between these 18 pairs. In spite of the differences in background, the similarity in meaning of the synthesised findings across the participant pairs was striking. There was remarkable consistency within and between groups. Other methodological work is occurring which attempts to combine and synthesise quantitative meta-analyses and qualitative meta-syntheses (see, for example, Roen *et al.* 2004; Pluye *et al.* 2004). Accordingly, while it remains the case that quantitative methods still hold the dominant position within health science research (especially if one adopts an international perspective and examines the funding/publication patterns in different countries), there are very clear signs that there is movement within the academic community towards methodological pluralism; and a parallel recognition that the health care research academe needs both paradigms in order to achieve the most complete understanding possible.

Evaluating clinical supervision: qualitative and quantitative data

Attempts to evaluate the effect of CS on client outcomes must include both qualitative and quantitative data (Severinsson 1995; Butterworth *et al.* 1996). Each research paradigm provides particular types of knowledge and can thus answer certain research questions. Quantitative methods provide 'know that' knowledge, where as qualitative methods provide 'know how' knowledge. Therefore, with regards to evaluating the relationship between receiving CS and effects on client outcomes, qualitative methods would provide answers to such questions as: how does receiving CS affect the care provided by the supervisee? How does receiving CS affect the emotional state of the supervisee? How does the emotional state of the practitioner affect the care they subsequently provide? Quantitative methods would provide answers to such questions as: how many nurses experience the identified benefits of receiving CS? How many clients experience improvements in the care provided by nurses who receive CS? What are the differences, as experienced by clients, of care provided by nurses who receive CS and nurses who do not? While at a stage of relative infancy, there exists an emerging literature of quantitative research reports that show how CS can have an effect on client outcomes (see for example, McKee and Black 1992; Fallon *et al.* 1993; Gennis and Gennis 1993; Sox *et al.* 1998). Other (earlier) research appeared to centre around a hypothesis of CS effecting client outcomes; this hypothesis suggests that 'a happy nurse is a healthy nurse, and a healthy nurse is an effective nurse'. Thus, if qualitative data can be induced that shows how receiving CS makes nurses feel 'happier' and healthier, then our knowledge base pertaining to CS and improved client outcomes has been advanced. One such way of obtaining that qualitative research evidence would be to undertake some case studies.

Justification for case studies: the case for the idiographic

Considering the need for qualitative research the author suggests that one method of addressing this issue is case studies. Yin (1989: 23) defined a case study as an empirical inquiry that 'investigates a contemporary phenomenon within its real-life context'. Janesick (1994) added to this definition suggesting that case studies allow the writer/researcher to focus on the naturalistic, holistic, cultural and phenomenological (e.g. the lived experiences) elements of a given situation. They enable readers to juxtapose their own practice and experiences with those described in the studies, creating parallels between the case and their own actual experiences. Stake (1994) highlighted how case studies serve an epistemological function, allowing the reader to learn from actual 'real' cases. Furthermore, case studies provide detailed insight into these real situations, and enable understanding of how theoretical constructs have been applied within them. Therefore, case studies of CS provided to practitioners offer insights into the dynamics and processes involved in the 'lived world' of the supervisor, supervisee and the clients they care for. They enable readers to ask: 'How is CS making a difference to the practice of the supervisee?', 'How is the practice of the supervisee changing as a result of the CS they receive?' and 'How is the care the client receives altered by this changed practice?' Case studies can then reveal interesting patterns and commonalities; particularly, how receiving CS can influence the ways practitioners think, feel and behave and thus how the subsequent care they deliver to the clients is different, and hopefully improved. In order to have clarity and rigour, a researcher using a case study method should consider the following: the boundaries of the inquiry, the purpose/question, what unit of analysis is to be used, the design, the method of data collection and what method of analysis is to be used. Accordingly, the author will describe how each of these issues was addressed for the case studies reported on in the remainder of the chapter.

The purpose/question

The purpose of the case studies was to investigate the lived-experiences of psychiatric/mental health (P/MH) nurses as they engaged in CS.

The boundaries of the inquiry

In accordance with Stake's (1994) guidelines, the cases needed to be bounded units. Consequently, the boundaries of the inquiry corresponded with the boundaries of the CS sessions. Whatever the supervisee introduced into the session would thus also constitute legitimate data for inclusion in the case study analysis.

The unit of analysis

The unit of analysis was the CS session. In this instance each session needed to be conducted on a one-to-one basis, last for at least one hour, and needed to be facilitated by a supervisor who had a minimum experience of two years as a clinical supervisor.

The design

Yin (1989) identifies two basic types of design: the single case design and the multiple case design. Since single case designs are suggested when the case represents a typical case, a critical case, an extreme or unique case or a revelatory case, and given the current depth of understanding of the nature of what would constitute a 'typical' or 'critical' supervision session, it was prudent and appropriate to have used a multiple case design.

The method of data collection

Data was collected by audio recording the accounts of the supervisors each of whom described a recent CS session. In order to respect and maintain confidentiality, no client's or supervisee's real names were used.

The method of analysis

According to Yin (1989) there are two basic strategies for analysing case study data:

1 developing a case description;
2 employing the theoretical propositions on which the study is based to explain the case.

Consequently, since the author was concerned with obtaining an understanding of the lived-experiences of P/MH nurses and how these experiences appear to influence their practice, a phenomenological, hermeneutic analysis was undertaken.

Case study one

Terry was a 42-year-old gentleman with anxiety-related problems. During his one-to-one counselling sessions he would often bring up his concerns and worries. Whenever any move to address these concerns was initiated Terry would be silent for a while and then move on to another of his concerns. This pattern was repeated over several sessions with Terry often bringing up the same problems again and again. This pattern was raised in CS and the supervisor and supervisee focused on the process of communication rather than the content.

The supervisor encouraged the supervisee to take a step back and attempt to view the whole of the situation (taking a more global view, sometimes termed a 'helicopter' view) rather than focusing on the dynamics or issues of one session. Even though Terry asked for help and information he did not appear to be willing to accept it when offered. Therefore, they explored the possibility that perhaps airing these concerns was therapeutic in itself and that erudite answers and clever solutions were not necessary at this particular time. Perhaps the most important issue for Terry was that he needed to feel someone was listening to him.

A brief strategy was negotiated and agreed upon, that in the next session with Terry, the supervisee would be more concerned with listening and hearing rather than talking. The supervisor summed up this issue by suggesting that 'Sometimes the hardest thing to do is nothing.'

In the next session the supervisee did not attempt to provide any solutions to Terry's problems but concerned himself with communicating his interest and empathy non-verbally. Again, Terry spoke of the issues that were bothering him and his feelings and exasperation became evident. The supervisee did not say a great deal but assured Terry that he was there for him and encouraged Terry to ventilate his frustrations. At the end of the session Terry looked visibly calmer, displayed far less evidence of agitation and said 'Thanks for listening. I've been having an angry day and sometimes you just need to know that someone is hearing you.'

Case study two

Sid was a staff nurse working on a challenging behaviour unit, a feature of which was the potentially violent clinical situations that he encountered. Sid had been involved recently in a particularly stressful, violent incident where property had been damaged and the client had needed to be physically restrained. Following this incident, Sid raised the matter in CS as he was concerned about the anger he felt towards the client. He felt he would have to disengage from his role as the client's primary nurse. Sid said he could no longer work with this individual given the way he now felt about him.

The supervisor encouraged Sid to talk openly about the feelings he experienced during, and subsequent to, the incident. Sid spoke of a wide range of emotions including fear, anger, disappointment and guilt. The supervisor first offered Sid some support and reminded him that such a response to a violent situation is completely reasonable. Such intense violent situations often produce a response in the nurse that makes close interpersonal work with the client more difficult. Whittington and Wykes (1994) argued that, following such incidents, it is not unusual for the nurse to feel the need to withdraw. The supervisor felt that Sid maybe needed to give himself permission to experience these feelings and that it was okay to express them.

The supervisor and Sid then explored the value of having a formal debriefing process in place in order to allow ventilation of the feelings provoked by such incidents. This would also allow Sid (and other practitioners) to view each such incident as an opportunity for learning, both for them and for the client. Sid said he would talk to the ward staff about debriefing on his return. Importantly, as his feelings had been expressed and accepted, Sid said he felt less stressed. As his reaction had been validated as a reasonable response, not a response that should provoke feelings of guilt, he was able to avoid distancing himself or erecting barriers, and once more engage the client. The consequences of this, according to Whittington and Wykes (1994), would be to lessen the likelihood of further violent incidents and in this instance Sid was able to go on working therapeutically with the client in question.

Case study three

Nancy was a 31-year-old lady with low self-esteem who had recently separated from her long-term boyfriend. This event had a debilitating effect on her, eroding her self-confidence and further challenging her already compromised hope levels. The supervisee had chosen to adopt a humanistic approach when working with Nancy. At the same time he was keen to help Nancy move through her own process of bereavement. To this end, the supervisee was concerned with creating a safe, comfortable environment in which Nancy would be more likely to feel able to express any painful emotions.

In the early sessions very little progress was made with Nancy expressing predominantly negative self-expressions of hopelessness. The absence of any evidence of, or sense of, progression caused the supervisee to become doubtful and question whether or not he was using the appropriate approach. This was discussed in the supervision session. The supervisor encouraged the supervisee to explore and explain his rationale for choosing this particular approach over an alternative approach. Consequently, as Powell (1989) suggests, such exploration ushered the supervisee into a process of reflection. Without feeling threatened, the supervisee could consider the philosophical and theoretical constructs that were guiding his practice.

The supervisee believed that Nancy would begin to move through her own process of bereavement, in her own time, and that such a process could not be forced or coerced. The self-development and personal growth of the client was mirrored in the supervision whereby the supervisor creating the appropriate environment e.g. warmth, empathy and unconditional positive regard (Rogers 1952; Heron 1990) necessary for the supervisee's personal and professional development.

The supervisee subsequently found his own answers and moved through his own phases of development, just as he believed, given the appropriate environment, Nancy would do the same. Further sessions with Nancy thus took a similar approach, being non-directive, supportive and client-centred. When she began to feel safe enough, Nancy began to take her first steps towards resolving her bereavement, challenging some of her negative self-assumptions and adopted a more hopeful outlook.

Findings

The analysis and description of the data produced three key themes of the lived experiences of receiving CS on the practice of P/MH nurses. The findings are represented in diagramatic form by Figure 27.1. Each of these key themes is then discussed in more detail.

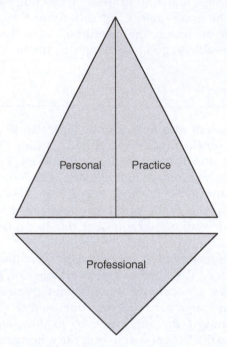

Figure 27.1 Personal, professional and practice development: the effect of receiving clinical supervision on the practice of mental health nurses.

Personal development

The essence of this key theme is the development of the practitioner as a person. It identifies that the lived experiences of engaging in CS were characterised by concerns with how the practitioner developed and refined certain qualities. Perhaps best expressed in terms of the 'lived-relations' (van Manen 1997), the interpersonal support was described by the participants as underpinning all the other processes and dynamics in supervision. This element of the lived-experiences is particularly highlighted by case study two. Just as Heron (1990) writes that his six categories of intervention need to be carried out with a supportive underpinning and that the client's well-being is paramount, this was also described as an essence of the experience of receiving CS. Data provided in the case studies indicated that CS conducted without support ceased to be enabling and started to become disabling and restrictive. Self-awareness is a pre-requisite for P/MH nursing (Peplau 1988) and thus it can be argued that any activity that enhances the development of self awareness in P/MH nurses, has the potential to enhance the nurses' practice. The lived-experiences described in case study two demonstrates the growth of self-awareness in the supervisee. In this case, as a result of engaging in CS, the supervisee realises that it is entirely understandable and reasonable to have reactions to clients and their behaviour. This supervisee developed an increased understanding that the issue is not that one has feelings, but moreover, what one actually does with (or how one manages) them that is key. According to Cutcliffe (2000: 354):

To admit that one finds things difficult, or that one's feelings are provoked, essentially, that one is human, is no crime or case for misconduct. Quite the opposite, it is only when such feelings and issues are brought 'into the light' that they can be explored, understood and learned from.

Professional development

The essence of this key theme is the development of the P/MH nurse as a professional. It identifies that the lived experiences of engaging in CS were characterised by helping the P/MH nurse examine, reflect on and address professional issues. The case studies illustrate a dynamic which is described by Hawkins and Shohet (1989) as 'mirroring'. Supervisees' experiences of CS described how some of the processes occurring in the CS mirrored those processes that occurred in the interaction with clients. Participants described how supervisors acted as a role model in demonstrating ways that the supervisee can develop as a professional. For example, the supervisors model the use of 'challenging skills' (see Cutcliffe and Epling 1997). Accordingly, supervisees experienced the therapeutic potential of such interventions and simultaneously were encouraged to think about how they might use these interventions to challenge restrictive and/or disabling aspects of their client's thoughts, feelings and behaviours. The cases also indicate a further theme of the lived experience, namely how the supervisee can draw upon the supervisor's experience in order to consider professional issues. That is not to suggest that the supervisor provides answers to each of the supervisee's concerns about professional issues; rather, it was experienced as a resource which the supervisee can draw upon.

Practice development

The essence of this key theme is the development of the P/MH nurse's practice. It identifies that the lived experiences of engaging in CS were characterised by helping the P/MH nurse examine particular practice problems (and successes). This theme of the lived experience is concerned with the process(es) of reflection practice (Hawkins and Shohet 1989). Indeed, without reflection, growth cannot occur (Schön 1984); without growth there is stagnation and this can only hinder the development of practice. This theme of the lived experiences describes how supervisees were encouraged to explore the possible reasons why some approaches or interventions work and when others sometimes do not. This theme is also concerned with how within supervision attempts were made to strengthen the links between theory and practice. The case studies show that having reached an impasse, the process of CS highlighted other options. Consequently, the problem was addressed, less time was spent searching for solutions, the practitioners had sound rationale for their interventions and the client consequently received a better service.

Discussion

Each of these case studies provides an example of how clinical practice can be influenced (indirectly) by engaging in CS. They do not generate a wealth of numerical data but the lived experiences do offer a deeper insight into, and evidence of, specific areas of growth and development. They indicate how the supervisee (and supervisor) can experience change as a direct result of CS and how real clinical problems were overcome. It is possible that other variables may have affected the outcome of the care. The clients could have received effective help from another source or experienced more support from their significant others. Alternatively, additional changes of the practice of the supervisee not brought about by the CS may have had an influence. Nevertheless, the case studies provide further qualitative evidence that supports the argument that receiving CS can affect the care provided by the nurses, and thus the clients can receive a better service.

If a nurse is developing as a person, as a professional and as a practitioner, her/his range or tool box of skills, attitudes and interventions is increased. The nurse is better able to engage with people, and better able to deal with her/his emotional reactions provoked by engaging with the client. Additionally the nurse has an increased ability to monitor the effect she/he is having on the client. Therefore, given all these changes and developments, it is not unreasonable to argue that the client is going to receive a better service from a nurse who has experienced these developments when compared to a nurse who has not.

As stated previously, evaluating the effectiveness of supervision requires both qualitative and quantitative data, and the use of case studies represents one way of obtaining qualitative data. Morse (1991) suggests that case studies allow an understanding of the meanings people ascribe to their particular experience and situations. Schultz (1967) states that phenomenological enquiry brings explicit clarity to the structures of the client's world; consequently, it is this clarity and understanding enabled by the case studies that highlights some of the processes of CS. Any argument used to convince sceptics of the benefits of CS would be more cogent if it included not only evidence that demonstrates that CS improves clinical practice, but in addition, evidence that explains *how* CS makes a difference to practice. Before quantifying how many supervisors and supervisees experience development and growth as a result of receiving CS, one first needs to establish what the nature of this growth is, and furthermore, how this growth and development actually occurs.

Dickoff and James' (1968) work on theory generation suggests that there are four levels of theory: factor isolating; factor relating; situation relating; and situation producing. Situation producing theory is described as the highest level of theory because the preceding levels of theory exist, in part, to enable higher level theory to be produced. Dickoff and James (1968) posit that situation producing theory can be described using the equation:

Variable A causes variable B in the presence of variable C.

The current level of theory, induced from the case studies, appears to be factor relating theory, in that the factors, CS, clinical practice and client outcomes appear to relate. Having induced this level of theory, the next logical step would be to test out the theory, and hopefully obtain quantitative evidence that then validates the relationships between these variables (and thus moving the theory to the level of situation producing theory).

Accordingly, nursing intervention (variable A) in the presence of CS (variable B) causes improved client outcome (variable C).

The qualitative data produced from each case study illustrates that the benefits to P/MH nurse practice (and consequently benefits to clients), as a result of receiving CS do not occur in isolation. Once a qualitative meta-synthesis is undertaken, enhanced practice arising out of engaging in CS may well be shown to be a widespread phenomenon. Additionally, the qualitative data paves the way for quantitative study to examine and determine how many practitioners and clients have experienced these benefits in practice.

Conclusions

Case studies can clearly add to the accumulating qualitative evidence that supports the widespread introduction of CS. They provide unique insights into the dynamics which occur, deepen our understanding of the processes and provide some tentative evidence of improved client care. The author suggests that is a need for more idiographic findings; more case studies of this nature which could produce a wealth of information about CS. Such information and data strengthen the links between receiving CS and improved client outcomes. Furthermore, each case study could then be included in a qualitative meta-synthesis of the effects of receiving CS which would then enable a solid mid-range theory to be induced.

Note

1 Though it would be inaccurate to posit the existence of only one, unified view of what the evidence-based (informed) movement actually entails.

References

Butterworth, T., Bishop, V. and Carson, J. (1996), First steps towards evaluating clinical supervision in nursing and health visiting: 1: theory, policy and practice development, a review, *Journal of Clinical Nursing*, 5(2): 127–132.

Cutcliffe, J.R. (2000), To record or not to record: documentation in clinical supervision *British Journal of Nursing*, 9(6): 350–355.

Cutcliffe, J.R. and Burns, J. (1998), Personal professional and practice development: clinical supervision, *British Journal of Nursing*, 7(21): 1319–1322

Cutcliffe, J.R. and Epling, M. (1997), An exploration of John Heron's confronting interventions within supervision: case studies from practice, *Psychiatric Care*, 4(4): 174–180.

Denzin, N.K. and Lincoln, Y.S. (1994), Part three: strategies of inquiry, in N.K. Denzin and Y.S. Lincoln (eds), *Handbook of Qualitative Research*, London: Sage, pp. 199–208.

Dickoff, J. and James, P. (1968), A theory of theories: a position paper, *Nursing Research*, 17(3): 197–203.

Evidence-Based Medicine Working Group (1992), Evidence-based medicine: a new approach to teaching the practice of medicine, *Journal of the American Medical Association*, 268(17): 2420–2425.

Fallon, W.F., Wears, R.L. and Tepas, J.J. (1993), Resident supervision in the operating room: does this impact on outcome? *The Journal of Trauma*, 35(4): 556–560.

Fenton, W.S. (2000), Evolving perspectives on individual psychotherapy for schizophrenia, *Schizophrenia Bulletin*, 26(1): 47–72.

Florence, Z., Schulz, T. and Pearson, A. (2005), Inter-reviewer agreement: an analysis of the degree to which agreement occurs when using tools for the appraisal, extraction and meta-synthesis of qualitative research findings, *The Cochrane Collaboration*, online, available at: www2.cochrane.org/colloquia/abstracts/melbourne/O-69.htm [accessed 2009].

Gennis, V.M. and Gennis, M.A. (1993), Supervision in the outpatient clinic: effects on teaching and patient care, *Journal of General Internal Medicine*, 8(7): 378–380.

Greene, J.C. (2007), *Mixed Methods in Social Inquiry*, San Francisco, CA: Wiley & Sons.

Greenhalgh, T. (1999), Narrative based medicine in an evidenced based world, *British Medical Journal*, 318(7179): 323–325.

Hawkins, P. and Shohet, R. (1989), *Supervision in the Helping Professions*, Milton Keynes: Open University Press.

Heron, J. (1990), *Helping the Client: A Creative Practical Guide*, London: Sage.

Janesick, V.J. (1994), The dance of qualitative research design: metaphor, methodolatry and meaning, in N.K. Denzin and Y.S. Lincoln (eds), *Handbook of Qualitative Research*, London: Sage, pp. 209–219.

McKee, M. and Black, N. (1992), Does the current use of junior doctors in the United Kingdom affect the quality of medical care? *Social Science and Medicine*, 34(5), 549–558.

McKibbon, K.A. and Walker, C.J. (1994), Beyond ACP Journal Club: how to harness Medline for therapy problems, *Annals of Internal Medicine*, 121(1): 125–127.

Mueser, K., Bond, G., Drake, R. and Resnick, S.G. (1998), Models of community care for severe mental illness: a review of research on case management, *Schizophrenia Bulletin*, 24(1): 37–74.

Muir Gray, J.A. (1997), *Evidence-Based Health Care*, Edinburgh: Churchill Livingstone.

Peplau, H. (1988), *Interpersonal relations in Nursing*, 2nd edn, New York: GP Putnam.

Pluye, P., Grad, R., Dunikowski, L. and Stephenson, R. (2004), *A Challenging Mixed Literature Review Experience*, 12th Cochrane Colloquium, The International Cochrane Collaboration, Ottawa, formerly online and available at: www. cochrane.org/colloquia/abstracts/ottawa/0–088.htm [accessed 2009], abstract online, available at: www.imbi.uni-freiburg.de/OJS/cca/index.php/cca/article/view/2610.

Powell, J.H. (1989), The reflective practitioner in nursing, *Journal of Advanced Nursing*, 14(10): 824–832.

Roen, K., Rodgers, R., Arai, L., Petticrew, M., Popay, J., Roberts, H. and Sowden, H. (2004), *Narrative Synthesis of Qualitative and Quantitative Evidence: An Analysis of Tools and Techniques*, 12th Cochrane Colloquium, The International Cochrane Collaboration, Ottawa, formerly online and available at: www.cochrane.org/ colloquia/abstracts/ottawa/0–058.htm [accessed 2009], abstract online, available at: www.imbi.uni-freiburg.de/OJS/cca/index.php/cca/article/view/2580.

Rogers, C. (1952), *Client Centred Therapy: Its Current Practice, Implications and Theory*, London: Constable.

Sackett, D.L., Rosenberg, W.M., Gray, J.A., Haynes, R.B. and Richardson, W.S. (1996), Evidence-based medicine: what it is and what it isn't, *British Medical Journal*, 312(7023): 71–72.

Sackett, D.L., Richardson, W.S., Rosenberg, W.M. and Haynes, R.B. (1997), *Evidenced-Based Medicine: How to Practice and Teach EBM*, London: Churchill Livingstone.

Schön, D. (1984), *The Reflective Practitioner*, New York: Basic Books.

Schultz, A. (1967), *The Phenomenology of the Social World*, Evanston, IL: Northern Western University Press.

Severinsson, E. (1995), The phenomenon of clinical supervision in psychiatric health care, *Journal of Psychiatric and Mental Health Nursing*, 2(5): 301–309.

Sox, C.M., Burstin, H.R., Orav, E.J., Conn, A., Setnik, G., Rucker, D.W., Dasse, P. and Brennan, T.A. (1998), The effect of supervision of residents on quality of care in five university-affiliated emergency departments, *Academic Medicine*, 73(7): 776–782.

Stake, R.E. (1994), Case studies, in N.K. Denzin and Y.S. Lincoln (eds), *Handbook of Qualitative Research*, London: Sage, pp. 236–247.

Van Manen, M. (1997), *Researching Lived Experience: Human Science for Action Sensitive Pedagogy*, New York: State University of New York Press.

Whittington, R. and Wykes, T. (1994), An observational study of associations between nurse behaviour and violence in psychiatric hospitals, *Journal of Psychiatric and Mental Health Nursing*, 1(2): 85–92.

Yin, R.K. (1989), *Case Study Research: Design and Methods*, Newbury Park: Sage.

Part V

International perspectives and developments in the state of the science of clinical supervision

28 The state of the science of clinical supervision in Australia and New Zealand

Lisa Lynch, Kerrie Hancox and Brenda Happell

In this chapter the authors draw attention to the relatively short history of clinical supervision in Australia and New Zealand. The chapter illuminates the development of clinical supervision and guidelines in the different jurisdictions since publication of *Fundamental Themes in Clinical Supervision*. The authors discuss the importance of a clearly defined concept, of leadership to expand the availability of clinical supervision to all nurses and of the need for evaluation research in order to systematically assess clinical supervision during its development. Contemporary research efforts are also featured.

We believe that this chapter is very interesting for educators, administrators and clinical supervisors. The authors focus on describing the core elements and challenges regarding the development and evolution of clinical supervision within a short time-frame. A reader can also find similarities between the authors' experiences with valuable learnings described in this chapter and occasions when clinical supervision is first introduced in an organisation unfamiliar with the concept.

Introduction

Clinical supervision (CS) for nurses in Australia and New Zealand in many ways has mirrored the experience of our nursing colleagues in the United Kingdom. Synergies can be found in the literature, in policy statements from the Departments of Health, nursing boards, peak professional and industrial bodies, from individual organisations and nurses' lived experience. Our struggles to universally define, implement and evaluate CS are not unique; similar struggles have been identified throughout the world – CS for nurses remains a global challenge (Lynch and Happell 2008; White and Winstanley 2009).

An overview of CS in Australia and New Zealand is an interesting but relatively brief experience – CS was almost non-existent in the local nursing literature until the late 1990s where a smattering of publications were found (Ryan 1998; Yegdich 1999). Since that time CS gained momentum in the mental health nursing field with a significant increase in the volume of literature since 2000.

Much of the early literature on CS for nurses in Australia focused on trying to define what was and was not meant by CS. A lack of clear definition had led to the perpetuation of myths and different meanings of CS attributed to it across practice settings. Many nurses perceived CS as *'clinical snoopervision'* or a process linked with line management (Faugier 1994; Mackereth 1996; Platt-Koch 1986; Riordan 2002;

Ryan 1998; Yegdich 1999) and often saw a clinical supervisor as someone 'who directs, inspects, controls, and evaluates the nurses' work' (Platt-Koch 1986: 4).

There is also the added issue of other words being used interchangeably with CS, the most common being preceptorship and mentorship. However additional terms include management supervision, buddy systems, reflective practice, clinical education and more recently practice development (Lynch *et al.* 2008). A clear distinction between these terms and CS is a necessary precursor to the successful introduction of CS. However a recent review of the literature in Australia from 2000 until today using PUBMED, MEDLINE EbscoHost, MEDLINE OvidSP, CINAHL and E-Journal demonstrated that there is still considerable confusion regarding descriptors for CS. A search on the key word CS uncovered a vast array of different articles and texts on CS that may or may not be applicable to the topic. In light of this, the literature search included the following key words: CS, preceptorship, mentorship, clinical education, practice development and psychiatric/mental health nursing.

In this chapter the Australian experience of CS will be explored using the following framework:

- rationale and purpose
- leadership
- implementation and evaluation.

Rationale and purpose: why clinical supervision for Australian nurses?

Much attention has been drawn to the crisis in the recruitment and retention of nurses in Australia. This current nursing crisis is based on research and anecdotal evidence, which suggests that all nations are facing a serious nursing shortage (Daly *et al.* 2004). In addition to the concern regarding global shortages, extensive local studies such as the Australian Institute of Health and Welfare (AIHW 2009) *Report on the Australian Nursing and Midwifery Labour Force* and the Australian Institute of Health and Welfare (AIHW 2008) *Report on Mental Health Services in Australia 2005–2006* highlight that the nursing workforce continues to age. Nurses working in mental health are more likely to work full time, are slightly older on average, and much more likely to be male than nurses in the general workforce (AIHW 2008). There has been a 1.4 per cent average annual increase in the average age of mental health nurses since 2001. The average age of employed mental health nurses in 2005 was 46.4 years. Female nurses working in mental health nursing were younger, on average, than their male counterparts (45.8 years compared with 47.7 years). These reports clearly highlight the reality facing Australian nurses as a substantial proportion of the nursing workforce is moving closer to retirement age.

The Australian studies also identified that nursing work is highly stressful and there is poor job satisfaction, linked to high staff turnover. Nursing workloads, stress and burnout, workplace violence and aggression, for example, are frequently identified as major factors contributing to nurses leaving the profession (Daly *et al.* 2004; White and Winstanley 2009).

CS has been identified as one possible solution to the nursing crisis. It is considered to be an important strategy in recruiting and retaining high quality staff and decreasing stress and burnout (Ashmore and Carver 2000; Akerjordet and Severinsson 2004; Lynch and Happell 2008; Walker 2009; White and Winstanley 2009; Winstanley 2000).

Parker (2004) describes the complex and extraordinary pressure that impinge upon nurses working in medical areas on a daily basis. She draws upon psychoanalytic theories to investigate some of the seemingly straightforward and taken for granted areas of a medical nurse's work, and considers the valuable role CS could play in supporting medical nurses.

The importance of CS for nurses within the primary care setting has recently emerged. Daly and Bryant (2007) and Keleher *et al.* (2007) highlight the expanding nurse role in primary care with practice nurses being employed in approximately 60 per cent of all general practices and being allocated an increasing number of items in the Medicare Benefits Schedule, including in the area of mental health. *The authors note the need for appropriate and effective CS to ensure quality nursing care and optimal health outcomes and advocate for the development of guidelines for practice nurse supervision.*

Leadership

An exploration into the introduction of CS in Australia identifies a number of jurisdictions that began the process of implementing CS in the early 2000s. A review of official documents and websites suggests that, rather than a coordinated Australia-wide strategy of implementing CS led by government and peak nursing bodies, the leadership in this area appears to have originated from academic clinicians and professional and industrial bodies. *Consistency across Australia is therefore more likely to reflect the networking and information sharing efforts of key nursing leaders than a clearly developed and systematic implementation plan.*

The authorities responsible for the registration of nurses in Australia and New Zealand have no guidelines on CS of their own. When we first made the enquiry, they started to talk about developing guidelines for CS; it quickly became apparent that the understanding of CS we have was not held by the registering bodies. Each of the registering boards spoke of CS as the direct observation, critique and assessment of nurses doing their work. Some of the Boards indicated that they felt the responsibility for providing guidelines lay with organisations – that they should provide the guidance for their employees. *What was most apparent was the lack of a shared understanding as to what CS is.* CS is a term widely used in both generalist and mental health nursing, but it seemed the Boards were more familiar with the generalist understanding. Every conversation we had with a Registering body required a clarification of terms as they all related CS to teaching, direct observation and assessment of skill.

In Victoria, as a result of Enterprise Bargaining Agreements, the Mental Health Branch of the Department of Human Services announced the injection of considerable funds to support mental health nursing within the state. CS was identified as a key strategy. The implementation of CS was left to individual organisations rather than to a centralised/coordinated approach. Clinicians began to look to the Centre for Psychiatric Nursing Research and Practice (CPNRP), now called the Centre for Psychiatric Nursing (CPN) for key directions and guidance, and at the request of the senior nurses struggling with the task of implementing supervision, the CPNRP formed a working party consisting of key nursing leaders in the field to develop guidelines for CS in Victoria. This document was not published but became the catalyst for the Department of Human Services, Victoria to develop guidelines.

The resulting Clinical Supervision Guidelines (2006) state that CS refers to

> a formal, structured process of professional support. Supervision assists staff to understand issues associated with their practice, to gain new insights and perspectives, and to develop their knowledge and skills while supporting staff and improving consumer and carer outcomes. Clinical supervision may involve individual, group or peer approaches and can be informed by a variety of theoretical perspectives.
>
> (Department of Human Services, Victoria 2006: 1)

It is essential to note that, in addition to a definition, the guidelines from the Department of Human Services, Victoria attempt to address some of the identified myths about CS. They separate CS from line management supervision by highlighting that the focus is on professional development and not on monitoring performance. They also compare and contrast other forums that are often confused with CS such as preceptorship and mentorship.

Being able to define CS is considered essential to nurses' understanding of and participation in CS. Adopting a clear definition that dispels the myths and misconceptions should therefore form the basis for all implementation strategies (Mackereth 1996). This was a very positive aspect to the Victorian Guidelines that should be commended and acknowledged.

However despite the robust definition and clear description of what CS is and is not, the document then only provides a vague philosophical overview supporting the benefits of CS for nurses. Rather than providing guidance, the document delegated the responsibility for selecting and developing models of CS to individual mental health services. This document has not been expanded on since its release: as a result the leadership in Victoria is not clear and support for those implementing CS in their organisation is limited.

In some jurisdictions guidelines are being developed to support the understanding and implementation of CS. The first set of guidelines were published in 2005 in Western Australia, and provided a much more comprehensive document than the brief communiqué published by the Department of Human Services in Victoria. The Western Australian (Department of Health 2005) document provides a definition and an overview of the value of CS. It delineates the roles of supervisor and supervisee, suggests some preferred models of supervision and describes how the supervisory relationship should be initiated and developed. Ethical issues and procedural matters (such as how to deal with conflict should it emerge) are addressed. Examples of supervision agreements, schedules and record notes are included. However, it does not address the broader issue of how CS can be implemented.

Queensland Health released guidelines for CS within Mental Health Services in October 2009. This is a bold and comprehensive document that applies to medical staff, mental health nurses, allied health, indigenous mental health staff, consumer and carer workforce and other clinical staff working in Mental Health Services. This document clearly states the expectations of Queensland Health to support CS; CS is mandatory but supervisees do have input (with assistance if required) to find a clinical supervisor. They insist that the supervisors receive educational preparation for the role and receive their own CS. They also provide parameters as to the level of experience and training required to become a clinical supervisor. However, similar to the Western Australian document, the process of implementation is not considered and guidelines to assist this process are absent.

The Queensland document is detailed and it includes an approach to evaluation as well as a broad guide as to the frequency with which CS should take place, based on clinical complexity, clinician experience and role changes. The only concern relates to the assumption that an 'experienced clinician' with more than five years' practice (a mental health practitioner) only requires low frequency CS. With this comes the assumption that they are more capable of reflecting on their practice than less experienced colleagues. According to Cutcliffe and Lowe (2005) CS should be as an important career-long activity, supported by government and nursing governing bodies.

The South Australian Office of the Chief Nurse informed us that their guidelines were due to be released in December 2009; the latest position known is that a document is available internally only, the *SA Health Guideline Clinical Supervision Policy – Mental Health Nurses*, effective from March 2010. The Tasmanian office of the Chief Nurse indicated that they do not currently have specific guidelines and have devolved this responsibility to the local service. The chief nurses in the Australian Capital Territory (ACT) and New South Wales were not aware of any CS guidelines. In the ACT, CS was well established in the culture within mental health. They had invested money in providing education for their supervisors, follow up education a year after the initial beginning and used the same educators to provided organisational support for their implementation strategy. The Office of the Chief Nurse ACT had a good understanding of CS and is very keen to introduce the same level of education and support within the acute sector. The Office of the Chief Nurse in Northern Territory is currently developing guidelines. The Office of the Chief Nurse in New Zealand referred to its Registration Board who also do not have guidelines.

The Royal College of Nurses referred to CS as the direct observation, teaching and assessment of skills. They had no information on their website (www.rcna.org.au). The Australian College of Mental Health Nurses (ACMHN) had information on CS readily accessible posted on their website, under 'Career Resources', demonstrating support for CS (www.acmhn.org). The information reads like a position statement although it is not identified as one. It provides some clarification of terms and provides some guidance about the boundaries this formal relationship needs to have in order to differentiate it from other relationships. The ACMHN also has a credentialing programme that encourages nurses to take up CS through allocating points for nurses engaging in the process.

Te Ao Maramatanga – New Zealand College of Mental Health Nurses – does not have information on the website (www.nzcmhn.org.nz) but there is a link to Te Pou website that has National Guidelines for Professional Supervision for nurses working in addiction (Te Pou 2010). The information is difficult to find in part because they called CS professional supervision in the document and there are no indicators as to where the information can be found. It is also written specifically for addiction nurses even though the principles would be relevant for all.

Whilst we need to acknowledge the financial support provided by government and the efforts to establish guidelines, communications with nurses with direct involvement with the implementation of CS for nurses, suggests the process has not been carefully considered, planned and/or evaluated. *While there is significant anecdotal evidence to suggest that CS is now better understood and more available as a result of this initiative, the absence of formalised guidelines and systematic evaluation makes it difficult to estimate how successful the Australia-wide implementation of CS has been.*

The experience in New Zealand is similar to that in Australia. From 2003 to 2009 there was a large increase in the number of senior nurse positions in district health boards and non-government organisations providing nursing education and professional development. One of the roles of these senior nurses is that of clinical supervisor. Despite the New Zealand's Nursing Organisation's *Professional and Clinical Supervision Position Statement* (NZNO 2008), supervision is not readily available to all nurses. The main reasons provided for this includes resource constraints within nursing services and competing priorities (Walker 2009).

Implementation and evaluation

The absence of clear leadership and guidelines from government and nursing professional (registration) bodies is one factor that contributed to the many difficulties associated with the implementation of CS (Riordan 2002; Lynch *et al.* 2008; Spence *et al.* 2002).

The importance of a planned, systematic approach to the implementation of supervision has been described in the scholarly literature. This has been observed to be crucial to the successful introduction of CS and CS texts have included chapters addressing the implementation process (Bond and Holland 1998; Driscoll 2000; Lynch *et al.* 2008; Riordan 2002; Spence *et al.* 2002).

Despite the obvious importance of evaluating the implementation of CS there have only been a handful of studies exploring implementation in Australia. Each of these studies has examined the implementation of CS from a slightly different perspective. Other Australian studies that specifically explore implementation of note will be explored briefly below in relation to the key findings (Walsh *et al.* 2003; White and Roche 2006; White and Winstanley 2009).

A project in north-west Sydney was developed to improve access for all clinical staff and managers to CS (Lifiton *et al.* 2005). The mission statement for the project is for all clinical (medical, allied health and nursing) and management staff to have CS for at least 50 minutes once per month. Using a clinical practice methodology the diagnostic phase commenced in 1998 and concluded in February 2004.

Baseline data was collected from a phone survey to ascertain the number of staff receiving supervision and number of staff trained. The results highlighted that only 36 per cent of staff received CS, 16 per cent were trained in supervision and only 10 per cent of staff provide supervision. The team explored the possible reasons for the poor uptake of CS and devised two main strategies as possible solutions to the problems. These were:

1   Increase education about CS.
2   Increase the number of trained clinical supervisors.

A subsequent survey indicated that there had been some improvement by May 2005: 43 per cent of staff were receiving supervision, 39 per cent were trained and 11 per cent were providing CS. The team also reported a noticeable change in culture across the service and is keen to maintain the momentum for acceptance and commitment to CS. A more detailed project plan was developed but no further progress has been documented at this time.

Walsh *et al.* (2003) describe the development of a group model of CS to meet the needs of community mental health nurses. The initial impetus for a new model of CS arose from a group of nurses who were dissatisfied with the models of supervision they had been exposed to, including models that appeared to resemble line management supervision. Group supervision was determined to be the most appropriate starting point and the Proctor Model (Proctor 1986) provided the framework for each CS session. The group sessions were monthly and one and half hours in duration. The group started closed but agreed to admit new members as new staff joined the team.

The implementation of the six-month pilot group CS sessions was evaluated using a questionnaire (Walsh *et al.* 2003) The overall findings were positive and the group displayed a high degree of commitment with nearly 100 per cent attendance at all sessions. It was noted, following the formal evaluation, that perhaps the group in their attempt to be 'extra' supportive did not sufficiently challenge each other. The group was intending to explore ways to supportively challenge themselves and their peers within the CS sessions.

White and Roche (2006) conducted a scoping study of the implementation of CS for mental health nurses in the state of New South Wales. Scoping CS for mental health nurses in NSW presented the authors with a number of significant challenges, the first of which was trying to identify how to access all mental health nurses. The Registration Board did not keep a separate register and Area Mental Health Nurses could not easily identify all their mental health nurses. A sample of mental health nurses (n = 601) provided data for the study.

All Area Mental Health Services reported that some or all of their staff had CS (White and Roche 2006). However this was not widespread – in fact over two-thirds stated they did not have access to CS. The remaining third had supervision for less than two years. The majority of time in supervision was focused on reflecting on clinical work, with some time being used for organisational issues. Increased confidence, insight and more positive working relationships were the main positive outcomes, and the appropriateness and credibility of the available supervisors the main barriers.

White and Winstanley (2006) conducted a comprehensive overview of CS in Australia. The authors aggregated previous unreported anonymised data from four independent evaluations on the effectiveness of CS in Australia and New Zealand, using the Manchester CS Scale (Winstanley 2000). The results of all four studies were similar in relation to the effective scores on the Manchester Scale which indicated supervision was effective. The average cost of CS represented about 1 per cent of a nurse's salary. The authors argue that CS is cost effective given the benefits in reducing stress and burnout.

White and Winstanley (2009) are currently conducting a randomised control trial (RCT) funded by the Queensland Treasury/Golden Casket Foundation. The authors refer to the lack of evidence demonstrating the impact of CS on patient care. The preparation for the RCT included a clinical supervisor training programme: this ensured preparation for the clinical supervisory role. Selection of the participants included clinicians who are well respected by their potential supervisees and local managers. The outcome measures encompass the general profile of the hospital, ward, and nurses engaging in the process. The workplace had the sickness, absence rate and staff turnover recorded; they also captured complaints and perceptions of the unit. Finally they used the Service Attachment and Psychiatric Care Satisfaction Questionnaires to capture the patient's experience. The article describes the process for conducting the RCT rather than its outcomes. The final report was due to be released in mid 2009. However no publicly available information could be accessed at the time of writing.

In addition to studies measuring the effectiveness of CS using the Manchester CS Scale (Brunero and Stein-Parbury 2008; Winstanley 2000; White and Roche 2006; White and Winstanley 2006, 2009), Hancox *et al.* (2004) conducted an in-depth evaluation into an educational programme for CS. Whilst also providing a detailed context of CS in Australia, this article explores the development of the CS for Health Care Professionals Course. The course developed by Hancox and Lynch was offered at that time through the Centre for Psychiatric Nursing Research and Practice (now the Centre for Psychiatric Nursing).

The primary aim of the course was to develop knowledge and skills in CS. The participants in the evaluation were the 63 mental health nurses who had completed the CS course. More than 500 mental health nurses have attended training with Hancox and Lynch since this study. The authors developed an evaluation instrument that consisted of two separate parts, the first section a 12 question, five point Likert scale survey. These questions sought participants' attitudes to and opinions about receiving and providing clinical supervision, their level of knowledge and confidence, and the extent to which it is important to practice. The second part included four open-ended questions. Participants were asked to describe what they considered the most helpful and least helpful aspects of the course, suggestions for improvement and how they felt completing the course would impact on their practice.

The overall findings were positive with 90 per cent reporting an increased understanding in supervision, 89 per cent stating they now consider CS to be necessary for nursing practice and are likely to seek it in their practice. Participants felt more conformable providing (87 per cent) and receiving supervision (89 per cent) and a total of 95 per cent considered their level of confidence had increased at completion of the course. Answers to the open-ended questions regarding the most helpful aspects (110 specific responses) highlighted the value of role plays, videos and group discussions. A total of 41 responses were provided the least helpful aspects of the course section with the majority commenting on the venue and facilities.

The findings from this evaluation suggest that the CS for Health Care Professionals Course made a valuable contribution to existing knowledge by highlighting the preference for a CS course that is interactive and practical. The education and training provided at the rural mental health service is now provided privately through Clinical Supervision Consultants (www.clinicalsupervision.com.au).

Conclusion

CS has become a focus of considerable attention and activity in Australia and New Zealand in recent years. Despite this there remains a paucity of formal guidelines to maintain quality standards, and a paucity of published research and evaluation to demonstrate the effectiveness of this strategy. If nurses do not become informed about clinical supervision, embrace the opportunities that are currently provided and push from the ground up it may fall off the nursing agenda. We as nurses have the responsibility to ensure that clinical supervision remains our priority – for us and for our patients/consumers.

References

AIHW (Australian Institute of Health and Welfare) (2008), *Mental Health Services in Australia 2005–06*, Mental Health Series No. 10, Cat no. HSE 56, Canberra: AIHW.

AIHW (Australian Institute of Health and Welfare) (2009), *Nursing and Midwifery Labour Force 2007*, National Health Labour Force Series No. 43, Cat. no. HWL 44, Canberra: AIHW.

Akerjordet, K. and Severinsson, E. (2004), Emotional intelligence in mental health nurses talking about practice, *International Journal of Mental Health Nursing*, 13(3): 164–170.

Ashmore, R. and Carver, N. (2000), Clinical supervision in mental health nursing courses, *British Journal of Nursing*, 9(3): 171–176.

Bond, M. and Holland, S. (1998), *Skills of Supervision for Nurses*, Oxford: Open University Press.

Brunero, S. and Stein-Parbury, J. (2008), The effectiveness of clinical supervision of nursing: an evidence based literature review, *Australian Journal of Advanced Nursing*, 25(3): 86–94.

Cutcliffe, J.R. and Lowe, L. (2005), A comparison of North American and European conceptualizations of clinical supervision, *Issues in Mental Health Nursing*, 26(5): 475–488.

Daly, J. and Bryant, R. (2007), Professional organisations and regulatory bodies: Forging and advancing the role of nurses in Australian primary care, *Contemporary Nurse*, 26(1): 27–29.

Daly, J., Speedy, S. and Jackson, D. (2004), *Nursing Leadership*, Marrickville, NSW: Elsevier.

Department of Health, Western Australia (2005), *Clinical Supervision, Framework for WA Mental Health Services and Clinicians*, pp. 1–9, online, available at: www.health.wa.gov.au/docreg/Education/Population/Health_Problems/Mental_Illness/HP3095_Clinical_supervision_framework_for_WA_mental_health.pd.

Department of Human Services, Victoria (2006), *Clinical Supervision Guidelines*, online, available at: www.health.vic.gov.au/mentalhealth/pmc/clinical-super.pdf.

Driscoll, J. (2000), *Practicing Clinical Supervision: A Reflective Approach*, London: Balliere Tindall.

Faugier, J. (1994), Thin on the ground, *Nursing Times*, 90(20): 64–65.

Hancox, K., Lynch, L., Happell, B. and Biondo, S. (2004), An evaluation of an educational program for clinical supervision, *International Journal of Mental Health Nursing*, 13(3): 195–203.

Keleher, H., Joyce, J., Parker, R. and Piterman, L. (2007), Practice nurses in Australia: current issues and future directions, *Medical Journal of Australia*, 187(2): 108–110.

Lifiton, B., Ovenden, J., James, P., Stone, C., Codd, A., Bains, J., Revson, K. and McMahon, L. (2005), Clinical supervision for clinical and management staff, *The Australian Resource Centre for Healthcare Innovations* (ARCHI), online, available at: www.archi.net.au/e-library/awards/baxter05/competence/ management_supervision.

Lynch, L. and Happell, B. (2008), Implementing clinical supervision: Part 1 Laying the ground work, *International Journal of Mental Health Nursing* 17(1): 57–64.

Lynch, L., Hancox, K., Happell, B. and Parker, J. (2008), *Clinical Supervision for Nurses*, Oxford: Wiley-Blackwell.

Mackereth, P. (1996), Clinical supervision for 'potent' practice, *Complementary Therapies in Nursing and Midwifery*, 3(2): 38–41.

NZNO (New Zealand Nursing Organisation) (2008), *Professional and Clinical Supervision*, online, available at: www.nzno.org.nz/Portals/0/publications/ 79Professional and Clinical Supervision.pdf.

Parker, J.M. (2004), Nursing on the medical ward, in J.M. Parker, *A Body of Work: Writings on Nursing*, Bournemouth: Nursing Praxis Press International.

Platt-Koch, L.M. (1986), Clinical supervision for psychiatric nurses, *Journal of Psychosocial Nursing*, 24(1): 7–15.

Proctor, B. (1986), Supervision: a cooperative exercise in accountability, in M. Marken and M. Payne (eds), *Enabling and Ensuring*, Leicester: National Youth Bureau, pp. 21–23.

Queensland Health (2009), *Clinical Supervision Guidelines for Mental Health Services*, Queensland Government, pp. 1–37.

Riordan, B. (2002), Why nurses choose not to undertake CS: the findings from one ICU, *Nursing in Critical Care*, 7(2): 59–66.

Ryan, T. (1998): *Clinical Supervision in Mental Health Nursing*, online, available at: www.clinical-supervision.com.

Spence, C., Cantrell, J., Christie, I. and Samet, W. (2002), A collaborative approach to the implementation of clinical supervision, *Journal of Nursing Management*, 10(2): 65–74.

Te Pou (2010), *Professional Supervision*, online, available at: www.tepou.co.nz/page/ 289.

Walsh, K., Nicholson, J., Keough, C., Pridham, R., Kramer, M. and Jeffery, J. (2003), Development of a group model of clinical supervision to meet the needs of a community mental health nursing team, *International Journal of Nursing Practice*, 9(1): 33–39.

Walker, J. (2009), Examining the benefits of professional clinical supervision, *Kai Tiaki Nursing New Zealand*, 15(5): 12–14.

White, E. and Roche, M. (2006), A selective review of mental health nursing in New South Wales, Australia, in relation to clinical supervision, *International Journal of Mental Health Nursing*, 15(3): 209–219.

White, E. and Winstanley, J. (2006), Cost and resource implications of clinical supervision in nursing: an Australian perspective, *Journal of Nursing Management*, 14(8): 628–636.

White, E. and Winstanley, J. (2009), Clinical supervision for nurses working in mental health settings in Queensland, Australia: a randomised controlled trial in progress and emergent challenges, *Journal of Research in Nursing*, 14(3): 263–276.

Winstanley, J. (2000), Manchester clinical supervision scale, *Nursing Standard*, 14(19): 31–32.

Yegdich, T. (1999), Clinical supervision and managerial supervision: some historical and conceptual considerations, *Journal of Advanced Nursing*, 30(5): 1195–1204.

29 The state of the science of clinical supervision in Europe

Ingela Berggren and Elisabeth Severinsson

This chapter focuses on the state of clinical supervision science in various parts of Europe based on an extensive literature review. The authors draw the reader's attention to the research evidence regarding concept, theories and models applied in clinical supervision. They also synthesise the literature regarding: the different styles used by supervisors; ethical issues; and effects of clinical supervision. At the end the authors provide the contextual description of clinical supervision. This extensive work was accomplished by utilising a systematic approach inspired by Burns and Grove (2001).

We believe that this chapter is valuable for researchers and clinical supervisors and supervisees conducting research. It is very important in terms of the number of papers which the authors have reviewed and synthesised. And it is interesting in terms of the number of papers that are published today on clinical supervision and also their predominant locus in the UK and Scandinavia rather than throughout Europe. Still, the activities of those conducting research on clinical supervision are providing a rich body of knowledge that is very valuable to the profession as a whole.

Background

Over the past two decades there has been an increase in research on clinical supervision (CS) both in Scandinavia and other parts of Europe. *This chapter presents a critical synthesis of the published literature related to CS from a European perspective.* We searched for literature on CS in different electronic databases for the period 2000–2009. In this chapter we will describe the concept of CS, the different styles used by supervisors, the ethical issues involved and the effects of CS. In order to critically analyse the state of knowledge on the topic of CS, the following research questions were addressed:

1. What evidence can be found in the literature about how CS is described, defined and measured?
2. What theoretical perspectives, models, ethical issues and contextual descriptions of practice are reported?
3. Is there evidence that CS affects clinical practice?

A search of the Ovid online health databases including Academic search Elite, Medline, PubMed, CINAHL and PsychInfo was performed in November 2008 and covered the period 2000–2008, with an additional search covering January–August 2009. The main keywords employed were clinical supervision and nursing.

The inclusion criteria were peer-reviewed studies dealing with CS and published in the English language. The exclusion criterion was CS related to nursing students. The literature review was carried out by means of skimming, comprehending, analysing and synthesising of sources inspired by Burns and Grove (2001). The skimming process included a review of 102 papers. We grouped and presented the authors, titles and aims in table form in order to obtain an overview of the most prevalent information. Comprehension presupposes an understanding of the papers' theories, the models discussed therein and evidence of the effects of CS. Thereafter we analysed the methods used and the findings of each paper to gain an overview i.e. a synthesis of the contents. This phase included formulating an additional table to present different aspects of the research questions.

The state of the science

A great deal of previous research consists of literature reviews on the *concept* of CS, e.g. Sloan, White and Coit (2000), Sloan and Watson (2001b), Sloan and Watson (2002), Cotrell (2002), Howatson-Jones (2003), Jukes *et al.* (2004), Bush (2005), Sloan (2005), Turner (2005), Coleman and Lynch (2006), Sirola-Karvinen and Hyrkäs (2006), Jones (2006a), Shanley and Stevenson (2006), Rice *et al.* (2007), Butterworth *et al.* (2007), Cummins (2009) and Buus and George (2009). In the *empirical studies*, qualitative methods (N=35) dominated over quantitative ones (N=16) and five employed mixed methods.

Definitions, different theories and models applied in CS

There are several *definitions* of CS in contemporary professional literature. Lyth (2000) proposes a definition in his concept analysis and underlines the difficulty of clarifying the concept, since nursing practice varies. However, the definition based on Lyth's analysis is as follows:

> Clinical supervision is a support mechanism for practising professionals within which they can share clinical, organizational, developmental and emotional experiences with another professional in a secure, confidential environment in order to enhance knowledge and skills. This process will lead to an increased awareness of other concepts including accountability and reflective practice.
>
> (Lyth 2000: 728)

Another concept analysis (Tveiten 2005) asserted that CS can be defined 'as a formal, pedagogical, relational enabling process, related to professional competence' (p. 17). However, Williams *et al.* (2005) and Rice *et al.* (2007) hold that there is confusion regarding the definitions of CS and, although there are similarities between them, no definition has been universally accepted.

The literature review revealed different *theories and models* applied in CS. In a quantitative study, Veeramah (2002) found that the CS framework consists of *theories of psychotherapy* (98 per cent), theories based on the *humanistic* (20 per cent) and the *behavioural* schools (19 per cent). According to Arvidsson and Fridlund (2005), nurse supervisors need to include more *nursing theory* in their supervisory methods. Berg and Kisthinios (2007) found that only three-quarters of approved clinical nursing supervisors stated that they employed a theoretical nursing perspective when supervising, hence there is obviously a need for further investigations in this area.

Several *models* used in CS are presented in the literature. Although the models are similar to each other, we will present them in some detail in order to illuminate various aspects of CS. While most CS models are based on the premise that the supervisor is a qualified nursing practitioner with expert knowledge relevant to the purpose of CS (Sloan *et al.* 2000), there is no universal agreement on a CS model (Barriball *et al.* 2004). According to Sloan and Watson (2001b), Heron's framework is a useful resource for clinical supervisors. It is a conceptual model developed for interpersonal relations containing six categories: prescriptive, informative, confronting, cathartic, catalytic and supportive. The first three categories are authoritative and the latter three facilitative. The six categories can be used as a supervision model, which according to Sloan and Watson (2001b), is an aspect that has been overlooked. Severinsson (2001) highlighted three theoretical core concepts in her CS model: confirmation, meaning and self-awareness. However, Sloan and Watson (2002) hold that no single supervision model suits all nursing contexts. The authors argued that those participating in CS should decide on the choice of framework. There is no empirical support for any of the supervision models referred to in the article. A quantitative study (Bradshaw *et al.* 2007) revealed tentative support for the development of new workplace-based CS models.

There is considerable variation in the frequency and duration of CS (Veeramah 2002; Barriball *et al.* 2004), which can be *organised* individually and/or in group sessions. In a group CS model with 4–6 members, the supervisor can employ an individual approach, even when the CS structure is based on group interaction (Barriball *et al.* 2004). Veeramah (2002) found that most CS was provided on a one-to-one basis (60 per cent) and that only 6 per cent comprised group CS. The sessions took place on a monthly (60 per cent) or bi-monthly (24 per cent) basis.

A *systematic structure* helps the supervisee to reflect, analyse, solve problems, plan actions and learn for future practice. In a quantitative study of CS methods, Veeramah (2002) found that nearly half (48 per cent) have a formal structure comprising contracts, rules and records. The nurses had received some initial training to prepare them for the role of supervisee (59 per cent), while 79 per cent of supervisors had been trained for their role. Thompson and Winter (2003) examined a National Health Service (NHS) Direct centre in the United Kingdom that provided facilities for nurses to take part in *telephone supervision* as a means of meeting their professional development requirements and reflecting on their practice in a structured way. The process is supported by a dedicated database. To some extent, the methods employed mirrored those used in contact with patients.

Different styles used by supervisors in CS

The clinical nurse *supervisor's style* is of importance for the outcome of CS and has been investigated by researchers including Sloan and Watson (2001a) and Berggren and Severinsson (2006). Sloan (2005) focused on the processes and attributes at the beginning of the supervisory relationship and claimed that this is a neglected aspect. In keeping with the different styles, some researchers have also extended the perspective focus on examining the supervisor's role. According to Sloan (2005), the characteristics of a good supervisor from the supervisee's perspective are an ability to form supportive relationships, relevant knowledge, clinical skills, a commitment to providing supervision and good listening skills. Furthermore, the supervisees considered their supervisor as a role model who inspired them and whom they held in high esteem due to his/her clinical practice and knowledge base. According to Sloan and Watson (2001a), the supervisors' role included reflecting on and conveying an understanding of client issues. According to Cerinus (2005), the development of the relationship is an essential component of effective CS. Furthermore, Knutton and Pover (2004) underlined the interdependence of honesty and challenge in CS. Similar findings were reported by Rice *et al.* (2007) in relation to mental health nurses. Cottrell (2002) highlighted the need for clarity, openness and collaboration during the CS introduction process as a means of preventing 'resistance, suspicion, tokenism or interpersonal difficulties' (p. 667).

According to Arvidsson and Fridlund (2005), nurse supervisors need to be aware of their own shortcomings and resources as well as have opportunities to discuss problems with a more experienced nurse supervisor. Sloan identified limitations in the supervisory process (2005), such as when the supervisees' manager is appointed their clinical supervisor, since a CS session documented by one's manager defeats the purpose of CS. However, Agélii *et al.* (2000) have pointed out that the supervisor–supervisee relationship may lead to an unusual set of ethical problems that arise from the supervisor's contradictory roles. The supervisor strives to preserve the rights and dignity of both patients and nurses and to take responsibility for the way in which supervision is carried out. Veeramah (2002) has pointed to the need for both supervisor and supervisee to attend CS training sessions.

Ethical issues related to CS

There is little previous research on *ethical issues* in relation to CS. However, CS is one way of creating a caring environment where ethical issues can be reflected upon (Lyth 2000). It has a systematic structure that: helps the supervisee to reflect, analyse, solve problems; plan actions and learn for future practice; and focuses on nurse–patient interaction. In CS the supervisors are morally responsible for applying the process and establishing a relationship with supervisees. Severinsson (2001) stated that the view of the human being includes an ethical aspect in the form of supervision norms and that supervisors should possess competencies such as self-awareness, an action repertory, motivation and skills. Bégat and Severinsson (2001) also pointed out the ethical dimension of CS, for example, in the supervisor's obligation to develop the supervisee's moral responsibility.

Determined efforts have to be made to influence organisations to give nurses the support they need in their everyday work, thereby enabling them to provide 'good care'. According to Magnusson *et al.* (2002), 'to do good' means making decisions for the patient when his/her health may be in danger. Berggren and Severinsson (2006) described nurse supervisors' different ethical decision-making styles and found that these are important for the outcome of CS, especially as the supervisors are role models. A genuine encounter, consciousness of one's own core values, confirmation and forming a relationship were described by nurse supervisors as the caring values of nursing supervision (Johansson *et al.* 2006). According to Berggren *et al.* (2005), the core ethical issues in CS are caring, dignity, responsibility and virtue. It can be assumed that one effect of studies of CS will be an increased understanding of ethical issues.

Effects of CS

CS has been investigated in terms of its *influence on the team* around the patient and *quality of care*. For example, Hyrkäs and Paunonen-Ilmonen (2001: 492) highlighted the effects of CS on multiprofessional teams and quality of care. Furthermore, Hyrkäs *et al.* (2002) conducted a qualitative study on the *effect* of CS aimed at describing the experiences of five pairs of supervisors engaged in *multiprofessional team supervision*. The findings revealed that the factors that influenced team supervision were: advanced knowledge of supervision and confidence of supervisors; commitment and motivation; interaction and collaborative relationships; and the organisation of team supervision. Team supervision had a positive influence on interaction and human relationships in the work environment, and also strengthened professional identity and the development of multiprofessional practice. Rice *et al.* (2007) stated that when nurses work in a multiprofessional team it is not necessary for the supervisor to be a nurse.

The effects of CS on *professional competence* have been studied by means of qualitative (Arvidsson *et al.* 2000; Nordentoft 2008; Pettifer and Clouder 2008), quantitative (Magnusson *et al.* 2002; Veeramah 2002; Edwards *et al.* 2005) and combined methods (Teasdale *et al.* 2001; Jones 2006b). A study by Magnusson *et al.* (2002) demonstrated that health care professionals who received CS perceived themselves as more certain in terms of decision making, safer in their relationship with the patient and having gained a deeper insight into the meaning of security for both patient and provider. According to Frankel (2008), supervision can encourage the supervisees' learning in practice by applying theory. Jones (2003, 2008) asserted that CS enhances reflective capacity and strengthens the readiness and ability to assume responsibility in palliative nursing. Arvidsson *et al.* (2000) also reported a sense of security in nursing situations and a feeling of personal development. CS can facilitate autonomy, develop professional identity and reduce the culture of shame. However, there is little evidence to suggest that CS can reduce stress. This does not necessarily mean that CS is not valuable, but rather that the evidence is not yet available. According to Rice *et al.* (2007), it is important for supervisors to feel valued and an increased sense of self-confidence in order for them to function as good supervisors. A significant number of supervisees and supervisors stated that they would appreciate some additional training in order to derive maximum benefit from the sessions (cf. Malin 2000; Robinson 2005; Kelly *et al.* 2001).

Three studies (Grant 2000; Howatson-Jones 2003; Rice *et al.* 2007) demonstrate, however, that despite research findings attesting to the advantages of CS, there is nevertheless resistance to its introduction in nursing settings. Grant (2000) provided explanations regarding the obvious gap between recommendations and practice around CS. The researcher claims that the gap appears to be due to the nature of the organisation itself, i.e. its hierarchy, which de facto impedes the proper implementation of CS. Thus, there is a need for a broader dialogue about CS in the organisation. The study by Howatson-Jones (2003) is an attempt to focus on the core of the problem(s) and it tries to determine how to remove the barriers to implementing CS and lifelong learning. Rice *et al.* (2007) performed an investigation in order to explore ways to make CS available to all mental health nurses and to improve and evaluate their contribution to patient care. The findings revealed that the nurses were apprehensive about participating in CS and that the definition of CS was unclear.

There are also empirical studies and findings that provide evidence of the *effects on nurses' competence development.* Hyrkäs and Paunonen-Ilmonen (2001) have stated that reflection on practice encourages nurses to assume realistic personal and professional responsibility. CS also creates the formation of independence and strengthens professional identity (Arvidsson *et al.* 2000).

Perceived reported benefits in the literature are: improved patient care, stress reduction, increased skills and job satisfaction (Hyrkäs *et al.* 2006, Rice *et al.* 2007). Edwards *et al.* (2006) and Hyrkäs *et al.* (2006) found evidence that effective CS is associated with lower levels of burnout. Bégat and Severinsson (2006) and Bégat *et al.* (2005) as well as Hyrkäs *et al.* (2006) investigated the positive influence of CS on job satisfaction and the psychosocial work environment. Team supervision (Hyrkäs and Paunonen-Ilmonen 2001; Hyrkäs *et al.* 2006) seems to have an impact on the quality of care (Wood 2004) and it can be considered a quality improvement intervention in nursing practice.

Nursing knowledge challenges the practical skills of supervisors and their ability to improve the quality of care for the benefit of the patient. According to Nordentoft (2008), CS may prevent stress and burnout in palliative care. CS benefits not only the personal and professional development of health care staff but also the terminally ill patients and their relatives.

Arvidsson *et al.* (2000) found that CS influenced nurses' professional competence in the following ways: a feeling of job satisfaction, acquisition of knowledge and competence, a sense of security in nursing situations and personal development. According to Teasdale *et al.* (2001), the clinical nurse supervisees appeared to use CS for reflection on actions but informal networks for more immediate support and advice. Moreover, while CS was seen as helpful for managing difficult events, informal support networks continued to be used and valued, even by those with access to CS.

Contextual description of CS

Cutcliffe and McFeely (2002) investigated the effects of CS on the practice of *primary care* nurses and found that it enhanced their engagement and thus had a positive effect on patient care. A quantitative study performed by Davey *et al.* (2006) revealed that few health care professionals are offered CS and that it is most common in the area of *psychiatric care.* Rice *et al.* (2007) explored ways to make CS available to all *mental health nurses* in Northern Ireland in order to improve and evaluate their contribution to patient care. The results indicated a willingness to assist healthcare providers in the development of local CS policies and procedures for practising mental health nurses. Williams *et al.* (2005) and Abbott *et al.* (2006) evaluated the implementation of CS for *community nurses* and found that there was a need for flexibility in the daily team discussions and the planning of CS. Team discussions were experienced as informal and the CS as formal. As there were many requests for individual CS, this was later firmly embedded in the organisation (Abbott *et al.* 2006). Another context in which CS has been examined is *the behaviour unit* (Carney 2005), and it appears that senior staff members seem to benefit more and experience greater satisfaction from regular supervision than junior staff. Furthermore, an investigation of learning disability nurses' perceptions of clinical supervision (Sines and McNally 2007) highlighted the importance of providing access to supervision and the need to separate it from line management. The context of Kilcullen's (2007) study was *renal and urological nursing*. Interviews with both supervisors and supervisees were analysed by means of content analysis. The greatest benefit of CS was stated as 'to provide a high standard of nursing care, it is necessary to feel supported' (p. 1036). The context of Turner's (2005) study was *neurology clinical nurse specialists*, where the evaluation of a group CS programme indicated that CS helped nurses to manage difficult clinical situations, recognise their limitations, cope with conflict, work more effectively both individually and as a group and maintain healthy behaviours. It also helped them to deal with professional isolation and made them realise that the time spent setting up ground rules was worthwhile. The study proposes that CS is an essential element of neurology nurse specialists' clinical responsibility to reach their full potential both personally and professionally.

In the Tveiten and Severinsson (2006) and Tveiten *et al.* (2005) studies, the context is *public health nurses* and client supervision. The findings revealed that it is important for the outcome to build a trusting relationship and to look beyond the current situation. The registered public health nurses' CS model seems to correspond to principles in the new strategies for health promotion initiated by the World Health Organization. In the Barriball *et al.* (2004) study the focus of CS was *primary care*, while in the Eriksson and Fagerberg (2008) study it was *the care of older people*. In a Swedish study (Fläckman *et al.* 2007) the aim was to describe *nursing home caregivers'* experiences while receiving education and clinical supervision over a two year period. Another focus of CS has been *nursing leadership* (Hyrkäs *et al.* 2005, 2008; Sirola-Karvinen and Hyrkäs 2006, 2008; Alleyne and Jumaa 2007), where CS was found to be beneficial for *nursing leaders* who appreciated its value. Pettifer and Clouder (2008) explored the potential of an alternative approach to the facilitation of CS in practice by focusing on academic staff members' experiences of providing CS for clinical colleagues. Finally, there are empirical studies showing that CS led to improved practice in an *acute paediatric ward* (Robinson 2005), in the context of *midwives* (Deery 2005) as well as in *perioperative care* (Wood 2004).

Conclusion and summary of the key points

In conclusion, the state of the science and contextual areas of CS demonstrate that it is an important and valuable way of creating a caring environment. The benefit of group CS is that the supervisees can reflect together with their colleagues. CS is pedagogical in the sense that it is a forum for sharing, learning and reflecting on clinical experiences of patient care and ethical issues. CS enhances the supervisees' professional development and leads to positive outcomes in the quality of patient care. Furthermore, the ethical dimension of CS promotes the supervisee's moral responsibility, which becomes visible in the care of individual patients and their relatives, as well as in their relationships with colleagues and other health care providers. The competence of the supervisor is vital due to his/her ability to influence the atmosphere within the CS group, in which the supervisee should be treated with respect and not made to feel guilty about not being good enough. The theoretical and conceptual framework is important for a better understanding of the underlying ethical issues involved in CS and also facilitates the understanding of caring. *Finally, the synthesis of the existing literature reveals that CS is applied in the UK and the Scandinavian countries but less in other parts of Europe.* From a contextual perspective, CS is primarily employed in psychiatric care but there are indications that it is spreading to other health care contexts.

References

Abbott, S., Dawson, L., Hutt, J., Johnson, B. and Sealy, A. (2006), Introducing clinical supervision for community-based nurses, *British Journal of Community Nursing*, 11(8): 346–348.

Agélii, E., Kennergren, B., Severinsson, E. and Berthold, H. (2000), Ethical dimensions of supervision: the supervisors' experiences, *Nursing Ethics*, 7(4): 352–359.

Alleyne, J. and Jumaa, M.O. (2007), Building the capacity for evidence-based clinical nursing leadership: the role of executive co-coaching and group clinical supervision for quality patient services, *Journal of Nursing Management*, 15(2): 230–243.

Arvidsson, B. and Fridlund, B. (2005), Factors influencing nurse supervisor competence: a critical incident analysis study, *Journal of Nursing Management*, 13(3): 231–237.

Arvidsson, B., Löfgren, H. and Fridlund, B. (2000), Psychiatric nurses' conceptions of how group supervision in nursing care influences their professional competence, *Journal of Nursing Management*, 8(3): 175–185.

Barriball, L., White, A. and Münch, U. (2004), An audit of clinical supervision in primary care, *British Journal of Community Nursing*, 9(9): 389–397.

Bégat, I. and Severinsson, E. (2001), Nurses' reflections on episodes occurring during the provision of care – an interview paper, *International Journal of Nursing Studies*, 38(1): 71–77.

Bégat, I. and Severinsson, E. (2006), Reflection on how clinical nursing supervision enhances nurses' experiences of well-being related to their psychosocial work environment, *Journal of Nursing Management*, 14(8): 610–616.

Bégat, I., Ellefsen, B. and Severinsson, E. (2005), Nurses' satisfaction with their work environment and the outcomes of clinical nursing supervision on nurses' experiences of well-being: a Norwegian study, *Journal of Nursing Management*, 13(3): 221–230.

Berg, A. and Kisthinios, M. (2007), Are supervisors using theoretical perspectives in their work? A descriptive survey among Swedish-approved clinical supervisors, *Journal of Nursing Management*, 15(8): 853–861.

Berggren, I. and Severinsson, E. (2006), The significance of nurse supervisors' different ethical decision-making styles, *Journal of Nursing Management*, 14(8), 637–643.

Berggren, I., Barbosa da Silva, A. and Severinsson, E. (2005), The core ethical issues of clinical nursing supervision, *Nursing and Health Sciences*, 7(1): 21–28.

Bradshaw, T., Butterworth, A. and Mairs, H. (2007), Does structured clinical supervision during psychosocial intervention education enhance outcome for mental health nurses and the service users they work with? *Journal of Psychiatric and Mental Health Nursing*, 14(1): 4–12.

Burns, N. and Grove, S.K. (2001), *The Practice of Nursing Research: Conduct, Critique and Utilisation*, 4th edn, London: WB Saunders Company.

Bush, T. (2005), Overcoming the barriers to effective clinical supervision, *Nursing Times*, 101(2): 38–41.

Butterworth, T., Bell, L., Jackson, C. and Pajnkihar, M. (2007), Wicked spell or magic bullet? A review of the clinical supervision literature 2001–2007, *Nurse Education Today*, 28(3): 264–272.

Buus, N. and George, H. (2009), Empirical studies of clinical supervision in psychiatric care. A systematic literature review and methodological critique, *International Journal of Mental Health Nursing*, 18(4): 250–264.

Carney, S. (2005), Clinical supervision in a challenging behaviour unit, *Nursing Times*, 101(47): 32–34.

Cerinus, M. (2005), The role of relationships in effective clinical supervision, *Nursing Times*, 101(14): 34–37.

Coleman, D. and Lynch, U. (2006), Professional isolation and the role of clinical supervision in rural and remote communities, *Journal of Community Nursing*, 20(3): 35–37.

Cotrell, S. (2002), Suspicion, resistance, tokenism and mutiny: problematic dynamics relevant to the implementation of clinical supervision in nursing, *Journal of Psychiatric and Mental Health Nursing*, 9(6): 667–671.

Cutcliffe, J.R. and McFeely, S. (2002), The development of practice nursing: the impact of clinical supervision: a pilot study, *The All Ireland Journal of Nursing and Midwifery*, 2(7): 40–45.

Cummins, A. (2009), Clinical supervision: the way forward? A review of the literature, *Nurse Education in Practice*, 9(3): 215–220.

Davey, B., Desousa, C., Robinson, S. and Murrells, T. (2006), The policy-practice divide: who has clinical supervision in nursing? *Journal of Research in Nursing*, 11(3): 237–248.

Deery, R. (2005), An action-research study exploring midwives' support needs and the effect of group clinical supervision, *Midwifery*, 21(2): 161–176.

Edwards, D., Burnard, P., Hannigan, B., Cooper, L., Adams, J., Juggessur, T., Fothergill, A. and Coyle, D. (2006), Clinical supervision and burnout: the influence of clinical supervision for community mental health nurses, *Journal of Clinical Nursing*, 15(8): 1007–1015.

Edwards, D., Cooper. L., Burnard, P., Hannigan, B., Juggessur, T., Adams, J., Fothergill, A. and Coyle, D. (2005), Factors influencing the effectiveness of clinical supervision, *Journal of Psychiatric and Mental Health Nursing*, 12(4): 405–414.

Eriksson, S. and Fagerberg, I. (2008), Supervisor experiences of supervising nursing staff in the care of older people, *Journal of Nursing Management*, 16(7): 876–882.

Fläckman, B., Fagerberg, I., Häggström, E., Kihlgren, A. and Kihlgren, M. (2007), Despite shattered expectations a willingness to care for elders remains with education and clinical supervision, *Scandinavian Journal of Caring Sciences*, 21(3): 379–389.

Frankel, A. (2008), Applying theory to practice through clinical supervision, *Nursing Times*, 104(30): 30–31.

Grant, A. (2000), Clinical supervision and organisational power: a qualitative paper, *Mental Health Care*, 31(12): 398–401.

Howatson-Jones, I.L. (2003), Difficulties in clinical supervision and lifelong learning, *Nursing Standard*, 17(37): 37–41.

Hyrkäs, K. (2008), Clinical nursing leadership: perspectives on current topics, *Journal of Nursing Management*, 16(5): 495–498.

Hyrkäs, K. and Paunonen-Ilmonen, M. (2001), The effects of clinical supervision on the quality of care: examining the results of team supervision, *Journal of Advanced Nursing*, 33(4): 492–502.

Hyrkäs, K., Appelqvist-Schmidlechner, K. and Haataja, R. (2006), Efficacy of clinical supervision: influence on job satisfaction, burnout and quality of care, *Journal of Advanced Nursing*, 55(4): 521–535.

Hyrkäs, K., Appelqvist-Schmidlechner, K. and Kivimäki, K. (2005), First-line managers' views of the long-term effects of clinical supervision: how does clinical supervision support and develop leadership in health care? *Journal of Nursing Management*, 13(3): 209–220.

Hyrkäs, K., Appelqvist-Schmidlechner, K. and Paunonen-Ilmonen, M. (2002), Expert supervisors' views of clinical supervision: a study of factors promoting and inhibiting the achievements for multiprofessional team supervision, *Journal of Advanced Nursing*, 38(4): 387–397.

Johansson, I., Holm, A.-K., Lindqvist, I. and Severinsson, E. (2006), The value of caring in nursing supervision, *Journal of Nursing Management*, 14(8): 644–651.

Jones, A. (2003), Clinical supervision in promoting a balanced delivery of palliative nursing care, *Journal of Hospice and Palliative Nursing*, 5(3): 168–175.

Jones, A. (2006a), Clinical supervision: what do we know and what do we need to know? A review and commentary, *Journal of Nursing Management*, 14(8): 577–585.

Jones, A. (2006b), Group-format clinical supervision for hospice nurses, *European Journal of Cancer Care*, 15(2): 155–162.

Jones, A. (2008), Towards a common purpose: group-format clinic supervision can benefit palliative care, *European Journal of Cancer Care*, 17(2): 105–106.

Jukes, M., Millard, J. and Chessum, C. (2004), Nurse prescribing: a case for clinical supervision, *British Journal of Community Nursing*, 9(7): 291–297.

Kelly, B., Long, A. and McKenna, H. (2001), A survey of community mental health nurses' perceptions of clinical supervision in Northern Ireland, *Journal of Psychiatric and Mental Health Nursing*, 8(1): 33–44.

Kilcullen, N. (2007), An analysis of the experiences of clinical nursing supervision on registered nurses undertaking MSc/graduate diploma in renal and urological nursing and on their clinical supervisors, *Journal of Clinical Nursing*, 16(6): 1029–1038.

Knutton, S. and Pover, J. (2004), Applied management: the importance of honesty in clinical supervision, Part 1: developing and maintaining honest relationships, *Nursing Management*, 10(9): 29–31.

Lyth, G. (2000), Clinical supervision: a concept analysis, *Journal of Advanced Nursing*, 31(3): 722–729.

Magnusson, A., Lützen, K. and Severinsson, E. (2002), The influence of clinical supervision on ethical issues in home care of people with mental illness in Sweden, *Journal of Nursing Management*, 10(1): 37–45.

Malin, N.A. (2000), Evaluating clinical supervision in community homes and teams serving adults with learning disabilities, *Journal of Advanced Nursing*, 31(3): 548–557.

Nordentoft, H.M. (2008), Changes in emotion work at interdisciplinary conferences following clinical supervision in a palliative outpatient ward, *Qualitative Health Research*, 18(7): 913–927.

Pettifer, A. and Clouder, L. (2008), Clinical supervision: a means of promoting reciprocity between practitioners and academics, *Learning in Health and Social Care*, 7(3): 168–177.

Rice, F., Cullen, P., McKenna, H., Kelly, B., Keeney, S. and Richey, R. (2007), Clinical supervision for mental health nurses in Northern Ireland: formulating best practice guidelines, *Journal of Psychiatric and Mental Health Nursing*, 14(5): 516–521.

Robinson, J. (2005), Improving practice through a system of clinical supervision, *Nursing Times*, 101(23): 30–32.

Severinsson, E. (2001), Confirmation, meaning and self-awareness as core concepts of the nursing supervision model, *Nursing Ethics*, 8(1): 36–44.

Shanley, M. and Stevenson, C. (2006), Clinical supervision revisited, *Journal of Nursing Management*, 14(8): 586–592.

Sines, D. and McNally, S. (2007), An investigation into the perceptions of clinical supervision experienced by learning disability nurses, *Journal of Intellectual Disabilities*, 11(4): 307–328.

Sirola-Karvinen, P. and Hyrkäs, K. (2006), Clinical supervision for nurses in administrative and leadership positions: a systematic literature review of the studies focusing on administrative clinical supervision, *Journal of Nursing Management*, 14(8): 601–609.

Sirola-Karvinen, P. and Hyrkäs, K. (2008), Administrative clinical supervision as evaluated by the first-line managers in one health care organization district, *Journal of Nursing Management*, 16(5): 588–600.

Sloan, G. (2005), Clinical supervision: beginning the supervisory relationship, *British Journal of Nursing*, 14(17): 918–923.

Sloan, G. and Watson, H. (2001a), Illuminative evaluation: evaluating clinical supervision on its performance rather than applause, *Journal of Advanced Nursing*, 35(5): 664–673.

Sloan, G. and Watson, H. (2001b), John Heron's six-category intervention analysis: towards understanding interpersonal relations and progressing the delivery of clinical supervision for mental health nursing in the United Kingdom, *Journal of Advanced Nursing*, 36(2): 206–214.

Sloan, G. and Watson, H. (2002), Clinical supervision models for nursing; structure, research and limitations, *Nursing Standard*, 17(4): 41–46.

Sloan, G., White, C. and Coit, F. (2000), Cognitive therapy supervision as a framework for clinical supervision in nursing: using structure to guide discovery, *Journal of Advanced Nursing*, 32(3): 515–524.

Teasdale, K., Brocklehurst, N. and Thom, N. (2001), Clinical supervision and support for nurses: an evaluation study, *Journal of Advanced Nursing*, 33(2): 216–224.

Thompson, S. and Winter, R. (2003), A telephone-led clinical supervision pilot for nurses in different settings, *Professional Nurse*, 18(8): 467–470.

Turner, K. (2005), Group clinical supervision: supporting neurology clinical nurse specialists in practice, *Journal of Community Nursing*, 19(9): 4–8.

Tveiten, S. (2005), Evaluation of the concept of supervision related to public health nurses in Norway, *Journal of Nursing Management*, 13(1): 13–21.

Tveiten, S. and Severinsson, E. (2006), Communication: a core concept in client supervision by public health nurses, *Journal of Nursing Management*, 14(3): 235–243.

Tveiten, S., Ellefsen, B. and Severinsson, E. (2005), Conducting client supervision in community health care, *International Journal of Nursing Practice*, 11(2): 68–76.

Veeramah, V. (2002), The benefits of using supervision, *Mental Health Nursing*, 22(1): 18–23.

Williams, B., French, B. and Higgs, J. (2005), Clinical supervision: community nurses' experience, *Primary Health Care*, 15(6): 35–39.

Wood, J. (2004), Clinical supervision, *British Journal of Perioperative Nursing*, 14(4): 151–156.

30 The state of the science of clinical supervision in the United States

A social work- and nursing-focused perspective

Carlean Gilbert and John R. Cutcliffe

This chapter focuses on a rigorous review of the clinical supervision literature emanating from social work and nursing in the US. It provides background to the inception and subsequent development of clinical supervision in both disciplines, looks at changes in terminology and trends over time, and draws attention to a number of perhaps disconcerting contemporary changes in supervision practices in social work. Similarly, it highlights how, according to the limited extant literature, the practices of clinical supervision appear to have 'morphed' over the years in US nursing; moving dramatically away from the original conceptualisations and tenets.

In the view of the editors, it is both interesting and somewhat disturbing to note a distinct similarity in so-called developments in clinical supervision that is evident across many countries. Namely, an apparent movement away from clinical supervision as a phenomenon that is concerned with professional growth and development, geared towards permissiveness and support, into something else that is more concerned with the administrative needs of the organisation. Perhaps more worryingly, in certain places, as this chapter reports, clinical supervision may even be displaced completely as it is perceived by some to have little value in terms of income generation and can be resource/cost intensive. Not only are such positions actually at odds with a more comprehensive understanding of the (international) literature that focuses on clinical supervision, in that there is some evidence indicating cost savings to an organisation that embraces clinical supervision for its clinicians; but it also completely fails to take account of the purported *enhancements in quality of care* that occur when clinicians receive clinical supervision.

Introduction

Clinical supervision has played a critical role in the development of health care professions and professionals in the United States (US). Changing societal conditions and clinical practices have been reflected in changes in clinical supervision as past concerns have given way to new challenges. Advances in biomedical technology, the shift from acute to chronic care, co-morbid disorders, regulatory requirements, managed care, poverty, cultural practices, pandemics, and migration are just some of the factors that affect patient care. To address these complexities many programs have sought the combined wisdom of multidisciplinary or interdisciplinary teams, composed of a variety of combinations of counsellors, nurses, physical and occupational therapists, physicians, psychologists, social workers, speech pathologists, and other health professionals.

Performing an exhaustive and comprehensive interdisciplinary literature review of US clinical supervision in health care is beyond the scope of this chapter. This chapter subsequently is limited to a rigorous review update of clinical supervision in nursing and social work in the US. For readers wishing to access US clinical supervision literature reviews of psychology and counseling the authors refer to these fine examples (see, for example, Borders 2005; Ellis 2010; Freitas 2002; Goodyear *et al.* 2005; Wheeler and Richards 2007), marriage and family therapy (Anderson *et al.* 1995; Lee *et al.* 2004), social work (Bogo and McKnight 2005; Pack 2009), and substance use counseling (Center for Substance Abuse Treatment 2009; Roche *et al.* 2007).

Examination of clinical supervision from the (combined) perspectives of nursing and health care social work is especially fitting. In 1905 Dr. Richard Cabot, a physician at Massachusetts General Hospital in Boston, established the first medical social work position (Cabot 1919; Cannon 1930, 1952) The following year he hired Ida Cannon, a registered nurse and graduate of the Boston School of Social Work (now Simmons College), who pioneered the field of medical social work. Trained in both nursing and social work and inspired by Jane Addams, Cannon collaborated with physicians and other health care professionals and demonstrated the interrelationships among the physical, social, and environmental conditions that affected patients.

Harbingers of changes in clinical supervision in health care in the US can be traced to the early 1980s when health care delivery and funding began to undergo radical transformations due to "managed care," whereby "managed care" is defined as a payment and delivery system that regulates, monitors, and coordinates health care usage of resources in order to contain costs and increase efficiency. In the early 1980s the Medicare capitated payment system, a form of managed care, was implemented in an effort to reduce spiraling health care costs. The Medicare prospective payment system shifted the financial risks from payer to provider, and health care revenues were reduced. Confronted with a rapidly changing environment and intense competition for dwindling resources, health care executives in both public and private sectors responded by forming alliances with other health care systems, merging with competitive institutions, and separating functions into independent, decentralized programs or teams (Lee and Alexander 1999; Weil 2003). The effects of reorganization have been to reduce operating costs by flattening organizational structures, consolidating management, integrating related operations, and shortening lengths of stay. Restructuring of health care organizations has affected changes in the amount and content, in sources of and in models of clinical supervision. Since the 1990s supervisors also have witnessed an emerging emphasis on ethical practice, risk management, and use of evidence-based practice.

Terminology and trends in clinical supervision social work terminology

Variations in use of three terms, supervision, field education, and clinical supervision, by social workers confound discussions, writings, and research both within the profession and within other disciplines like nursing. Understanding the extensive history of social work clinical supervision, which has its roots in organizational models, professional education, and practice, contributes to insight into contemporary practices and challenges of clinical supervision. Between the 1850s and 1890s the concept of supervisors was manifested in overseers of institutions such as asylums whose charge was to ensure humane and effective care of patients and efficient operations (Munson 2002). The Charity Organization Societies (COS) that began to emerge in the late 1800s used volunteers called "friendly visitors," predecessors of professional social workers, to help families in need. These almsgivers were engaged, trained, and directed by "paid agents" employed by the societies (Kadushin and Harkness 2002). Like contemporary supervisors, the paid agents performed educational and managerial functions by assigning visitors to families, reviewing their case records, advising visitors regarding their work, and serving as liaisons between the visitors and administratively oriented COS district committees.

Eventually evolving into the Columbia University School of Social Work, the first professional social work education was a six-week training program for 27 students offered in 1898 by the New York COS. By 1910 five schools of social work existed in the US. Since their inception the schools have regarded the primary responsibility for education to be academic coursework, but the signature pedagogy of the profession has been internships in agencies, community service organizations, and institutions. The first course for training supervisors was offered in 1911 by the Charity Organization Department, whose director was Mary Richmond, of the Russell Sage Foundation. In 1917 Mary Richmond published the classic social work textbook *Social Diagnosis*, a title that reflected her adaptation of the medical model to the conceptualization of social ills. Recognizing the need to develop a common knowledge base for the education and training of social case workers, Richmond hired two experienced case workers, a family worker and a medical worker, to analyze original case records from child welfare, medical, and social agencies in five cities. The systematically acquired findings that were presented in her book include descriptions of "a case supervisor who is responsible for the work of a group of social case workers" (Richmond 1917: 347).

As social work education and professional identity developed, scholars advanced theories and models of supervision. Kadushin's (1976, 1992) classic conceptualization of clinical supervision is based on three interrelated functions: administrative, educational (clinical), and supportive. The administrative function of supervisors is based upon authority delegated by their employers to maintain supervisees' job performance. Supervisors are charged to facilitate workers' abilities to deliver effective, efficient services to clients in ways that are consistent with the organizational policies, procedures, and structure as well as professional practice standards (Kadushin and Harkness 2002; Shulman 1993; Tsui 2005). These functions are accomplished through assignment of cases and service assignments, oversight of workers' assessments and interventions, and performance appraisal by the supervisor. Educational or clinical supervision improves the knowledge and skills of workers within the mandate of the employing agency (Munson 2002). Supportive clinical supervision reduces job-related stresses and fosters worker self-awareness to cope with them (Bogo and McKnight 2005; Kadushin and Harkness 2002; Tsui 2005).

Given that the original terminology of clinical supervision (within US social work) referred to agency-based practices with dominant administrative functions, social work educators have referred to "supervisors" of students and emphasize the distinction in roles and functions. In social work the signature pedagogy, the central form of instruction and learning in which professions socialize their students to carry out their roles of practitioners, is field education:

> The intent of field education is to connect the theoretical and conceptual contribution of the classroom with the practical world of the practice setting ... the two interrelated components of curriculum – classroom and field – are of equal importance within the curriculum and each contributes to the development of the requisite competencies of the professional practice. Field education is systematically designed, supervised, coordinated, and evaluated based on criteria by which students demonstrate the achievement of program competencies.
>
> (Council on Social Work Education 2008: Educational Policy 2.3).

Clinical social work clinical supervision is defined in a position paper under revision by the American Board of Examiners in Clinical Social Work (ABECSW) as clinical supervision that is provided by social workers with advanced training, years of practice experience, and mastery of competencies to assist a supervisee acquire knowledge, skills, and identity as a clinical social worker (American Board of Examiners in Clinical Social Work 2004). Competencies include: assessment and diagnosis; treatment planning; knowledge of clinical supervision processes such as parallel process, self awareness, and observational tools; and evaluation of practice and clinical supervision outcomes. The ABECSW paper distinguishes between clinical supervision, which is provided directly or subcontracted by the supervisees' employing institutions, and consultation, which occurs when supervisees independently hire individuals to help them develop competencies. Gibelman and Schervish (1997b) claimed that the growing emphasis on clinical social work in the US, including social workers who enter private practice, has altered the definition of clinical supervision. Their description of clinical supervision was not inevitably agency-based and focused on the client–clinician dynamics in accord ABECSW.

Trends in supervision

In 2004 researchers used a stratified random sample of approximately 10,000 licensed social workers from 48 states and the District of Columbia who were members of the National Association of Social Workers (NASW) to profile their roles and functions (Whitaker *et al.* 2006). Having 150,000 members, NASW is the largest organization of professional social workers in the world (NASW 2010). At the time of the study approximately 310,000 social workers were licensed in the US, a number that represented 38 percent of self-identified social workers according to the Bureau of the Census, 2000 (as cited by Whitaker *et al.* 2006). Findings from this NASW benchmark study revealed vital information about the primary practice areas, tasks, and employment settings of study participants, 79 percent with masters and 2 percent with doctoral degrees. Researchers found that the largest primary practice areas for social workers were mental health (37 percent) followed by health care practice (13 percent). Although aging was categorized as a discrete field of practice, it has much in common with health care. Gerontological social workers (9 percent) reported that the most general problem of older adults was chronic illnesses, which was followed by psychosocial stressors (67 percent), acute medical conditions (62 percent), and physical disabilities (61 percent).

When asked about their roles as clinical supervisors, 7 percent of respondents stated that they spent "20 hours or more" per week in clinical supervision (Whitaker *et al.* 2006), which was more than the 5.5 percent of NASW members who listed clinical supervision as their primary function in 1995 (Gibelman and Schervish 1997b). In 2004, 58 percent of respondents reported that they spent "any amount of time" in the role of clinical supervisor (Whitaker *et al.* 2006). One could deduce from the data of Whitaker *et al.* that 35 percent of social workers do not provide any clinical supervision. Unfortunately the data do not distinguish clinical supervision in health care from other practice(s) nor do they capture the percentages of social workers who receive clinicals. Their findings must be interpreted with caution because not all licensed social workers belong to NASW. Building upon findings from the benchmark data collected in 2004, Whitaker and Arrington (2008) invited NASW members to participate in a follow-up survey in 2007. Almost replicating the statistics of the 2004 study (Whitaker *et al.* 2006), the majority of respondents were licensed and identified their primary practice areas as mental health followed respectively by health, child and family welfare, and aging. Within three years, however, social workers reported that the amount of time that they spent in clinical supervision dropped from 7 percent to 5 percent. Although the findings of these self-selected participants cannot be generalized to the entire population of NASW members, who do not represent all degreed social workers, they may suggest a trend towards reduced clinical supervision.

Licensed social workers indicated increased barriers to effective service and decreased support systems in the two years preceding the 2004 data collection (Whitaker *et al.* 2006). They claimed that the primary impediments to effective practice were increased paperwork, increased severity of client problems, and increased caseloads; the smallest increase among the eight presented factors was availability of professional training, which is arguably a source of support. Approximately 2.5 percent of study participants also acknowledged that a decrease in clinical supervision, which was second only to reimbursement levels (approximately 4 percent), had a negative impact on their work. The diminishment of clinical supervision could be inferred as one of the reasons why 12 percent of the respondents revealed that they planned to leave the profession. Expressing concerns about retention, Whitaker *et al.* conclude that

> Although most social workers express satisfaction with their career choice and aspects of their practices, too many become discouraged by agency environments that are unresponsive to their needs for professional growth, respect and fair compensation.
>
> (Whitaker *et al.* 2006: 35)

Supervision trends in health care

Historically social work services have been provided in public and non-profit sectors, and the greater part of clinical supervision has been agency-based. The importance of working within bureaucratic structures is evidenced by the fact that one of the six standards in the NASW Code of Ethics, Standard 3: Social Workers' Ethical Responsibilities in Practice Settings, details guidelines for Supervision and Consultation (Standard 3.01) and Commitment to Employers (Standard 3.09) (NASW 1999). Health social workers (56 percent) reported working primarily in hospitals, 85 percent of which were located in metropolitan areas (Whitaker *et al.* 2006); they also can be found in outpatient clinics, home health agencies, nursing homes, assisted living facilities, hospices, and public health agencies. The majority of health social workers (55 per cent) were employed in private/non-profit sectors.

Given that the organization is a dominant influence on social work practice, changes in the organization impact the functions of practice and clinical supervision. Managed care strategies that took hold in the 1980s resulted not only in elimination of the positions of middle managers who provided supervision but also the amount of time afforded to it (Gibelman and Schervish 1997a; Kadushin and Harkness 2002). Paralleling these changes in the financing of health care organizations was the movement towards social work licensure, which gave states the power to enforce standards of practice. Since 1983 the American Association of State Social Work Boards has developed national examinations for social work credentialing (Biggerstaff 1995). In 2005 Michigan became the fiftieth state to provide social work licensure based upon a combination of education, performance on examinations, and hours of supervised experience, which for a license requires two years of post-Master's employment combined with weekly one-hour clinical supervision. Managed care organizations underplayed the functions of clinical supervisors and shifted reliance to state licensure as a measure of competence (Munson 2006). *Kadushin and Harkness (2002) suggest, furthermore, that because administrative supervision directly benefits the organization, it may be the sole form of supervision recognized by hospitals within a cost containment environment. They also hypothesized that clinical and supportive supervision, which are resource-intensive and non-revenue generating functions, may be devalued by hospital administrators within an environment of cost containment.*

Berger and Mizrahi (2001) examined clinical supervision from the perspective of supervisors in a national sample of 750 hospitals in 1992, 1994, and 1996 and found a decrease in clinical supervision by clinical social workers. As health care delivery systems flattened their organizational structures to decrease costs, clinical supervisor positions were eliminated and clinical social workers were often left to consult with peers, be supervised by other professionals such as nurses, or interdisciplinary teams (Berger and Mizrahi 2001; Giberman and Shervish 1997a). In the first study of hospital-based social work supervisees by Kadushin *et al.* (2009), social workers confirmed suspicions that clinical supervision is organizationally driven rather than focused on individual learning needs of supervisees. Seventeen social workers, 12 of whom were licensed, from various regions of the US participated in one of seven telephone focus groups. They reported that restructuring and resizing strategies had led to changes in supervisees' roles, elimination of social work directors, transfer of reporting relationships to non-social work personnel, and/or implementation of matrix models in which the clinical supervisor could be a nurse, a social work department director or a social worker at the corporate level. The participants reported that many social work clinical supervisors carried wide-ranging administrative responsibilities for corporate social work systems, entire geographic areas, or several hospital departments. Some supervisees who had social work supervisors reported difficulty in obtaining supervision because of clinical supervisors' administrative demands trumped those of clinical supervision and sometimes questioning their clinical competence. The study also confirmed anecdotal stories that even when practitioners are available to provide the required clinical supervision for licensure candidates, the supervisors were unwilling to do so because they lacked administrative sanction. Clinical supervision content was reported to be focused primarily on administrative issues. In contrast to the literature that identifies formal clinical supervision as the most widely used model (Bogo and McKnight 2005; Kadushin and Harkness 2002; Tsui 2005), focus groups participants reported that individual supervision was infrequent and supplanted by variety of supervision models. As individual clinical supervision became less frequent once supervisees obtained licensure, they reported seeking secondary on-site supervision from team leaders and senior workers, participating in group and team supervision, and contacting supervisors on an as-needed basis. Workers also relied on hospital-contracted and peer consultations for clinical guidance.

Findings from this study cannot be generalized because of the small sample size, the potential for partiality from using supervisors with membership in the Society for Social Work Leadership in Health Care to recruit participants, and bias from self-selection. Anecdotal accounts of practitioners acquiring clinical supervision at their own expense or using their personal therapists to discuss work-related cases raise accountability, ethical, and liability issues.

Clinical supervision in nursing in the United States

Literature search method

In order to make the most comprehensive effort possible to ascertain the state of the science of the clinical supervision emanating from nurses (or nursing) in the United States, the authors undertook a comprehensive search of the extant literature. Literature reviews are not spared from the vagaries of attention to method, in part as a way to indicate thoroughness and thus enhance the credibility of the findings of the search. Accordingly, it is important to set out the authors' approach to undertaking the search as a means of establishing the fidelity of the findings. The validity of the method was increased by ensuring that the literature search incorporated Booth's (1996) three principles: it was systematic, explicit, and reproducible. The literature search was conducted to encompass articles relating to clinical supervision and nurses/nursing, and included first an electronic (database) search and a hand search of United States nursing textbooks. To allow for both the provision of research findings as well as a discussion of conceptual ideas, the review included empirical studies (qualitative and quantitative) as well as theoretical/clinical review articles. The review was generated from two full searches. The first full search was executed by searching within the journal *The Clinical Supervisor*, the second by combining the databases of PsycINFO, PsycARTI-CLES, CINAHL, Academic Search Premiere, and Health Source: Academic/Nursing Edition. Criteria for inclusion in the review were: (a) published in English; (b) published between January 1980 and January 2010; and (c) clinical supervision was the main theme in the document. Editorials and brief items were omitted.

For both searches, key word search terms were clinical supervision as subject, and nursing and United States in default, producing three hits for the journal search and 35 hits for the database search. All abstracts were reviewed by the second author to determine if the articles met the aforementioned criteria. Articles that warranted inclusion were accessed/ordered and reviewed. This produced a total of six papers, four of which focused on nurse practitioners receiving supervision from physicians or other forms of supervising student performance in the clinical areas. One offered a review of Powell's approach to clinical supervision from substance use/misuse counseling and the other was Jones' (2005) fine review of clinical supervision in nursing in the United States.

The hand search of textbooks faired even less well, with most textbooks referring to the supervision of students in clinical settings (e.g. Varcarolis *et al.* 2006) or including no reference to clinical supervision (e.g. Kneisl and Trigoboff 2009; Fontaine 2009). It may be of particular note that the hand search included N-Clix revision manuals (e.g. Hogan *et al.* 2009) and no exam preparation/revision questions could be located that specifically referred to clinical supervision in the United States. However, Stuart and Laraia's (2005) fine text is worthy of particular note as the only US nursing textbook the authors could locate that included reference to clinical supervision as more than supervision of students in clinical areas. Key ideas from Stuart's (2005) chapter are incorporated below.

US nurses' contribution to the extant clinical supervision literature

The search of the extant US nursing literature, such as it is, appears to reinforce the findings of previously published papers such as Jones (2005) and Cutcliffe and Lowe (2005). It seems that little has changed in this substantive area over the last ten years in the United States, to the extent that Rounds' (2001) statement is still accurate today. Rounds points out that the term clinical supervision is used in nursing in the United States (in the main) to refer to relationships between an administrator or superior and a more junior "other" (the supervisee). Most commonly, according to the findings of our review, the term clinical supervision in nursing in the United States is used to refer to clinical performance monitoring of students (in a variety of different nursing programs). Varcarolis *et al.* (2006: 163) refer to it as the "validation of performance quality through scheduled supervisory sessions." Lysaker *et al.* (2009) similarly write of the CS of advanced students within a recovery model and asks how a clinical supervisor should assist students as they begin to try and apply their knowledge in a clinical context. Both Jones (2005) and Cutcliffe and Lowe (2005) illustrated how within the US nursing literature, the supervisor is often described as having a supervisory responsibility for the performance of the supervisee. Importantly, then, the authors here offer a list of some key aspects of US nursing representations of clinical supervision and it is noteworthy that these are very different from representations found in other parts of the world and in other related disciplines:

- US nursing clinical supervision is concerned with clinical performance and performance evaluation.
- There is always a significant power imbalance present between the expert/advanced clinician undertaking the performance evaluation (the supervisor) and the person being the subject of the performance evaluation (the supervisee).

- These "supervisory" performance evaluations are clearly at odds with the original and documented rationales for introducing clinical supervision in nursing the US (see below).
- There is no evidence to suggest these performance evaluations are driven by supervisee concerns, supervisee's reflection on action, or are tied to reflective journals.
- US nursing clinical supervision carries with it the possibility of "failure"; of receiving a "failing grade" (as any formal clinical performance evaluation would).
- US nursing clinical supervision most commonly but not always (due to the relatively recent model of student nurse practitioners receiving "supervision" from the physician colleagues) occurs between a senior nurse and a less senior nurse.

Our review of the literature (and tracking citations during the hand search) indicates that there are a handful of US nursing authors who not only describe clinical supervision in, shall we say, similar terms and ways to those other parts of the world where clinical supervision is established (e.g. the UK, Australasia, Europe); but there are some who even advocate for the adoption of these views of clinical supervision within the US. Stuart (2005) appears to have developed her view of clinical supervision from those depicted in her 2001 edition. In 2005, clinical supervision is distanced (somewhat) from clinical performance evaluation, is depicted as more than clinical case reviews and is posited as a phenomenon that can also serve as support system for nurses. Stuart draws upon Laskowski's (2001) paper (which did not show up in our electronic search, as it does not include the key words), which reported how clinical supervision was described as an essential component of outpatient mental health clinical nurse specialist practice, even by the more experienced study participants; and how receiving clinical supervision brought about positive experience such as an increased sense of validation, insight, and support. Billings' (1998) earlier opinion piece offers similar remarks regarding the utility of clinical supervision as a support system. It also captures something of the original US ideas behind or rationales for having clinical supervision for nurses, for example the wholesome atmosphere of informality (Wolf 1941), focused on professional growth and development (Day 1925; Schmidt 1926), geared towards permissiveness and support (Freeman 1952) and thus the key idea that nurses need to care or look after themselves before they are capable to care for others.[1]

In her fine and searching review article, Jones (2005) attempts to move the US nursing clinical supervision debate forward significantly and argues unabashedly that the US should adopt the UK approach to (or model of) clinical supervision. Jones (2005) purports that the empirical evidence highlighting the benefits arising from clinical supervision would appear to underscore this argument. Though it may also be worthy of note that some in the US do not always appear to endorse imports from the United Kingdom, even if the import is shown to have utility.[2] Accordingly, a solid evidence base alone may not be sufficient and the introduction of clinical supervision into nursing in the US might best be achieved if it can attach itself to a US endorsed, US product. Consequently, Jones[3] highlights the very clear linkages between UK-style clinical supervision and the Magnet status hospital program (see ANCC 2010; Center for Nursing Advocacy 2008). Space and word limits do not permit a thorough discussion of the overlap and linkages; however, a few key points are worthy of note.

Magnet status hospitals are concerned with demonstrating the strength and quality of their nursing (ANCC 2010; Center for Nursing Advocacy 2010), and this strength and quality is gauged according to a range of criteria. As a result, if it can be shown that engaging in high quality clinical supervision can produce the same (or closely related) criteria, then it is a logical step to introduce clinical supervision into those hospitals aiming to achieve Magnet status. These criteria include:

- where nurses have a high level of job satisfaction (Butterworth *et al.* 1997;[4] Winstanley 2001);
- where nurses have a low staff nurse turnover rate [and turn-over has been linked with burnout] (Butterworth *et al.* 1997;[5] Winstanley 2001);
- where nurses have an appropriate grievance resolution;
- nursing delivers excellent patient outcomes (see published work linking clinical supervision with improved client care e.g. Smith – Chapter 16 in the present volume; Holm *et al.* 1998; Sloan 1999; Lyth 2000; Kilminster and Jolly 2000; Winstanley and White 2003);
- where nurses are involved in evidence-based decision making for client care delivery – and thus integrate theory/evidence into practice (see Holm *et al.* 1998; Severinsson 1995, 2001).

Ethical and malpractice issues

Although professional ethics are of concern to practitioners in all fields of social work practice, they are a prime concern to social workers in health care. Health care social workers confront multifaceted cases in complex organizational settings, navigate among the different values, ethics, and priorities of multidisciplinary colleagues, and cope with the implications of cutting-edge advances in biotechnology. As the majority of health social workers were employed in agencies that received state or federal funding (Whitaker *et al.* 2006), they faced potential ethical dilemmas because the governments determined what entities can do in terms of efficiency, effectiveness, and adherence to performance measurements based upon Diagnosis Related Groups (DRGs) and most recently participation in Core Measures mandated by the Center for Medicare and Medicaid Services (CMS). Perhaps these factors account for health care social workers ranking the desire for more education and training in professional ethics highest (22.8 percent) in contrast to social workers from all other fields of practice in the NASW workforce study? Beginning in the 1990s, however, social workers also began to appreciate that their ethical judgments carried with them risk of ethics complaints to state licensing board, NASW, and law suits regarding such issues as privacy, release of confidential information, informed consent, and the right to refuse services.

Interdisciplinary clinical supervision

As US health care administrators implemented managed care programs designed to decrease expenses by consolidating management and eliminating duplicative services, hospitals frequently separated functions into independent, decentralized programs or teams (Lee and Alexander 1999; Bazzoli *et al.* 2004; Weil 2003). This strategy often dismantled social work departments and eliminated the positions of the social work managers and directors who traditionally provided supervision (Kadushin and Harkness 2002; Weissman and Rosenberg 2002) that included clinical and supportive functions. Kadushin and Harkness (2002) suggest that because the administrative function of supervision benefits the organization, administrative supervision may be dominant in a cost containment environment. Social workers who retained their management positions were challenged to provide clinically focused supervision because of their increased administrative obligations to multisystem social work networks and additional hospital programs such as interpretive services and pastoral care.

The restructuring strategies implemented in hospitals often led to interprofessional supervision due to changes in reporting relationships and/or implementation of matrix models for organizational structure. An artifact of the shift from centralized departments to interdisciplinary teams, for example, is that physicians, nurses, or other health professionals who lead the team may have supervisory authority over the other team members (Kadushin and Harkness 2002). Supervision in matrix structures could come from a social worker retained in management position, a nurse, or a social worker at the corporate level (Kadushin *et al.* 2009).

Although social workers, nurses, and occupational therapists reported valuing the supervision from persons in professions other than their own, they also expressed unenthusiastic reactions (Bogo *et al.* in press). Social workers who received inter-professional supervision felt that others did not understand the social work profession, and they expressed the desire for the profession-specific terminology, values, roles, and functions that were experienced in social work supervision (Bogo *et al.* in press; Kadushin *et al.* 2009). Researchers also found that both the intra-professional and inter-professional supervision in contemporary health care focused on administrative functions.

Concluding remarks

In drawing on both historical and contemporary literature, such as it is, regarding clinical supervision in the United States, this chapter highlights something of a counter-intuitive situation. The extant, historical literature indicates how the US was amongst the nations pioneering and leading the introduction and development of clinical supervision. This literature shows what the original purpose(s), philosophical stance and rationale for creating clinical supervision was. Yet the contemporary literature from several disciplines indicates that current clinical supervision practice in the United States is a long way from these original conceptualizations. One can conclude that clinical supervision has morphed, or perhaps more accurately, has been annexed (not sure by whom) by people that would rather focus on the economic needs of the organization. Furthermore, there is evidence to suggest that this is occurring across different disciplines; it is not limited or restricted to one discipline.

However, there is also a glimmer of hope emerging in the extant literature with a few "voices" making the case for movement towards a so-called UK/European model of CS. It should not be lost on US-based practitioners that such a movement would, not without a distinct sense of irony, return the US to its original (and some might say pioneering) conceptualization and operationalisation of CS. The authors therefore add their own voices to those already recorded in the extant literature in advocating for the introduction of CS within the US, that is concerned with creating a wholesome atmosphere of informality, focuses on professional growth and development of the practitioner, is geared towards permissiveness and support, and is cognizant of the truism that nurses need to care or look after themselves before they are capable to care for others.

Notes

1 For an excellent review of these historical positions and developments see Yegdich (1999).
2 For example, see the response of some to the suggestion of incorporating a British Parliamentary style "Prime Minister's Question Time" for the incumbent US president, despite the overwhelmingly positive response to President Obama's recent and historic televised "question time" with the Republican party in January 2010. In an MSNBC pole (accessed 2010), 74 percent of over a thousand respondents stated "yes" in response to the question, "Should Barack Obama make televised Q&A sessions with lawmakers of both parties a regular feature of his presidency?" However, despite these expressions of public support the Republican party refused to accept this proposal and no such development occurred.
3 And here Jones (2005) echoes the views of the editors of this book.
4 The study by Butterworth *et al.* (1997) reported that when supervision was withdrawn from supervisees during the second phase of the national project there was a significant decrease in levels of job satisfaction. The opposite effect was seen for the participants who had previously not been in receipt of supervision; that is, those who, in phase one of the study, had formed the control group. This group and the supervisors group showed a decrease in levels of satisfaction whilst not in receipt of clinical supervision and a stabilisation once supervision was introduced.
5 The study by Butterworth *et al.* (1997) found that levels of emotional exhaustion and depersonalization showed an increase for nurses on the evaluation study who had not been receiving clinical supervision. Once clinical supervision had been introduced the instrument also showed that levels had stabilized, and in some cases decreased. A Swedish study (Palsson *et al.* 1996) also analyzed levels of burnout amongst groups of district nurses before and after systematic clinical supervision. In contrast, they reported no significant change over time, within or between groups.

References

American Board of Examiners in Clinical Social Work (2004), *Clinical Supervision: A Practice Specialty of Clinical Social Work: A Position Statement of the American Board of Examiners in Clinical Social Work*, online, available at: www.abecsw.org/images/ABESUPERV2205ed406.pdf.

ANCC (American Nurses Credentialing Center) (2010), *ANCC Magnet Recognition Program*, online, available at: www.nursecredentialing.org/Magnet/ ProgramOverview/Magnet-Characteristics.aspx [accessed 2010].

Anderson, S.A., Rigazio-DiGilio, S.A., and Kunkler, K.P. (1995), Training and supervision in marriage and family therapy: current issues and future directions, *Family Relations: Journal of Applied Family and Child Studies*, 44: 489–500.

Bazzoli, G., Dynan, L., Burns, L., and Yap, C. (2004), Two decades of organizational change in health care: what have we learned? *Medical Research and Review*, 61(3): 247–331.

Berger, C. and Mizrahi, T. (2001), An evolving paradigm of supervision within a changing health care environment, *Social Work in Health Care*, 32(4): 1–18.

Biggerstaff, M.A. (1995), Licensing, regulation, and certification, in R.L. Edwards (ed.), *Encyclopedia of Social Work*, 19th edn, Washington, DC: NASW Press, pp. 1616–1624.

Billings, C. (1998), Professional insights: on peer feedback, *Journal of the American Psychiatric Nurses Association*, 4(3), 103–104.

Bogo, M. and McKnight, K. (2005), Clinical supervision in social work: a review of the research literature, *The Clinical Supervisor*, 24(1/2): 49–67.

Bogo, M., Paterson, J., King, R., and Tufford, L. (in press), Interprofessional clinical supervision in mental health and addiction: toward a universal approach, *The Clinical Supervisor*.

Booth, A. (1996), In search of the evidence: informing effective practice, *Journal of Clinical Effectiveness*, 1(1), 25–29.

Borders, L.D. (2005), Snapshot of clinical supervision in counselling and counsellor, *The Clinical Supervisor*, 24(1/2): 69–113.

Butterworth, T., Carson, J., White, E., Jeacock, J., Clements, A., and Bishop, V. (1997), *It is Good to Talk: Clinical Supervision and Mentorship: An Evaluation Study in England and Scotland*, Manchester: The School of Nursing, Midwifery and Health Visiting, University of Manchester.

Cabot, R.C. (1919), *Social Work: Essays on the Meeting-ground of Doctor and Social Worker*, New York: Houghton Mifflin Company.

Cannon, I.M. (1930), *Social Work in Hospitals: A Contribution to Progressive Medicine*, revised edition, New York: Russell Sage Foundation.

Cannon, I.M. (1952), *On the Social Frontier of Medicine: Pioneering in Medical Social Service*, Cambridge: Harvard University Press.

Center for Nursing Advocacy (2008), *What is Magnet Status and How's that Whole Thing Going?* online, available at: www.nursingadvocacy.org/faq/magnet.html [accessed 2010].

Center for Substance Abuse Treatment (2009), *Clinical Supervision and Professional Development of the Substance Abuse Counselor*, Treatment Improvement Protocol (TIP) Series 52. DHHS Publication No. (SMA) 09–4435. Rockville, MD: Substance Abuse and Mental Health Services Administration.

Council on Social Work Education (2008), *Educational Policy and Accreditation Standards*, Washington, DC: CSWE.

Cutcliffe, J.R. and Lowe, L. (2005), A comparison of North American and European conceptualisations of clinical supervision, *Issues in Mental Health Nursing*, 26(5): 475–488.

Day, G.A. (1925), Changing competencies of supervision, *The Modern Hospital*, 24(5): 469–470.

Fontaine, K.L. (2009), *Mental Health Nursing*, 6th edn, Upper Saddle River, NJ: Pearson Education.

Ellis, M.V. (2010), Bridging the science and practice of clinical supervision: some discoveries, some misconceptions, *The Clinical Supervisor*, 29(1): 95–116.

Freeman, R. (1952), Supervision in the improvement of nursing services, *Public Health Nursing*, 44(7): 370–373.

Freitas, G.J. (2002), The impact of psychotherapy supervision on client outcome: A critical examination of 2 decades of research, *Psychotherapy: Theory, Research, Practice, Training*, 39(4): 354–367.

Gibelman, M. and Schervish, P.H. (1997a), Supervision in social work: characteristics and trends in a changing environment, *The Clinical Supervisor*, 16(2): 1–15.

Gibelman, M. and Schervish, P.H. (1997b), *Who We Are: A Second Look*, Washington, DC: NASW Press.

Goodyear, R.K., Bunch, K., and Claiborn, C.D. (2005), Current supervision scholarship in psychology: a five year review, *The Clinical Supervisor*, 24(1/2): 137–147.

Hogan, M.A., Gaylord, C., Gruener, R., Rodgers, J., and Kameg-Zalia, K. (2009), *Mental Health Nursing: Reviews and Rationales*, Upper Saddle River, NJ: Prentice Hall.

Holm, A.K., Lantz, I., and Severinsson, E. (1998), Nursing students' experiences of continual process-oriented group supervision, *Journal of Nursing Management*, 6(2): 105–113.

Jones, J.M. (2005), Clinical supervision in nursing: what's it all about? *The Clinical Supervisor*, 24(1/2): 149–162.

Kadushin, A. (1976), *Supervision in Social Work*, New York: Columbia University Press.

Kadushin, A. (1992), Social work supervision: an updated survey, *The Clinical Supervisor*, 10(2): 9–27.

Kadushin, A. and Harkness, D. (2002), *Supervision in Social Work*, 4th edn, New York: Columbia University Press.

Kadushin, G., Berger, C., Gilbert, C., and de St Aubin, M. (2009), Models and methods in hospital social work supervision, *The Clinical Supervisor*, 28(2): 180–199.

Kilminster, S.M. and Jolly, B.C. (2000), Effective supervision in clinical practice settings: a literature review, *Medical Education*, 34(10): 827–840.

Kneisl, C.R. and Trigoboff, E. (2009), *Contemporary Psychiatric-Mental Health Nursing*, 2nd edn, Upper Saddle River, NJ: Prentice Hall.

Laskowski, C. (2001), The mental health clinical nurse specialist and the difficult patient: evolving meaning, *Issues in Mental Health Nursing*, 22(5): 5–22.

Lee, R.E., Nichols, D.P., Nichols, W.C., and Odom, T. (2004), Trends in family supervision: the past 25 years and into the future, *Journal of Marital and Family Therapy*, 30(1): 61–69.

Lee, S.D. and Alexander, J.A. (1999), Consequences of organizational change in U.S. hospitals, *Medical Care Research and Review*, 56(3): 227–273.

Lysaker, P.H., Buck, K.D. and Lintner, J.I. (2009), Addressing recovery from severe mental illness in clinical supervision of advanced students, *Journal of Psychosocial Nursing Mental Health*, 47(4): 36–42.

Lyth, G.M. (2000), Clinical supervision: a concept analysis, *Journal of Advanced Nursing*, 31(3): 722–729.

MSNBC (2010), *Should Barack Obama make Televised Q&A Sessions with Lawmakers of Both Parties a Regular Feature of his Presidency?* online, available at www.politics.newsvine.com/_question/2010/02/03/3848732-should-barack-obama-make-televised-qa-sessions-with-lawmakers-of-both-parties-a-regular-feature-of-his-presidency [accessed 2010].

Munson, C.E. (2002), *Handbook of Clinical Social Work Supervision*, 3rd edn, New York: The Haworth Press.

Munson, C.E. (2006), Contemporary issues and trends in social work supervision, in W.J. Spitzer (ed.), *Supervision of Health Care Social Work: Principles and Practice*, Petersburg, VA: The Dietz Press, pp. 1–29.

NASW (National Association of Social Workers) (1999), *Code of Ethics of the National Association of Social Workers*, Washington, DC: NASW.

NASW (National Association of Social Workers) (2010), from www.socialworkers.org/ swportal/nsites/ [accessed February 28 2010].

Pack, M. (2009), Clinical supervision: an interdisciplinary review of literature with implications for reflective practice in social work, *Reflective Practice*, 10(5): 657–668.

Palsson, M., Hallberg, I.R., Norberg, A., and Bjorvell, H. (1996), Burnout empathy and sense of coherence among Swedish district nurses before and after systematic clinical supervision, *Scandinavian Journal of Caring Sciences*, 10(1): 19–26.

Richmond, M.E. (1917), *Social Diagnosis*, New York: Russel Sage Foundation.

Rizzo, M.D. (2003), Clinical supervision: a working model for substance abuse acute care settings, *The Health Care Manager*, 22(2): 136–143.

Roche, A.M., Todd, C.L., and O'Connor, J. (2007), Clinical supervision in the alcohol and other drugs field: an imperative or an option? *Drug and Alcohol Review*, 26(3): 241–249.

Rounds, L. (2001), A North American perspective on clinical supervision, in J.R. Cutcliffe, T. Butterworth, and B. Proctor (eds.), *Fundamental Themes in Clinical Supervision*, London: Routledge, pp. 303–315.

Schmidt, E. (1926), Principles and practices of supervision, *American Journal of Nursing*, 27(2): 119–120.

Severinsson, E. (1995), *Clinical nursing supervision in health care*, doctoral dissertation at the Nordic School of Public Health, Göteborg, Sweden.

Severinsson, E. (2001), Confirmation, meaning and self-awareness as core concepts of the nursing supervision model, *Nursing Ethics*, 8(1): 36–44.

Shulman, L. (1993), *Interactional supervision*, Washington, DC: NASW Press.

Sloan, G. (1999), Good characteristics of a clinical supervisor: a community mental health nurse perspective, *Journal of Advanced Nursing*, 30(3): 713–722.

Stuart, G.W. (2001), Actualizing the psychiatric nursing role: professional performance standards, in: G.W. Stuart and M.T. Laraia (eds.), *Principles and Practices of Psychiatric Nursing*, 7th edn, St. Louis, MI: Mosby, pp. 199–213.

Stuart, G.W. (2005), Implementing the nursing process: standards of care and professional performance, in G.W.Stuart and M.T. Laraia (eds.), *Principles and Practices of Psychiatric Nursing*, 8th edn, St. Louis, MI: Elsevier-Mosby, pp. 183–205.

Stuart, G.W. and Laraia. M.T. (eds.) (2005), *Principles and Practices of Psychiatric Nursing*, 8th edn, St. Louis, MI: Elsevier-Mosby.

Tsui, M.S. (2005). *Social Work Supervision: Contexts and Concepts*, New York: Sage.

Varcarolis, E.M., Carson, V.B., and Shoemaker, N.C. (2006), *Foundations of Psychiatric Mental Health Nursing: A Clinical Approach*, 5th edn, St. Louis, MI: Elsevier-Saunders.

Weil, T.P. (2003), Hospital downsizing and workforce reduction strategies: some inner workings, *Health Services Management Research*, 16(1): 13–23.

Weissman, A. and Rosenberg, G. (2002), Health care and social work: dilemmas and opportunities, in R. Patti, (ed.), *The Handbook of Social Welfare Management*, Thousand Oaks, CA: Sage Publications, pp. 511–520.

Wheeler, S. and Richards, K. (2007), The impact of clinical supervision on counsellors and therapists, their practice and their clients: a systematic review of the literature, *Counselling and Psychotherapy Research*, 7(1): 54–65.

Whitaker, T. and Arrington, P. (2008), *Social Workers at Work: NASW Membership Workforce Study*, Washington, DC: NASW.

Whitaker, T., Weismiller, T., and Clark, E. (2006), *Assuring the Sufficiency of a Frontline Workforce: A National Study of Licensed Social Workers, Executive Summary*, Washington, DC: NASW.

Winstanley, J. (2001), Developing methods for evaluating clinical supervision, in J.R. Cutcliffe, T. Butterworth and B. Proctor (eds), *Fundamental Themes in Clinical Supervision*, London: Routledge, pp. 210–224.

Winstanley, J and White, E. (2003), Clinical supervision: models, measures and best practice, *Nurse Researcher*, 10(4): 7–38.

Wolf, L. (1941), Development of floor nursing and supervision, *Hospital*, March: 53–56.

Yegdich, T. (1999), Clinical supervision and managerial supervision: some historical and conceptual considerations, *Journal of Advanced Nursing*, 30(5): 1195–1204.

31 Clinical supervision in Canada

Bridging the education-to-practice gap
through interprofessional supervision and
lateral mentoring: a value added
approach to clinical supervision

Nancy Arthur and Shelly Russell-Mayhew

In this chapter, the authors focus on the introduction of interprofessional (IP) supervision as a key direction for advancing clinical supervision within the Canadian context. The authors discuss the advantages and challenges of IP supervision and they offer suggestions for enhancing clinical placements. A new perspective, lateral mentoring, is introduced as a supervision practice, through which trainees benefit from exposure to the perspectives of professionals from multiple disciplines. The authors propose that traditional approaches to clinical supervision may be enhanced by a shift in philosophy and practice towards lateral mentoring.

We believe that this chapter offers a new and important perspective for clinical supervisors and educators in the twenty-first century. The opportunities and benefits of interprofessional supervision are still to be uncovered, but it is possible to assume that this approach will enhance the quality of care, improve interprofessional collaboration and engage patients as active members in their care.

Introduction

Interprofessional collaboration (IPC) is premised on providing the best quality of health care to patients and matching the best expertise of health care professionals to patient needs. In order for IPC to be accepted as the preferred practice or common way that professionals and patients interact with one another, they need to be adequately prepared and supported. IPC calls for a shift in culture regarding how we educate professionals, how professionals interact with one another, and how organizations are structured around professional practice (Herbert 2005).

Although innovative models of interprofessional education and practice have emerged in the literature (e.g. D'Amour and Oandasan 2005), *there has been little attention paid to the ways in which clinical supervision can be leveraged to help professionals acquire interprofessional competencies for "learning with and from other each other to improve collaboration and the quality of care"* (Barr *et al.* 2005: 31). Clinical supervisors are important role models for trainees; supervisors need to be both confident and capable of modeling the value of collaborative practice and provide trainees with learning opportunities on interprofessional teams.

Context

Within Canada, there are a number of initiatives that have created considerable momentum in the field of interprofessional education and practice, only a few of which are highlighted in this chapter. Initiatives related to collaborative practice have been strongly supported by Health Canada during the previous five years, and are now considered to be an integral aspect of primary care (Herbert 2005). For example, in the landmark report entitled *Building on Values: The Future of Health Care in Canada* (Romanow 2002), Commissioner Roy Romanow emphasized the need for new models of service delivery and new ways of preparing health care professionals. The important relationship between interprofessional education and practice was articulated as follows: "If health care providers are expected to work together and share expertise in a team environment, it makes sense that their education and training should prepare them for this type of working arrangement" (p. 109).

A major initiative was launched through Health Canada's Interprofessional Education for Collaborative Patient-Centered Practice (IECPCP), aimed at ensuring that health care practitioners have the competencies to practice together through effective collaboration (Herbert 2005). Phase one of this research initiative involved a systematic review of national and international trends in IP education and practice. The results of this review were subsequently published as a special issue of the *Journal of Interprofessional Care* (Hammick 2005). Amidst discussion of relevant terms and concepts, a working definition of IPC was noted as:

> A way of health care professionals working together and with their patients. It involves the continuous interaction of two or more professionals or disciplines, organized into a common effort, to solve or explore common issues with the best possible participation of the patient ... It enhances patient- and family-centered goals and values, provides mechanisms for continuous communication among caregivers, optimizes staff participation in clinical decision making within and across disciplines, and fosters respect for disciplinary contributions of all professionals.
>
> (Herbert 2005: 2)

Phase two of the initiative focused on the advancement of knowledge through multi-year IECPCP learning projects to advance research and practice within the Canadian context.

Another example of initiatives in Canada demonstrates the importance of collaboration between professional associations. In 2006, the Enhancing Inter-disciplinary Collaboration in Primary Health Care (EICP) Initiative, a coalition of ten professional associations (e.g., Canadian Medical Association, Canadian Psychological Association, Canadian Nursing Association), released their *Principles and Framework for Inter-disciplinary Collaboration in Primary Health Care* (EICP 2006).

A central message emerging from these initiatives is that the future delivery of health care requires professionals to work together effectively. Health care policy that addresses IPC is being integrated into workforce planning and the operations of many organizations. However, there are wide variations in the degree to which practice sites are ready to engage in IPC. In turn, there appear to be varying levels of readiness in terms of professional attitudes that support collaborative practice, knowledge about best of practices, and skills to enact successful collaboration. The field of interprofessionality has made tremendous strides during the past decade in emphasizing the benefits and barriers for professional practice. Along with advances in conceptualization and models, there is emerging evidence to show the benefits of IPC (Barrett *et al.* 2007). *It is timely to consider the ways in which clinical supervision can be enhanced through incorporating fundamental principles and practices of IPC.*

Reasons for interprofessional collaboration

There are a number of reasons commonly cited to support an increased emphasis on IPC related to patient care, staff satisfaction, workforce optimization, and health care resources (Herbert 2005). First and foremost, the complexity of patient issues means that a variety of professional expertise is often required to address multilayered care. Correspondingly, a coordinated effort is needed to involve multiple professionals in service planning and delivery. Professionals may feel less overwhelmed with the complexity of patient needs if they can tap into a system of shared expertise. Professionals may also benefit if case planning allows them to use their best specialist skills. Therefore, it is proposed that both patients and professionals benefit from the availability of appropriate consultation, referral, and appropriate service resources. Coordinated care often requires bringing together available resources within or between service agencies. However, it is important to go beyond bringing people together; they need to be trained to work on professional teams and with competencies to maximize the effectiveness of collaborative care.

Financial issues and operating costs have prompted a spotlight on workforce optimization. The increasing costs of health care require innovative practices that optimize the roles and functions of professionals who provide services. The idea is to have the best person with the best skills providing the best services, and avoid duplication and "wasteful" use of professional expertise. A related issue is the predicted shortage of health care professionals, which has prompted examination of workforce utilization and scope of practice. Calls to reform health care have emphasized the necessity of IPC as a leading edge in future health care planning and implementation (Romanow 2002).

The call for a changing culture in health care must be matched with corresponding changes in the ways that we prepare trainees. It is recognized that health care practitioners do not work in isolation, but must be prepared to work on health care teams. It is increasingly common for health care staff to consult with, refer to, and seek resources for patients from professionals from various disciplines. Given the emphasis on team-based approaches to service provision, professional education curricula need to support the acquisition of competencies for IPC (Suter *et al.* 2009). However, there has been limited discussion in the literature about clinical supervision and ways that principles of IPC could be integrated into supervisory practices.

Infusing interprofessional collaboration into clinical supervision

Supervision has been defined as "a formal process of professional support and learning which enables practitioners to develop knowledge and competence, assume responsibility for their own practice and enhance consumer protection and the safety of care in complex situations" (Bailey 2004: 267). Supervision is seen as fundamental to the process of professionalization, and each profession has developed its own supervision history and literature (Clouder and Sellars 2004). One factor that appears to cut across professions is the importance of learning from practice. Yet, there appears to be wide variation in approaches, and little accountability regarding how supervision practices prepare trainees for working both within and across professional disciplines.

The key features of IP supervision are: (a) an interaction between at least two people; (b) one person is attempting to support the other in becoming better at helping people; (c) the process is about a relationship within which education, support and quality control can happen; and (d) there are two or more professional groups represented in the interaction (Davies *et al.* 2004). The importance of incorporating multiple perspectives is a common theme in the literature on IP collaboration (Peacock *et al.* 2001). A parallel process occurs at the level of IP supervision. For example, the roles we need to consider in supervision are, at minimum, the supervisee, the supervisor, and the patient(s) and perhaps also other team members, family members and academics. Intuitively, it makes sense that IP supervision might work because knowledge in real life settings is not applied in a "take turns" fashion but rather in an integrated holistic way.

There are many benefits associated with IP supervision. *The essence is that IP supervision provides opportunity for multiple perspectives and a wider knowledge base. Increased creativity, critical thinking, and decreased complacency have been theorized as advantages to IP supervision* (Bailey 2004). It has also been proposed that there are enhanced contributions to the transfer of learning from training to practice (Bailey 2004).

Although the focus of the discussion has been on the benefits of preparing professionals for IP collaboration, the potential benefits for patients need to be considered. To recap, one of the primary purposes of interprofessional collaboration is to improve patient-centered practice (D'Amour and Oandasan 2005). This requires professionals to look carefully at what patients need and ways to include them in determining the direction of their care. Patients are increasingly being called upon to be active members in managing their care, but their roles on interprofessional teams are not well defined. The extent to which patients define themselves as active members of IP teams or passive recipients of care varies considerably according to patient expertise and service provider practices (Pyle and Arthur 2009). As we look towards IPC as a means of improving health care, professionals will need to be informed about ways to empower their patients and relate to them as active decision makers. However, there appears to be variability in the extent to which professionals are willing and able to amend their traditional position of an expert, and share decision-making power with patients. In turn, *approaches to clinical supervision will need to shift from an emphasis on delivery of care to patients towards collaborative care with patients, and consider trainees as active collaborators in the learning process.*

Barriers to interprofessional supervision

Along with many of the positive assets associated with interprofessional collaboration, a number of common barriers have been identified related to professional knowledge and scope of practice, role clarity, power and status, and the rigidity of professional cultures (e.g. Baxter and Brumfitt 2008; Hall 2005; Kvarström 2008). In turn, a number of contentious issues appear as barriers for IP supervision. For example, different experiences and interpretations of what supervision means within each professional body sets up a system where protecting the autonomous nature of the home profession is commonplace (Hyrkäs and Appelqvist-Schmidlechner 2003; Larkin and Callaghan 2005). Professional codes of practice have traditionally required supervision within the individual profession itself and each professional brings a history and practice experience about supervision (Bailey 2004; Emerson 2004; Townend 2005). As such, a number of difficulties related to supervision in an IP context emerge as locations for learning about IP collaboration.

First, there are practical and logistical issues to address, such as time for case consultation and how to coordinate schedules so that professionals from various disciplines can come together for supervision sessions. These organizational constraints should not be viewed lightly or their importance minimized; our experience in attempting to shift traditionally uniprofessional education to shared classrooms and instructional time has proven that this is often a monumental task, requiring a high degree of commitment between academic departments and practice sites.

Second, there are a number of terms used between professions to describe what might traditionally have been considered the supervisor, including mentor, facilitator, clinical supervisor, practice teacher, fieldwork educator, peer reviewer, tutor, preceptor, and field/site supervisor. It should not be assumed that these terms can be used interchangeably, as the roles and functions may differ and the quality of supervision may suffer if key elements are lost (Yonge *et al.* 2007).

Emerson (2004) proposes that "placement educator" is a neutral term that could transcend the different professions. However, this issue is more than about semantics, it is important to consider what is meant by supervision, and how the functions, goals, and processes in common might be negotiated. Bailey (2004) proposes that "clinical supervision" be called "work-based supervision" because it is more inclusive of a number of professions. The emphasis on work-based supervision also acknowledges the emphasis on socialization to the workplace and preparing trainees for bridging education with workplace practices.

Third, the issue of language is connected to issues of professional identity and power between professional groups. The willingness to negotiate a commonly understood term for supervision might be an indication of the willingness to transcend traditional domains of practice. The bottom line is that power issues intrude on the possibility of IP supervision. Underlying issues of professional stereotypes and professional status need to be addressed, in order for IP supervision to be accepted as legitimate practice.

Fourth, ethical issues seem to pervade discussions about IP supervision, although the nature of such concerns is rarely specified. A notable exception is a study by Wall and Austin (2008) in which the dynamics of negotiating ethical practice in health care teams is detailed. The question of whose code of ethics prevails is posed as a barrier and traditional reporting relationships may lead some professionals to claim more authority and more liability than others. New ways of working that involve sharing of power and control can lead to strong emotional reactions. It is possible that anxiety and fear may be heightened when "other" professional groups are involved in supervision, due to concerns about revealing weaknesses to other professions (Hyrkäs and Appelqvist-Schmidlechner 2003; Townend 2005). Yet, these very concerns underscore the importance of supportive supervision practices that address such dynamics in the workplace.

Fifth, one of most contentious barriers is how professional associations recognize supervision hours for trainees who are attempting to meet requirements for licensure or registration in their own profession. It is one thing to have conceptual agreement that working together on IP teams is conducive for learning. However, until professional associations begin to recognize and legitimize this form of training, IP supervision will not likely be viewed by professionals or trainees as a necessary part of professional education.

We are heartened by the fact that discussion of these barriers has surfaced in the literature to encourage open dialogue about the structures and functions of interprofessional education and practice. Such discussions may serve the dual purpose of addressing traditional barriers, and also focusing on issues from which tremendous learning about IPC may occur (Kvarnström 2008).

Supporting interprofessional supervision

Given the discussion of the advantages of pursuing IP supervision and the existing barriers to doing so, we offer a key question to further the debate: What will it take to support IP supervision? To recap, there are encouraging signs that professional groups are more often working together through a commitment to patient-centered collaborative practice as a best practice in the delivery of health care services. Concurrently, we need to prepare health care professionals for the realities of professional practice in which they will need to perform as a member of the larger care team.

What becomes obvious is the need to prepare trainees to make the transition from a trainee to a competent and confident member of an interprofessional team. One of the key ways of addressing the gap between education and practice is through IP supervision. In order to enhance IP supervision practices, more research is required which addresses what makes these experiences effective and efficient for all involved, including supervisors, supervisees, and patients. For example, research has examined trainees' perceptions of the benefits of supervision through preceptorship in comparison to supervision provided through a collaborative learning unit in which trainees had access to a number of mentors within the nursing profession (Callaghan *et al.* 2009). Research could be extended to consider trainees' experiences with IP supervision.

One particularly successful endeavor in IP supervision involved different professionals all trained in cognitive behavioral therapy (CBT) (Townend 2005). Although each CBT practitioner may have been from different and diverse professions, the fact that they all had training in this particular approach to service delivery facilitated the IP supervision of the team. Pragmatically, common documentation systems (Larkin and Callagan 2005) such as the way patient files are managed and maintained, joint supervision policies (Larkin and Callaghan 2005) such as the required number of individual versus group supervision hours, and a developmental approach to improving practice (Bailey 2004) have also been shown to facilitate successful IP supervision experiences.

Research has articulated competencies that may be addressed through supervision to enhance trainees' capacities for collaborative practice. In particular, role clarity and effective communication are highlighted (Suter *et al.* 2009). Research has also informed the development of frameworks in which core domains of interprofessional practice are defined with requisite competencies (e.g., Wood *et al.* 2009). In Canada, a national interprofessional competency framework (Canadian Interprofessional Health Collaborative 2010) has been developed. This framework is intended to guide the interprofessional education curriculum, and the competencies can be used to set standards for interprofessional practice. It is also a beneficial document to chart the course for IP supervision. Supervisors and trainees could use the competencies as a foundation from which to direct supervision planning, trainee learning activities, and debriefing of practice experiences.

Some key debates in the field remain. For example, when is the optimal time to introduce trainees to interprofessional practice: alongside the development of their professional identity or post-licensure? We would argue that exposing trainees early in their professional education programs has tremendous benefits for learning about their own disciplines and the disciplines of other health professionals. Part of the challenge, however, is creating learning opportunities for collaborative practice. The practicum component of professional education is a key time from which to foster IP supervision. However, it is of concern that it is left up to the individual interests and expertise of faculty and site supervisors to determine learning objectives and practice activities. Integrating interprofessional competencies into professional education, and particularly practicum training, would be a starting point. This could open the door for a coordinated approach with both faculty and site supervisors about how opportunities for interprofessional learning could be integrated into practicum experiences.

A related implication is that faculty and site supervisors need to be adequately prepared to design and deliver IP supervision initiatives. The extent to which supervisors are chosen for their supervisory versus clinical experience remains a concern. It should not be assumed that an experienced clinician has the requisite skills for supervision. Literature suggests that the success of supervision is highly dependent on the skills and qualities of the supervisor (Hyrkäs and Appelqvist-Schmidlechner 2003). Recent research has suggested that there are notable gaps in both the perceived competencies of supervisors for engaging in clinical supervision and their confidence for doing so (Heale *et al.* 2009). *It is evident that in order to promote effective IP supervision, the preparation of both supervisors and trainees needs to be taken into account.* In a previous publication (Arthur and Russell-Mayhew in press) we described a workshop designed for site supervisors in the fields of psychology, nursing, and social work to come together to learn more about interprofessional practice in general, and about ways to specifically foster IP supervision.

Although there are examples of research that address the perspectives of supervisors and trainees (Bailey 2004; Hyrkäs and Appelqvist-Schmidlechner 2003; Hyrkäs *et al.* 2002), the links between IP supervision and patient outcomes have not been researched. Again, we need to keep in mind that the purpose of IP supervision is about more than fostering the education of future practitioners; it is about providing quality care. *The extent to which IP supervision contributes to positive patient outcomes requires future examination through research.*

Recasting supervision as interprofessional mentorship

The discussion in the previous section outlines some of the benefits and challenges for advancing IP supervision. One of the most promising directions is the opportunity for supervisory practices to be revised, based on current knowledge about IPC. If we accept the notion that trainees may be better prepared for their future practice roles through exposure to the practices of professionals from multiple disciplines, then that idea should translate into future directions in supervision. It has been proposed that traditional supervision models could be expanded to an IP mentorship approach, in which trainees would have opportunities to "learn with and from staff and trainees from other disciplines" (Lait *et al.* 2010: 1). The concept of lateral mentoring is based on the premise of shared expertise that could be used to guide supervisory practices for clinical and work-based placements. *The key idea is that supervision would be enhanced by moving away from reliance on the expertise of only one supervisor, to incorporating the expertise of several practice site mentors, from various disciplines.* Trainees could still be assigned a primary supervisor or preceptor in their professional discipline in order to preserve the key teaching and learning functions of that role (Yonge *et al.* 2007). *However, trainees would also have the advantage of learning from a team of professionals assigned to their supervision.*

Preliminary research has identified a number of potential advantages to lateral mentoring (Lait *et al.* 2008). First, the main advantage of lateral mentoring is that trainees have the opportunity to learn from a range of professionals. That means they are exposed to multiple disciplinary perspectives and multiple approaches to supervision. Second, lateral mentoring supports trainees to find out areas of commonality and effective team practices (Mullarkey and Playle 2001). Third, at the same time, through recognizing differences, trainees acquire appreciation for the unique contributions to be made by their own profession and by members of other professional groups. Fourth, lateral mentoring activities can be used to support trainees to gain a multitude of competencies (e.g. problem-solving, teamwork, professional behavior) that are not profession-specific. Mentors do not have to be from the same professional discipline in order to enhance trainees' competency development. Fifth, a point that deserves to be reiterated is the necessity of preparing trainees for the realities of practice they will face in the workforce. Lateral mentoring provides early exposure to working with other professionals and helps trainees to develop competencies that builds their capacity for future IPC. To summarize, lateral mentoring involves enhancing trainees' understandings about their own profession, other professionals, and how to work together collaboratively for future practice.

A final point is warranted about the implementation of lateral mentoring. These suggestions can be implemented without major changes to the educational curriculum, but through leveraging available opportunities in practice settings (Lait *et al.* 2008). It may be necessary to address some of the attitudinal barriers that continue to set limits on professionals working together. However, willingness to share expertise, including supervisory expertise, has been shown to have major benefits for trainees from a wide variety of academic disciplines (Lait *et al.* 2008). If resources are coordinated in more effective ways, trainees and professionals may benefit from the learning that occurs through interactions with one another. Ultimately, this should translate to trainees developing competencies to enhance patient care in ways that are not possible through supervision from only one discipline. *In order to shift the emphasis from hierarchical models of supervision, lateral mentoring offers the advantage of incorporating many of the foundational premises of IPC that exemplify best of practices in health care.*

Conclusion

The field of interprofessional education and practice has emerged as a key direction for the future of health care. IPC is based on the premise of improving patient care through bringing together the best people to provide the best care. However, the call for IPC must be matched with curriculum reform, including approaches to supervision. This chapter has outlined several benefits of adopting IP supervision as a value-added model for enhancing the competency development of trainees. Based on the notion of learning with and from each other, IP supervision affords trainees the opportunity to be exposed to the practices of other professionals. We would encourage professionals in practice sites to become more than contacts for trainees, and take on the role of mentors in fostering their professional growth and development. Lateral mentoring provides unprecedented opportunities for trainees to experience the roles and responsibilities of their own profession in relation to other professions they will inevitably work with in the future. If we consider work-based supervision as a bridge between education and practice, trainees would benefit from having a number of mentors to help them cross that bridge. Learning from the expertise of multiple professionals provides a foundation of practice from which trainees can develop their sense of professional identity and foster interprofessional practice competencies. Advancing clinical supervision approaches to incorporate lateral mentoring will support the preparation of professionals who are ready, willing, and able to engage effectively in IPC.

References

Arthur, N. and Russell-Mayhew, S. (in press), Preparing counsellors for interprofessional collaboration through supervision and lateral mentoring, *Canadian Journal of Counseling*.

Bailey, D. (2004), The contribution of work-based supervision to interprofessional learning on a masters programme in community mental health, *Active Learning in Higher Education*, 5(3): 263–278.

Barr, H., Koppel, I., Reeves, S., Hammick, M., and Freeth, D. (2005), *Effective Interprofessional Education: Argument, Assumption and Evidence*, Oxford: Blackwell.

Barrett, J., Curran, V., Glynn, L., and Godwin, M. (2007), *CHSRF Synthesis: Interprofessional Collaboration and Quality Primary Healthcare*, Ottawa, ON: Canadian Health Services Research Foundation.

Baxter, S.K. and Brumfitt, S.M. (2008), Professional differences in interprofessional working, *Journal of Interprofessional Care*, 22(3): 239–251.

Callaghan, D., Watts, W., McCullough, D., Moreau, J., Little, M., Gamroth, L., and Durnford, K. (2009), The experience of two practice education models: collaborative learning unit and preceptorship, *Nurse Education in Practice*, 9(4): 244–252.

Canadian Interprofessional Health Collaborative (2010), *A National Interprofessional Competency*

Framework. Vancouver, BC: CIHC, online, available at: www.cihc.ca/files/CIHC_IPCompetencies_Feb1210.pdf [accessed June 21, 2010].

Clouder, L. and Sellars, J. (2004), Reflective practice and clinical supervision: an interprofessional perspective, *Journal of Advanced Nursing*, 46(3): 262–269.

D'Amour, D. and Oandasan, I. (2005), Interprofessionality as the field of interprofessional practice and interprofessional education: an emerging concept, *Journal of Interprofessional Care*, 19(Suppl. 1): 8–20.

Davies, E.J., Tennant, A., Ferguson, E., and Jones, L.F. (2004), Developing models and a framework for multi-professional clinical supervision, *The British Journal of Forensic Practice*, 6(3): 36–42.

Emerson, T. (2004), Preparing placement supervisors for primary care: An interprofessional perspective from the UK, *Journal of Interprofessional Care*, 18(2): 165–182.

EICPC (Enhancing Inter-disciplinary Collaboration in Primary Care) (2006), *Principles and framework for inter-disciplinary collaborative practice in primary health care*, Ottawa, ON: EICPC.

Hall, P. (2005), Interprofessional teamwork: professional cultures as barriers, *Journal of Interprofessional Care*, 19(Suppl. 1): 188–196.

Hammick, M. (ed.) (2005), Interprofessional education for collaborative patient-centred care: Canada as a case study (editorial), *Journal of Interprofessional Care*, 19 (Suppl. 1).

Heale, R., Mossey, S., Lafoley, B., and Gorham, R. (2009), Identification of facilitators and barriers to the role of a mentor in the clinical setting, *Journal of Interprofessional Care*, 23(4): 369–379.

Herbert, C. (2005), Changing the culture: interprofessional education for collaborative patient-centred practice in Canada, *Journal of Interprofessional Care*, 19(Suppl. 1): 1–4.

Hyrkäs, K. and Appelqvist-Schmidlechner, K. (2003), Team supervision in multiprofessional teams: team members' descriptions of the effects as highlighted by group interviews, *Journal of Clinical Nursing*, 12(2): 188–197.

Hyrkäs, K., Appelqvist-Schmidlechner, K., and Paunonen-Ilmonen, M. (2002), Expert supervisors' views of clinical supervision: a study of factors promoting and inhibiting the achievements of multiprofessional team supervision, *Journal of Advanced Nursing*, 38(4), 387–397.

Kvarnström, S. (2008), Difficulties in collaboration: a critical incident study of interprofessional healthcare teamwork, *Journal of Interprofessional Care*, 22(2): 191–203.

Lait, J., Suter, E., Arthur, N., and Taylor, E. (2010), *Interprofessional Mentorship: Enhancing Students' Clinical Learning*, manuscript submitted for publication.

Larkin, C. and Callaghan, P. (2005), Professionals' perceptions of interprofessional working in community mental health teams, *Journal of Interprofessional Care*, 19(4): 338–346.

Mullarkey, K. and Playle, J.F. (2001), Multiprofessional clinical supervision: challenges for mental health nurses, *Journal of Psychiatric and Mental Health Nursing*, 8(3): 205–211.

Peacock, J.R., Bradley, D.B., and Shenk, D. (2001), Incorporating field sites into service-learning as collaborative partners, *Educational Gerontology*, 27(1): 23–35.

Pyle, N. and Arthur, N. (2009), Service user positioning in interprofessional practice, *Journal of Interprofessional Care*, 23(5): 531–533.

Romanow, R. (2002), *Building on Values: The Future of Health Care in Canada*, final report of the Commission of the Future of Health Care in Canada, November 2002, online, available at: www.cbc.ca/healthcare/final_report.pdf.

Suter, E., Arndt, J., Arthur, N., Parboosingh, J., Taylor, E. and Deutschlander, S. (2009), Role understanding and effective communication as core competencies for collaborative practice, *Journal of Interprofessional Care*, 23(1): 41–51.

Townend, M. (2005), Interprofessional supervision from the perspectives of both mental health nurses and other professionals in the field of cognitive behavioral psychotherapy, *Journal of Psychiatric and Mental Health Nursing*, 12(5): 582–588.

Wall, S. and Austin, W. (2008), The influences of teams, supervisors, and organizations on health care practitioners' abilities to practice ethically, *Nursing Leadership*, 21(4), 85–99.

Wood, V., Flavell, A., Vanstolk, D., Bainbridge, L., and Nasmith, L. (2009), The road to collaboration: developing an interprofessional competency framework, *Journal of Interprofessional Care*, 23(6): 621–629.

Yonge, O., Billay, D., Myrick, F., and Luhanga, F. (2007), Preceptorship and mentorship: not merely a matter of semantics, *International Journal of Nursing Education Scholarship*, 4(1), 1–13.

32 A comparison of US and European conceptualisations of clinical supervision

John R. Cutcliffe

This chapter compares the extent of United States and European nursing literature that focuses on substantive clinical supervision (CS) matters. Examination of this body of work indicates (at least) two principal, differing conceptualisations of the purpose and resultant practice of CS. The chapter points out how the US conceptualisation creates the need for all supervisors to be more 'expert' in the particular specialty of nursing than the supervisee; the European conceptualisation posits supervision as a forum for considering the personal, interpersonal and clinical aspects of care so as to develop and maintain nurses who are skilled and reflective practitioners. In such a conceptualisation, this creates the need for supervisors to be effective at supporting nurses in self-monitoring, identifying difficulties in practice and finding the proper place to make good the deficit, not necessarily to be more expert in the particular nursing speciality. The chapter concludes by highlighting and discussing two key issues that emerged from this comparison: does the clinical supervisor of a nurse have to share the same specialty background as the supervisee (the recipient of the CS) and, what are the advantages of cross-discipline supervision?

The editors note how this chapter draws attention to several important points/questions. Clearly, there are multiple interpretations and/or versions of CS; in different parts of the world, the same term has very different meanings. The resultant confusion and difficulty in international, translation (or exporting) of CS should not come as a surprise. The persistent confusion surrounding the term continues to bedevil our academe's research efforts; it inhibits clinicians' attempts to grapple with and subsequently embrace CS; it enables a variety of practices which bear little passing resemblance to the original conceptualisations of CS to be 'passed off' as CS. Movement towards an agreed (and, the editors would argue, international) shared conceptualisation of CS (and an associated nomenclature) can then be regarded as one of the most pressing issues facing the CS academe.

This chapter is adapted from the paper which was originally published as Cutcliffe, J.R. and Lowe, L. (2005) A comparison of North American and European conceptualisations of clinical supervision, *Issues in Mental Health Nursing*, 26(5), 475–488.

Introduction

Anyone who is conversant with the significant developments within psychiatric/mental health (P/MH) nurse education and practice over recent decades will have a familiarity with clinical supervision (CS). The importance of P/MH nurses engaging in CS has been formalised in a number of United Kingdom (UK) policy documents. The 1994 review of P/MH nursing *Working in Partnership* (Department of

Health 1994) explicitly stated the need for all P/MH nurses to receive regular CS. The Department of Health documents, *The New NHS* (National Health Service) and *A First Class Service* (Department of Health 1997, 1998) both highlight how engaging in CS must be a career-long activity. Further, the then governing body of United Kingdom nurses, the United Kingdom Central Council (now re-formed into the Nursing Midwifery Council) issued a position statement on CS in 1996 and added their support to the principle of P/MH nurses entering into CS throughout the duration of their career. Most recently, the Chief Nursing Officer's review of P/MH nursing once more highlighted the centrality of clinical supervision to practice stating: 'Clinical supervision was seen as being essential to underpin good practice' (Department of Health: Chief Nursing Officer 2006: 2).

Indeed, it is heartening to see that within the UK, more than any other specialty of nursing, P/MH nursing has embraced CS (Bishop 1998; Bulmer 1997; Butterworth 1997). Bishop's (1998) nationwide survey determined that, of all the nursing specialties, P/MH nurses had the highest level of engagement in CS. More recent studies repeatedly verify that a very high proportion of P/MH nurses continue to view CS as important, valuable and highly beneficial, and not surprisingly they continue to engage in CS (Kelly *et al.* 2001).

Despite the well-established interest in and continuing practice of CS that P/MH nurses have shown, the conceptualisations and resultant operationalisation of CS across different groups of P/MH are far from consistent. Indeed, such is the extent of the lack of unanimity that what one group might recognise and call CS, another group might not. Pivotal differences in conceptualisation can be seen between US and European perspectives on CS. As a result, this chapter focuses on some of the key differences in conceptualisation (and resultant operationalisation) of CS between Europe and the US. In so doing, it draws attention to the particular issues that arise out of such conceptualisations and asks a number of questions (see Box 32.1).

A US conceptualisation of clinical supervision

According to Rounds (2001), in the main, the term clinical supervision is used in nursing in the United States to refer to relationships between an administrator or superior and a more junior 'other' (the supervisee). The term implies the idea of the supervisor having a 'supervisory responsibility' for the performance of the supervisee. The term is not synonymous with equity within the relationship, nor is it

---

Box 32.1 Key questions arising out of a comparison of European and United States conceptualisations of clinical supervision

1a Does the clinical supervisor of a nurse have to share the same specialty background as the supervisee (the recipient of the CS)?

1b Does the clinical supervisor of a nurse have to be more experienced than the supervisee (the recipient of the CS)?

1c Does the clinical supervisor of a nurse even have to be a nurse at all?

2 Are there advantages to cross-discipline clinical supervision?

necessarily indicative of a relationship between peers or colleagues. Rounds (2001) offers the example of how the nurses who care for patients in a formal care setting will report problems or concerns to 'their supervisor', seek guidance in administrative matters, and receive performance evaluations from 'their supervisor'. Interestingly, many of the dynamics and principles of 'European' conceptualisations of CS can be found in both the education and practice of nurses in the US but, most often, these exist under the banner of a different title. The procedure of assigning a preceptor to undergraduate nursing students for the clinical placements that occur during the later stages of a programme is common (Hagopian *et al.* 1992; Meng and Morris 1995). The preceptor–student relationship is a formal one, it can have a one-on-one format; it is driven by the principle that working closely with the preceptor will give the student the opportunity to function more fully in the nursing role. It should be pointed out, though, that often the relationship has an inherent power imbalance, with the preceptor being partly responsible for assigning grades to the student.

Another recent development in some parts of the US, that similarly echoes the 'European' model of CS, involves assigning preceptors and 'mentors' to new graduates, in order to help them adjust to the realities of practice. Rounds (2001) points out that this can also involve a one-on-one relationship, most often with a more experienced (and often more senior) nurse who provides guidance, support, and instruction as needed. Such developments have been expanded to advanced nursing practice programmes, most notably, nurse practitioner programmes. The above-mentioned notions of performance appraisal remain very much evident in Stuart's (2001) conceptualisation of CS; and Varcarolis tenders a conceptualisation of CS that is highly congruent with Stuart's. She states that CS involves: 'validation of performance quality through regularly scheduled supervisory sessions' (Varcarolis 2002: 231). In scenarios such as those depicted by Stuart (2001) and Varcarolis (2002) CS is conducted either by a more experienced clinician or through discussion with the nurse's peers in professionally conducted supervisory session.

Very few voices within the US nursing CS literature could be located that offer a different view to the one outlined above; a notable exception being Billings' (1998) opinion piece.[1] Billings suggests that in addition to reviewing (and appraising) the supervisee's clinical care, CS can also be used as a support system. Billings' insightful comments regarding the need for P/MH nurses to take care or look after themselves before they are capable to care for others adds an important dimension to CS, and one which is relatively absent in US conceptualisations of CS.

A European conceptualisation of clinical supervision

The European CS literature is replete with multiple definitions and conceptualisations of CS; consequently it is extremely difficult to find one definition/conceptualisation that captures all of the key elements of CS. Nevertheless, much of this literature shares commonality and congruence and there remain pivotal differences with the US conceptualisations of CS. In *Fundamental Themes in Clinical Supervision*, Cutcliffe *et al.* (2001: 3–4) produced and put forward a comprehensive list of parameters that, when considered collectively, could be seen to underpin the 'European' conceptualisation of CS. These parameters can be found in Chapter 1 of the current volume.

In the largest review of CS literature undertaken in the United Kingdom to date, Gilmore's (2001) summary of the nature (and purpose) of CS adds credibility to the parameters proffered by Cutcliffe *et al.* (2001). Gilmore found that the main purposes of CS are professional development and support for the practitioner. Some European conceptualisations of CS focus primarily on case reviews, caseload issues and treatment/care delivery (Gilmore 2001). There are some obvious similarities here with some US conceptualisations such as Stuart's (2001). More prominent within Gilmore's review is the conceptualisation of CS that focuses on supervisee-led issues. Rather than having to be case specific, the range of issues to be considered is much broader, e.g. conflict with colleagues and how this impacts on care; issues arising from interactions with clients and/or relatives; or how to deal with the 'emotional baggage' that results from engaging in demanding interpersonal work.

An important difference between European and US conceptualisations of CS goes to the issue of the supervisor occupying a position of power and authority over the supervisee. Original conceptualisations of CS for nurses in Europe highlighted that the roles of 'line manager' and 'clinical supervisor' should not be blurred. In his seminal work with Faugier, Butterworth was quick to allude to the problems that would ensue if CS were conflated with managerial supervision. Indeed, he was eager to disassociate CS with ideas of authority and power, and declared:

> People at work tend to think of their supervisor as authoritarian and that the whole concept of supervision is linked conceptually to an authority figure. This is a pity, because CS is much wider and more generous in its intention.
>
> (Butterworth 1992: 9)

He continued:

> Supervision is often negatively associated with more traditional disciplinary dealings between managers and their staff ... this is a narrow definition and more generous interpretations are available.
>
> (Butterworth 1992: 9)

When CS is conflated with managerial supervision, it ceases to be an emancipatory process and becomes analogous to Bentham's 'Panopticon'; a process more concerned with surveillance (Clouder and Sellars 2004) and Foucault's (1980) notion of 'the gaze.' Given these original conceptualisations it is not entirely surprising that for some there is continued resistance to CS when it is conflated with managerial supervision (Cutcliffe and Proctor 1998; Malin 2000).

Key questions and matters for discussion 1: does the clinical supervisor of a nurse have to share the same specialty background as the supervisee (the recipient of the CS)?

Issues relating to disciplinary congruence within CS relationships are prefaced by a preliminary question, namely: is the supervisee afforded the option of choosing his/her supervisor? The consensus within the European CS literature appears to be that wherever possible, the supervisee should have the chance to choose his/her own supervisor. Yet the limited availability of suitable, qualified and trained supervisors, logistical difficulties and to some extent, the conflation of the nature/purposes of CS with another form of management-led surveillance systems (Yegdich 1999; Kelly *et al.* 2001; Clouder and Sellars 2004), has led to the situation where many supervisees do not get the opportunity to choose their own supervisors. Dictating the identity and at the same time, the discipline (or profession) of the supervisor, sets the tone and establishes the dynamic of the supervision relationship. Such impositions reflect the power dynamic whereby the supervisee has less (or no) control of what happens in his/her own supervision. The selection of a supervisor and imposing this person on the supervisee as a fait accompli communicates a clear message that CS is something that is done unto the supervisee, whether he/she wants it or not. Impositions such as these are a direct contradiction of the emancipatory and enabling ethos that drove the introduction of CS into European nursing; after all: 'Clinical supervision is about empowerment – not control!' (Smith 1995: 1030).

The issues concerning choice/no choice of supervisor notwithstanding, the matter of disciplinary congruence between the supervisor and supervisee requires attention. An examination of the extant literature shows that, for some, the supervisor and supervisee should both belong to the same discipline. Power (1999: 36) purports that 'no nurse who has never had experience in your area of clinical practice' should supervise nurses.

Interestingly, no evidence is provided to substantiate this position. Furthermore, such a position appears not to take account of the historical inception of CS in nursing, wherein given the paucity of trained supervisors with a nursing background, the common model was cross-discipline (Gilmore 1973; Hadfield 2001; Proctor 2001). A less concrete position is asserted by Bond and Holland (1998: 18), who argue that supervisors 'should usually (although not always) be from the same clinical area or with sufficient recent experience of relevant clinical practice'. They continue: 'These clinical supervisors need to undergo further training in order to equip them for this role'.

What begins to become clear here is that is a relationship between one's particular conceptualisation of CS and supervisor/supervisee disciplinary congruence. If one holds the view that CS should focus *only or exclusively* on clinical performance evaluation, case reviews, and critique of treatment/care delivery choices (the orthodox conceptualisation within the US), then it becomes clear that one's supervisor will need to be more experienced (and knowledgeable) about the supervisee's substantive clinical area. Ergo – the supervisor needs inevitably to be from the same discipline. However, if one holds the perception that CS goes beyond such narrow, restricted views and is an opportunity to help and support nurses (practitioners) reflect on their dilemmas, difficulties and successes; a chance to explore how they reacted to, solved or achieved them; a forum for considering the personal, interpersonal and practical aspects of care so as to develop and maintain nurses who are skilled, reflective and healthy practitioners (Cutcliffe and Proctor 1998), then the choice of supervisor is predicated by wishing to work with an effective supervisor – not by supervisor/supervisee disciplinary congruence.

Accordingly, there is a need for aspirant supervisees to give some thought to their own conceptualisation of CS, as this is likely to influence their ultimate choice of supervisor. Epling and Cassedy (2001: 200) state:

It is the authors' experience from running training courses in CS that when first embarking on the concept, the supervisee initially wants someone from the same discipline and background to supervise him or her.

Findings from Kelly *et al.*'s (2001) study lend support to these views. Up to 40 per cent of their sample strongly disagreed/disagreed with the statement 'other disciplines can give supervision'. Given the range of conceptualisations of CS that exist, and the well-documented confusion that many practitioners have concerning the nature/purpose of CS (Clouder and Sellars 2004; Gilmore 2001), it is not unforeseen or unexpected that many supervisees hold the belief that only another individual with the same disciplinary background could supervise them. There is certainly some merit in sharing disciplinary congruence with one's supervisor; the familiarity with certain scenarios and dynamics can help the supervisee feel listened to and understood (Butterworth *et al.* 1997; Cutcliffe and Burns 1998). Having a supervisor from the same discipline would give the supervisee access to valuable experiential material and sometimes supervisees gain immense support in knowing that they are experiencing common, normal processes and reactions; an awareness they can gain through appropriate self-disclosure on the part of the supervisor (Butterworth *et al.* 1997; Cutcliffe and Burns 1998). It has been shown that increased technical competence can be an outcome of supervision where there is supervisor/supervisee disciplinary congruence (Paunonen 1991; Hyrkäs 2005).

An important element of this argument, and one that is rarely examined, is that of the theoretical (and practical) orientation of the supervisor and supervisee. While the supervision dyad may have the supervisor/supervisee disciplinary congruence this in no way guarantees congruence in theoretical/practical orientation. Accordingly, the supervisory direction will undoubtedly reflect theoretical orientation of the supervisor, which begs questions about, for example, how would a P/MH nurse help/guide a supervisee who has a completely different theoretical background, personal philosophy and/or orientation? Inevitably, the supervisee would be given 'fixes' and/or advice to client-based problems that are based in the particular theoretical orientation of the supervisor not that of the supervisee. For example, what would a P/MH nurse supervisee who, for want of a simplistic comparison, holds a humanistic view of P/MH nursing do with advice given to him/her by a supervisor with a biomedical or cognitive behavioural orientation?

In addition, considerations around supervisor/supervisee disciplinary congruence would be incomplete without giving attention to the issue of experiential congruence. If one accepts the view that CS should focus on clinical performance evaluation, case reviews, and critique of treatment/care delivery choices, then it is difficult to imagine an effective CS relationship where the supervisor/supervisee have no experiential congruence. Questions need to be asked about the veracity and accuracy of any performance evaluation, case review or treatment choice undertaken by a superivisor who has no experience of the clinical scenario being considered. For example, the supervisee wishes to receive performance evaluation on how he managed a violent client. Yet, the clinical supervisor has never had the experience of having to de-escalate a potentially violent situation or restrain a violent client. Such incongruity in experiential background is likely to impede, if not thwart, the supervisory process.

Matters for discussion 2: the advantages of cross-discipline supervision

Any argument about cross-discipline approaches to CS is prefaced by the need to acknowledge that during the formative years of introducing CS into nursing in Europe, this was the norm. Drawing on her experience of providing CS to a variety of health care professionals during the 1970s and 1980s, Proctor (2001: 27) declares:

> Supervisors seldom had experience in the core work and contexts of the practitioners they were working with, only usually in the interpersonal aspects of their work.

There simply were too few nurses who had received any training in CS to meet the needs of the workforce. Accordingly, the majority of CS of nurses was carried out by people with a psychology, psychotherapy and/or counselling background (Gilmore 1973; Proctor 2001). The body of empirical evidence which illustrates a wide variety of positive outcomes arising out of high quality CS continues to grow (for recent reviews see Gilmore 2001; Hyrkäs 2005), though it should be noted that, as yet, no comparisons between cross and uni-disciplinary CS outcomes could be located in the extant literature. There are, however, findings embedded within the literature emanating from empirical studies which underscore the positive outcomes that occur from cross-discipline CS (see Hyrkäs 2005). Furthermore, there is some evidence to indicate that cross-disciplinary approaches to CS are by their inherent nature more conducive to enabling supervisee-led rather than supervisor-led CS. The tendency of some supervisors to default to offering 'expert opinion and advice'; to default to traditional teacher-student power dynamics is well documented (see Epling and Cassedy 2001; Holloway and Poulin 1995). Such relationships maintain the supervisor in the position of the 'dominant knower' and the supervisee in the subservient position. However, if a potential supervisor lacks the expert knowledge specific to the discipline of the supervisee then clearly, he/she is less (un)able to act in the role of 'disciplinary expert' or 'dominant knower':

> ... it has been frequently reported by Supervisors that the tendency to act in the role of expert advisor diminishes when their own orientation and experience is different from that of the Supervisee ... some of the Supervisors have reported that the role of being an expert can get in the way of supervision. The tendency to encourage a more reflective style of supervision is almost forced by the virtue of not having a similar orientation to that of the supervisee.
>
> (Epling and Cassedy 2001: 77)

A further element of this argument is situated within the educational component of CS. Examination of the CS literature emanating from both sides of the Atlantic indicates that there is widespread agreement that CS, in whatever form it is manifest, inevitably contains an educational component. The pedagogical ideologies of emancipatory learning (van Manen 1997), which are in keeping with the nature and purpose of (European) CS, are epitomised by encouraging learners to find their own solutions and thus develop in a number of ways. The learning scenario becomes one less concerned with imparting knowledge from the expert to the learner, and more concerned with facilitating the (holistic) development of the learner. The author would argue that there is obvious and transferable utility in embracing the same (similar) emancipatory models of development in our CS, that we appear to embrace and uphold within our education/training systems. Moving from the position of expert knower to one of facilitator, in CS, requires a radical shift in philosophy and CS style. Engaging in CS in this manner (or approach) has a specific skill set, and while some interpersonal skills may well be transferable from nursing and/or psychotherapeutic education/training these would serve only as the foundation. Now while the precise nature and composition of this skill set (or more likely sets) remains a matter of debate (see Kilminster and Jolly 2000), the accepted wisdom is that some additional training/education is needed; particularly if one wishes to engage to move from the conceptualisations and practices of US CS to a more 'European' approach.

Conclusion

Examination of the extant substantive CS literature highlights the existence (broadly speaking) of two separate perspectives on the purpose of CS. One view, perhaps more commonly associated with US CS literature, appears to conceptualise CS as an opportunity for a more experienced nurse to monitor, educate and support a less experienced nurse in how they do clinical skills. Such a conceptualisation clearly creates the need for all supervisors to be more 'expert' in the particular specialty of nursing than the supervisee. Further, it requires a significant degree of experiential and theoretical supervisor/supervisee congruence. Alternatively, there is another view, perhaps more commonly associated with European CS literature, that appears to conceptualise CS as an opportunity to help and support nurses reflect on their dilemmas, difficulties and successes, and to explore how they reacted to, solved or achieved them. This view posits supervision as a forum for considering the personal, interpersonal and practical aspects of care so as to develop and maintain nurses who are skilled and reflective practitioners (Cutcliffe and Proctor 1998). This situation creates the need for supervisors to be effective at supporting nurses in self-monitoring, identifying difficulties in practice and finding the proper place to make good the deficit, not necessarily to be more expert in the particular nursing specialty.

Note

1 It is also worthy of note that outside of the nursing literature, in related disciplines, alternative views can quite easily be located, see for example the journal *The Clinical Supervisor: A Journal of Interdisciplinary Research, Theory, and Practice*.

References

Billings, C. (1998), Professional insights: on peer feedback, *Journal of the American Psychiatric Nurses Association*, 4(3): 103–104.
Bishop, V. (1998), Clinical supervision: what's going on? Results of a questionnaire, *NT Research*, 3(2): 141–149.
Bond, M. and Holland, S. (1998), *The Skills of Clinical Supervision*, Oxford: Oxford University Press.

Bulmer, C. (1997), Supervision: how it works, *Nursing Times*, 93(48): 53–54.

Butterworth, T. (1992), Clinical supervision as an emerging idea in nursing, in T. Butterworth and J. Faugier (eds), *Clinical Supervision and Mentorship in Nursing*, London: Chapman & Hall, pp. 3–17.

Butterworth, T. (1997), Clinical supervision … or a honey pot, *Nursing Times*, 93(44): 27–29.

Butterworth, T., Carson, J., White, E., Jeacock, J., Clements, A. and Bishop, V. (1997), *It is Good to Talk. Clinical Supervision and Mentorship: An Evaluation Study in England and Scotland*, Manchester: School of Nursing, Midwifery and Health Visiting, University of Manchester.

Clouder, L. and Sellars, J. (2004), Reflective practice and clinical supervision: an interprofessional perspective, *Journal of Advanced Nursing*, 46(3): 262–269.

Cutcliffe, J.R. and Burns, J. (1998), Personal, professional and practice development: clinical supervision, *British Journal of Nursing*, 7(21): 1318–1322.

Cutcliffe, J.R. and Lowe, L. (2005), A comparison of North American and European conceptualisations of clinical supervision, *Issues in Mental Health Nursing*, 26(5), 475–488.

Cutcliffe, J.R. and Proctor, B. (1998), An alternative training approach in clinical supervision: Part One, *British Journal of Nursing*, 7(5): 280–285.

Cutcliffe, J.R., Butterworth, T. and Proctor, B. (2001), Introduction, in J.R. Cutcliffe, T. Butterworth and B. Proctor (eds), *Fundamental Themes in Clinical Supervision* London: Routledge, pp. 1–5.

Department of Health (1994), *Working in Partnership: A Collaborative Approach to Care. Report of the Mental Health Nursing Review Team*, London: HMSO.

Department of Health (1997), *The New NHS: Modern and Dependable*, London: HMSO.

Department of Health (1998), *A First Class Service: Quality in the New NHS*, London: HMSO.

Department of Health: Chief Nursing Officer (2006), *Chief Nursing Officer's review of Mental Health Nursing: Summary of Responses to Consultations*, www.dh.gov.uk/prod_consum_dh/groups/dh_digitalassets/@dh/@en/documents/ digitalasset/dh_4131015.pdf [accessed 2008].

Epling, M. and Cassedy, P. (2001), Clinical supervision: visions from the classroom, in J.R. Cutcliffe, T. Butterworth and B. Proctor (eds), *Fundamental Themes in Clinical Supervision*, London: Routledge, pp. 64–83.

Foucault, M. (1980), *Power/Knowledge: Selected Interviews and Other Writings 1972–1977*, London: Harvester-Wheatsheaf.

Gilmore, A. (2001), Clinical supervision in nursing and health visiting: a review of the UK literature, in J.R. Cutcliffe, T. Butterworth and B. Proctor (eds), *Fundamental Themes in Clinical Supervision*, London: Routledge, pp. 125–140.

Gilmore, S. (1973), *The Counselor-in-Training*, Englewood Cliffs, NJ: Prentice-Hall.

Hadfield, D. (2001), Implementing clinical supervision: a personal experience, in J.R. Cutcliffe, T. Butterworth and B. Proctor (eds), *Fundamental Themes in Clinical Supervision*, London: Routledge, pp. 112–124.

Hagopian, G., Ferszt, G., Jacobs, L. and McCorkle, R. (1992), Preparing clinical preceptors to teach master's-level students in oncology nursing, *Journal of Professional Nursing*, 8(5): 295–300.

Holloway, E.L. and Poulin, K. (1995), Discourse in supervision, in E.L. Holloway (ed.), *Clinical Supervision: A Systems Approach*, London: Sage.

Hyrkäs, K. (2005), Clinical supervision, burn out, and job satisfaction among mental health and psychiatric nurses in Finland, *Issues in Mental Health Nursing*, 26(5): 531–556.

Kelly, B., Long, A. and McKenna, H.P. (2001), A survey of community mental health nurses' perceptions of clinical supervision in Northern Ireland, *Journal of Psychiatric and Mental Health Nursing*, 8(1): 33–44.

Kilminster, S.M. and Jolly, B.C. (2000), Effective supervision in clinical practice settings: a literature review, *Medical Education*, 34(10): 827–840.

Malin, N.A. (2000), Evaluating clinical supervision in community homes and teams serving adults with learning disabilities, *Journal of Advanced Nursing*, 31(3): 548–557.

Meng, A. and Morris, D. (1995), Continuing education for advanced nurse practitioners: preparing nurse-midwives as clinical preceptors, *The Journal of Continuing Education in Nursing*, 26(4): 180–184.

Paunonen, M. (1991), Education and clinical supervision in developing nursing care, *Hoitotiede [Nursing Science]*, 3(3): 90–95.

Power, S. (1999), *Nursing Supervision: A Guide for Clinical Practice*, London: Sage.

Proctor, B. (2001), Training for the supervision alliance, in J.R. Cutcliffe, T. Butterworth and B. Proctor (eds), *Fundamental Themes in Clinical Supervision*, London: Routledge, pp. 25–46.

Smith, J.P. (1995), Clinical supervision: a conference by the National Health Service Executive, *Journal of Advanced Nursing*, 21(5): 1029–1031.

Stuart, G.W. (2001), Actualizing the psychiatric nursing role: professional performance standards, in G.W. Stuart and M.T. Laraia (eds), *Principles and Practices of Psychiatric Nursing*, 7th edn, St Louis, MI: Mosby, pp. 199–213.

United Kingdom Central Council for Nursing, Midwifery and Health Visiting (1996), *Proposed Position Statement on Clinical Supervision for Nursing and Health Visiting*, London: UKCC.

Van Manen, M. (1997), *Researching Lived-Experience: Human Science for Action Sensitive Pedagogy*, New York: State University of New York Press.

Varcarolis, E.M. (2002), Developing therapeutic relationships, in E.M. Varcarolis (ed.), *Foundations of Psychiatric Mental Health Nursing: A Clinical Approach*, 4th edn, Philadelphia, PA: W.B. Saunders.

Yegdich, T. (1999) Clinical and managerial supervision: some historical and conceptual considerations, *Journal of Advanced Nursing*, 30(5): 1195–1204.

33 Clinical supervision for the twenty-first century and beyond

Successes, challenges and the road ahead

John R. Cutcliffe and John Fowler

This final chapter draws together some of the threads or themes which run throughout this book and then uses these as the basis for informing a possible research agenda for clinical supervision for the next ten years and beyond. Furthermore, again with reference to the preceding chapters, it highlights a number of unresolved issues/debates within the substantive area of clinical supervision and it offers some editorial comments.

In considering the future of clinical supervision the editors argue that the overall picture is an optimistic one; though one punctuated with the need for much hard work and further study. Clinical supervision as a practice is inextricably linked to health care, and thus is subject to the same vagaries as any other health care matter: most notably the evidence-based (informed) practice movement and a challenging (currently constricting) global economy. Accordingly, many of the debates that need to occur and studies that need to be undertaken will be influenced directly or indirectly by these two over-arching issues. And in the view of the editors, therein lies some of the optimism or hope for clinical supervision over the next decade and beyond. Our current and emerging evidence has already indicated the potential for clinical supervision to be highly cost effective (though more robust and international evidence pertaining to this would be most welcome). Extrapolating from this evidence base, we have good cause to be confident that in an increasingly cost-conscious world, high quality clinical supervision will continue to be shown as being very cost effective; giving a lot of 'bang for one's buck'. Furthermore, the shifting sands of the evidence-based movement and perhaps more especially, a distinct and well-documented shift towards more pluralistic approaches to evidence, means that the research-based knowledge base of clinical supervision will be able to expand exponentially as multi-method and/or mixed methods designs produce accurate and authentic findings. As multiple ways of knowing and multiple ways of generating knowledge are seen as legitimate, the range of currently un- or partially answered questions can be tackled and our evidence base can expand (and deepen).

Introduction

In the epoch of the evidence-based practice (EBP) movement, an honest appraisal of the 'state of the science' of clinical supervision (CS) indicates that the evidence base for CS should be described or categorised as incomplete, emerging or developing (see Part V of this book). This incomplete evidence base may cause a degree of discomfort to some; for others it may even be (and has been posited as) reason enough not to endorse or embrace CS. However, if we were to adopt this somewhat dogmatic and rigid approach to applying EBP, and the same categorisation were to be applied to describe the state of the science of the Western health care system (i.e. its knowledge and practices) per se, then the entire system would be placed in an untenable position. Even the most conservative of estimates assert that the percentage of health care practices currently utilised in contemporary health care which have a solid evidence base is less than 50 per cent (see for example, US Department of Health and Human Services, US Preventative Services Task Force, recovered 2010). Other estimates posit an even more disconcerting situation with figures as low as 15 per cent of current practitioners using evidence to drive clinical decisions and 85 per cent continuing to rely on 'traditional practices' and the clinician's own experience rather than research (according to data provided at the 2009 conference held at the Center for the Advancement of Evidence-Based Practice, University of Arizona). As a result, when the evidence base of CS is considered in the context of the evidence base of Western health care per se, then the state of the science of CS is comparable with many other practices (and better developed than others). While the authors cannot argue, with any legitimacy, that CS has a fully developed, robust evidence base, certain aspects of or issues within CS do indeed have supporting evidence and others have an emerging evidence base. Accordingly, mindful of what has been written in the preceding chapters in this book, this chapter will focus on a selection of these key areas/issues and such questions might help inform the CS research agenda for the next decade and beyond. In no order of priority these are:

1   The existence of robust qualitative evidence pertaining to many issues and aspects of CS.
2   The body of evidence relating to adequate/appropriate education and/or preparation of supervisors (and supervisees to a much lesser extent) in order to have effective CS.
3   The well-developed body of evidence which has repeatedly shown how the efficacy of CS is diminished when it is inappropriately conflated with managerial supervision.
4   The need for a growing evidence base which points to improved outcomes for clients when they receive care from practitioners who receive and engage in high quality CS.

The preceding chapters in this book also highlight a range of issues and unresolved debates within the formal area of CS and this chapter seeks to offer some editorial comments on each of these, as a means to advance the associated debates. In no order of priority these are:

1   Should the academe attempt to produce an agreed definition of clinical supervision and the creation of an accepted nomenclature?
2   Cross-disciplinary (inter-professional) clinical supervision or clinical supervision only within one's own discipline?
3   What records, if any, should be maintained regarding clinical supervision and who should be responsible for these?
4   The creation (or otherwise) of a minimum set of core competencies for supervisors.

Key areas/issues and questions that might help inform the clinical supervision research agenda for the next decade and beyond

1. The existence of robust qualitative evidence pertaining to many issues and aspects of clinical supervision

As pointed out above, we are now living and functioning within the epoch of the so-called 'evidence-based practice' (EBP) movement and though beleaguered with hitherto unresolved issues, the editors accept and embrace this situation wholeheartedly. A key component within the EBP movement, though far from an uncontested matter, is that of hierarchies of evidence. In essence, some authors have sought to create taxonomies or ranked lists of different forms of evidence; suggesting that certain forms of evidence are more valuable, reliable, 'hard' and scientific than others (see for example, Muir Gray 1997; Peat 2001; Petticrew and Roberts 2003; Evans 2003; Glasziou *et al.* 2004). Almost inevitably, these authors rank the findings or results produced from quantitative research (and more commonly, syntheses of multiple quantitative studies) as the so-called 'Gold Standard' of evidence (see for example, Appleby *et al.* 1995; Peat 2001; Petticrew and Roberts 2003; Evans 2003; Glasziou *et al.* 2004). Furthermore, even a cursory examination of the relevant CS-focused empirical literature will indicate that the same views are evident and some might argue, pervasive in this literature. For example, unless it can be shown that quantitative studies have been undertaken to examine a certain CS focused-/related-question, hypothesis or issue, then the evidence is seen as either weak or non-existent.

However, if one delves a little deeper into the EBP extant literature, one will find that more pluralistic perspectives with regards to the nature (and value) of evidence exist (see for example, Sackett *et al.* 1996, 1997; McKibbon and Walker 1994; McKenna *et al.* 2000; Greene 2007). In these and similar texts, the hegemony of hierarchies of evidence is contested. Alternative, and well-accepted, views posit that research methods within quantitative and qualitative paradigms can be regarded as a toolkit; a collection of methods that are purposefully designed to answer specific questions and discover particular types of knowledge. To attempt to place these designs (and the evidence they produce) into some artificial and linear hierarchy only serves to confuse and obfuscate. If what is needed to answer a particular problem (e.g. the therapeutic effects on the supervisee of two approaches to CS) is a meta-analysis of the current studies in one particular area, then for that particular problem, that is clearly the best form of evidence. Concomitantly, if what is required to answer a particular problem (e.g. what are the lived experiences of receiving CS from someone who is also your line manager) is a deep, thorough, sophisticated understanding, then for that particular problem, methods and studies that produce qualitative phenomenological data are going to produce the best form of evidence.

Moreover, examination of the extant methodological literature and, perhaps more significantly, the systematic review literature, will show that methodological pluralism is becoming the latest orthodoxy (see Greene 2007). Inextricably linked to this development is the growing recognition and valuing of findings from qualitative studies. Moreover, the criticisms that qualitative studies can sometimes be isolated and parochial in nature is being addressed by means of a number of processes, not least the development of methods for systematic review of qualitative studies and the increasing attention given to qualitative meta-synthesis (see for example the work emerging from the various international Cochrane Centres, such as Florence *et al.* 2005; Roen *et al.* 2004; Pluye *et al.* 2004). Work on the systematic review of qualitative studies using the Joanna Briggs Institute Qualitative Assessment and Review instrument (Florence *et al.* 2005) perhaps illustrates the nature of idiographic generalisable findings. Individual researchers from UK, Spain, the US, Canada, Thailand, Hong Kong, China and Australia independently produced a meta-synthesis of qualitative studies; with 18 pairs of reviewers from diverse cultures and contexts. The results of the meta-synthesis exercise were analysed to identify the degree to which inter-reviewer was achieved between these 18 pairs. In spite of the differences in background, the similarity in meaning of the synthesised findings across the participant pairs was striking. There was remarkable consistency within and between groups. Other methodological work is occurring which attempts to combine and synthesise quantitative meta-analyses and qualitative meta-syntheses (see for example, Roen *et al.* 2006; Pluye *et al.* 2006). Accordingly, while it remains the case that quantitative methods still hold the dominant position within CS focused-/ related-research (especially if one adopts an international perspective and examines the funding/publication patterns in different countries), there are very clear signs that there is movement within the academic community towards methodological pluralism; and a parallel recognition that the CS research academe needs both paradigms in order to achieve the most complete understanding possible.

Moreover, if one accepts the validity and cogency of, for want of a better term, the methodological pluralist stance, then the evidence base for CS becomes far more extensive and robust than if one holds to, for want of a better term, the hegemonic view of quantitative (or positivistic) research. The chapters in this book (and literature cited in the chapters) show that the following issues/areas have some solid, qualitative evidence:

- Multiple narrative and case study accounts exist which report improved outcomes for clients as a result of the practitioner receiving effective and high quality CS (e.g. Smith 2001).
- Practitioners can feel a much-needed sense of support when they experience high quality CS (e.g. Cutcliffe and McFeely 2001; Jones 2003, 2009).
- Stress management (and reduction) by means of engaging in small group CS (e.g. Alleyne and Jumaa 2007).
- Increased self-awareness (e.g. Cutcliffe and Epling 1997; Severinsson 2001; Holm *et al.* 1998, 2003).
- Small group CS as a forum for learning from others (e.g. Jones 2009).
- Relief of intra-personal angst such as feelings of guilt and inadequacy (e.g. Severinsson 2001; Holm *et al.* 1998, 2003).
- CS as a mechanism to improve an organisation's recruitment and retention of clinical staff (e.g. Akerjordet and Severinsson 2004; Lynch and Happell 2008; Walker 2009; White and Winstanley 2009).

Similarly, an argument can be constructed that the existence of a fairly extensive and growing body of qualitative evidence related to the substantive area of CS should not be surprising, given that many of these questions/issues require qualitative methods to elicit the evidence. Accordingly, the editors are of the view that this evidence can serve multiple purposes including (but not limited to):

- inform future research studies;
- highlight additional research questions;
- underpin CS course/training curricula;
- guide organisational CS policy; and by no means least,
- steer and inform practice.

2. The body of evidence relating to adequate/appropriate education and/ or preparation of supervisors (and supervisees to a much lesser extent) in order to have effective clinical supervision

Chapters in this book and the literature cited therein have made explicit reference to the wide variation in training/education/preparation of CS (this is explored in more detail below). Evidently, this wide variation also tolerates, if not actually permits, similar variation in curricula (course) content within these courses. While not wishing necessarily to homogenise preparation in/for CS, such documented wide variation can quite easily account for (at least some) differences in the findings vis-à-vis the efficacy of CS (see Cutcliffe 1997). Intuitively, it seems logical that there is a relationship between the quality of the CS preparation experience and the efficacy of CS subsequently offered by the practitioner. On a related note, given both the (ever increasing) empirical and theoretical literature that needs to be mined, in addition to the well-rehearsed argument regarding improvements in CS resulting from experiential learning, it seems likely that very short CS preparation courses are very unlikely to produce well-prepared, highly effective supervisors. While the editors acknowledge that this is a somewhat simplistic proposition, and the efficacy of the preparation will clearly be influenced by a range of variables, there exists some evidence that supports this proposition (Butterworth *et al.* 1997; see also evidence in the preceding chapters).

Now this is not to suggest that there is no utility or value in one-day workshops on CS. The editors are aware that such educational experience can whet the appetite for more, can provide a brief though interesting glimpse into the world of CS, and can help dispel some of the more common miscomprehensions and misunderstandings. Yet we would argue, and the limited evidence would appear to support our view, than such one-day workshops are not sufficient to produce fully prepared and effective supervisors.

Perhaps what is necessary is a range of CS preparatory 'courses' of different sizes, lengths and intensities, aimed at different groups and with very clearly articulated different goals? In considering this argument the editors are mindful of the seminal work of Bloom (1956) (and the many fine scholarly works that this original work spawned). Bloom described so-called 'higher level' thinking skills and, importantly, that such higher level thinking skills require prior learning (acquisition) of basic skills which, according to Bloom, are then integrated into higher order skills. Further, Bloom declared that skills at different levels must be taught (and evaluated) in different ways. Such central tenets then indicate that course designers and instructors need to take these differences into account when designing and running educational courses. As a result, if one accepts the cogency of Bloom's position and applies these tenets to CS courses/preparation and training, then there is a strong pedagogical case for having a range of different CS 'courses', some focused on 'basic skills' and others on 'higher level CS skills'. There are additional pedagogical lessons and rationales to support the argument for having a range of courses when one considers related (specialist) clinical practices and the different courses available to practitioners. To draw on the example of courses for (in) Cognitive Behavioural Therapy, introductory in-house overviews and study days, short courses and full-time master's level courses at university are available. While no doubt each deserving of merit, and each serving a particular purpose, the editors sincerely doubt that the receipient of an in-house study day, or short course would claim to be proficient (and the editors would argue – safe) as a Cognitive Behavioural Therapist.

The editors are also mindful, particularly in the post-2009 international economic meltdown, that any consideration of providing education/training in/for CS will inevitably have to be cognizant of the costs. Interestingly, the costs associated with providing adequate and appropriate training/education in CS were mentioned with conspicuous regularity during the 1990s (see, for example, Smith 1995). However, the editors would caution against possible short cuts in CS preparation, expecting disproportionate outcomes to financial support and course length. Furthermore, the editors argue that it is a false economy to short cut on CS preparation when there is body of evidence that shows how receiving high quality CS can keep clinical staff healthy and 'happy' (e.g. recipients of CS have lower burnout scores, depersonalisation scores, lower sickness (absence) rates etc.). Organisations therefore need to be thoughtful about allocating their limited training budgets to CS preparation, perhaps designing strategic plans to provide different courses to different practitioners; i.e. while in an ideal world it may be advantageous to provide intensive CS preparation to all clinicians, this is likely to be cost-prohibitive and thus offering a combination of courses to 'train the trainers' and introductory workshops might be a more realistic proposition.

Currently the preparation of supervisors and supervisees for their role(s) within CS appears to vary from no preparation at all to in-depth postgraduate level studies. To evaluate any such preparation, attention needs to be paid to validity issues, e.g. making sure that what is measured is an accurate indicator of any subsequent claims. For this reason, the editors suggest that evaluation of CS preparation must be undertaken at three levels. First, is the evaluation of the 'course' of preparation. This is typically carried out by end of course student evaluations and pre- and post-tests, which provide evidence of the students' learning. The next level of evaluation would focus on the students' subsequent application of the course to their practice; seeking to evaluate if they were applying the various elements of the course into their practice of CS. For this, the CS sessions would need to be audited in terms of frequency, structure and supervisee satisfaction. The third evaluative level is a far more complex issue to untangle, it relates to trying to measure the effects of the clinical supervision on the supervisees' clinical practice and whether it has changed, at least in part, as a result of the CS they receive. The first two levels of evaluation are relatively easy to undertake: variables can be defined, isolated and measured. However, the third level of evaluation, that of the relationship between a course of preparation and the subsequent effect(s) on the supervisees' clinical practice involves numerous confounding variables and attempt to isolate such variables has proved extremely difficult.

Where does this leave the evaluation of CS preparation/courses and any subsequent statements that one might want to make regarding the length, content, structure and academic level of such preparation? First is the need to identify the learning outcomes relating to the course of preparation. Once such learning outcomes have been agreed, then different course structures can be developed which aim to deliver the outcomes in different ways. Thus one could design six courses which differ in length, teaching style, mode of delivery and academic level etc. Such courses can then be evaluated in terms of the first two levels identified above in relation to the core learning outcomes. Such evaluations would require multisite studies, considerable planning, support and personnel if the results are to be recognised as valid and reliable, this equates to considerable financial cost. In many parts of the world and many health care organisations there is currently no obvious funding source for CS and even less for its ongoing development and evaluation. Thus if the academe is to further develop the body of evidence relating to the preparation of supervisors the following will be required:

- agreed learning outcomes for the preparation of supervisors;
- multisite co-operation;
- multilevel evaluation;
- funding.

3. The well-developed body of evidence which has repeatedly shown how the efficacy of clinical supervision is diminished when it is inappropriately conflated with managerial supervision

Numerous chapters in this book and literature cited within these chapters repeatedly shows the overall efficacy of CS is diminished when it is inappropriately conflated with managerial supervision. Such findings are not limited to certain geographical areas or certain disciplines (see Chapter 24). Furthermore, these findings are not new; the issue of managers also acting as supervisors and the resultant conflicts and confusion that this can (and does) create has been well documented in the literature (see White 1996; Butterworth *et al.* 1997; Cutcliffe and Proctor 1998a, 1998b; Deery 1999; Yegdich 1999; Cutcliffe 2003; Hyrkäs *et al.* 2005; 2006).

The editors of this book find the conflation of CS with managerial supervision (MS) to be a puzzling situation. As we have pointed out previously, such a conflation was never posited, implicitly or explicitly, in original conceptualisations and justifications for CS that emanated from the United States, the United Kingdom, or Scandinavian countries. Countries that based their CS on these initial conceptualisations (such as Australia, New Zealand) should not have confused CS with MS. Similarly, position statements from key policymakers, governing bodies and leading academics also make the distinction between CS and MS. The United Kingdom Central Council's position (2006) could not be clearer about the delineation between CS and MS (see also the recommendations of the Finnish Ministry of Health and Social Services 1983). In response to the rhetorical question, 'What is clinical supervision', the UKCC states:

1. Clinical supervision is not a managerial control system. It is not, therefore:
12.1 the exercise of overt managerial responsibility or managerial supervision;

12.2 a system of formal individual performance review or

12.3 hierarchical in, nature.

Despite the unequivocal nature of this literature (even acknowledging its recognised vintage in some situations), and despite the clarity of the policy statements, evidence reported in this book continues to show that CS often is arranged in a hierarchical, top-down or pyramidal way, with managers also acting as CS for the staff they manage and resulting in the most obvious conflation of CS and MS (see Wolsey and Leach 1997; Teasdale *et al.* 2000; Kelly *et al.* 2001; Barriball *et al.* 2004). Somewhat surprisingly there are also examples within the literature of those whom advocate *for* the conflation of CS with MS (see Teasdale *et al.* 2000). Indeed, though not an empirical finding, top-down, hierarchical or cascading models of CS (where the most senior practitioner within a unit supervises the next tier down, and the next tier down supervises the practitioners in the tier below them etc., etc.) appear to be, if not the most common approach, then one of the most common approaches to organising CS. When this approach is considered within the context of evidence-based practice, it becomes even more difficult to sustain/support. The empirical evidence that does exist, as Malin (2000) so eloquently points out (and see the findings detailed in Chapter 30), the outcomes of the CS in these cases, indicates that the activity now primarily serves the needs of the organisation (and the managers) – not the needs of supervisee (and supervisor to a lesser extent).

Now, the editors are mindful that such amalgamation of CS with MS appears to be linked to:

- an increased concern in health care policy and subsequent practice around the notions of safeguarding the patient (and public), quality of care, professional accountability (aka *normative issues*); and furthermore,
- (not least) as a means to 'prevent' further nursing 'disasters' such as those indicated in the Allitt inquiry (Department of Health 1994; Yegdich 1999).

The editors are also mindful that these are real issues, they deserve and require appropriate attention and in no way are the editors advocating a cavalier attitude towards such matters. However, multiple mechanisms for safeguarding against such clinical disasters already exist. Findings from inquiries into such disasters inevitably offer even more mechanisms for (for want of a better expression) 'defensive practices, policing and internal monitoring'. Related observations and associated critiques have been purported regarding mental health care, where more and more policies inevitably focus on control and containment. Within such discourses the solution to health care problems are inevitably couched in terms of greater 'policing', stricter adherence to rules, regulations, and tighter controls.

As a result, an argument can be made that even more policing, even stricter rule enforcement and creation, even tighter controls are unlikely to guarantee and/or safeguard *all* possible practice scenarios or situations. Metamorphosing CS into yet another organisational surveillance system then seems even more ill-advised. In place of this, the editors argue that there is space for the original conceptualisation of CS to be (re)accepted; there is space for CS to be conceptualised as an opportunity to help and support practitioners reflect on their dilemmas, difficulties and successes and to explore how they reacted to, solved or achieved them. There is space for CS to be used as a forum for considering the personal, interpersonal and practical aspects of care so as to develop and maintain practitioners who are skilled and reflective practitioners. There is a space for CS to be (one of) the mechanisms whereby practitioners can become effective in self-monitoring; identifying difficulties in practice and finding the proper place to make good the deficit. In this way, perhaps ironically, the practitioner becomes safer, more effective, more thoughtful, and more self-aware. When one considers that there already exist innumerable mechanisms for surveillance and professional accountability in health care, yet there are few enough existing opportunities for personal/practice development in an entirely safe, yet challenging and supportive, yet stimulating interpersonal environment; then the need for CS as it was originally conceptualised becomes abundantly clear.

4. The need for a growing evidence base which points to improved outcomes for clients when they receive care from practitioners who receive and engage in high quality CS.

In an ideal evidence-based, research world the evaluation of the effect(s) of CS on client outcomes is straightforward. A randomised, controlled trial study would be organised in which clients with exactly the same conditions, lifestyles, family backgrounds etc. are randomly selected into one of three identical clinical areas. Each of these clinical areas would also have exactly the same clinical staff in terms of experience, qualifications, social standing, personalities etc. In the first of these clinical areas staff would have regular CS according to standard criteria. In the second clinical area the staff would have the same time out from their clinical duties as those receiving CS, but during that time they would have a coffee on their own. The third group would act as a control group and continue without any time out, carrying on as normal. Then using multiple high validity client outcome measures, the study researchers would compare the client outcomes over a period of several months.

Having done this the researchers would then be in a position to make reasonably valid statements regarding the efficacy of clinical supervision on client outcomes. (Even then we are making the assumption that clinical supervision is only occurring during that set time out period and that the elements of clinical supervision are not occurring in all three clinical areas during 'normal' clinical exchanges!)

If we really want to measure the effects of CS on client outcomes then all of those confounding variables, and there are literally thousands in the above scenario, need to be controlled – arguably this is an unrealistic (and maybe even impossible task).

Any research project that aims to establish a causal relationship between CS and client outcomes, which does not control for the confounding variables as above, is naïve. Likewise, any request for such evidence reflects a poor understanding of both the components of CS and research methodology. What then can be measured with any degree of true validity and reliability?

1   We can measure the effects of receiving or participating in CS; with the caveat that due to limitations with controlling extraneous variables, these studies will most likely be undertaken using *quasi-experimental designs, not randomised control trials*.

2   We can measure the nurses' 'perceived' effects of clinical supervision on client outcomes.
3   We can measure the preparation of supervisors and supervisees.
4   We can measure the ongoing support that supervisors receive.
5   We can measure what percentage of staff receive supervision.

Nevertheless, it is regarded as axiomatic that even imperfect studies can yield solid and useful evidence. Indeed an often-cited statement is that there is no such thing as the 'perfect study'; a study, it is argued, will always have some limitations. Accordingly, while a 'pure' controlled study may not be possible, valuable evidence can be obtained from quasi-experimental and qualitative designs (to name but two). The editors argue that while there is some useful evidence pertaining to this issue to be mined, one of the more pressing epistemological needs here is more data from clients, patients: the recipient(s) of care. Data that would speak to, for instance, the client's experiences (satisfaction, views, etc.) of receiving care from a practitioner who engages in CS. Studies could be created with cross-over designs, and/or pre- and post-test designs, all with the objective of showing differences (where they exist) between care delivered by those who do engage in CS and those who do not. Not only is this methodologically possible (and quite practicable) it is entirely in keeping with the broader 'movement' vis-à-vis service user input to health care evaluation studies. It maybe worth reminding ourselves of this context by drawing on some of the associated literature; and we use the example of the formal area of mental health care.

The views of service users: hard to ignore

It is increasingly difficult for mental health practitioners to ignore the service user movement and its associated voice (Wallcraft 2003; Boardman 2005). In the UK, since the 1980s, there is compelling evidence of the growth and influence of the service user movement. This movement brings an increasing emphasis on the central position of the service user and his/her views on the planning, delivery and subsequent evaluation of public mental health care services (including CS); it understandably brings a corresponding erosion of the hegemony of the 'professionals'. Accordingly, maybe the views of mental health services users can shed some light on the question of the effects of CS on the care provided and the client experience of satisfaction with care received; especially if, as some literature purports, service users' perceptions of their needs and the help they would like to receive do not necessarily correspond with mental health care providers' views (see Barker 1994; Shepherd *et al.* 1995; Murray 1997; Forrest *et al.* 2000). Rather than adopt a cross-sectional view, if one examines the service user views literature over time, a number of key themes appear repeatedly and consistently.

These first of such themes refers to high value that service users place on inter-personal relationships with their practitioners particularly if such relationships are natural, warm and human rather than distant, cold and professional; if they are founded on respecting the person's dignity, treating him/her with due respect, and providing emotional support (see for example, Gordon *et al.* 1979; Weinstein 1979; Elbeck and Fecteau 1990; Avis *et al.* 1994; Beech and Norman 1995; Cutcliffe *et al.* 1997). As a result, the nature of the relationship between client and practitioner, and reflection on how this is effecting the care experience, could very easily be explored (as indeed they often are) in good CS. Findings focusing on the nature and value of the interpersonal relationship continue to appear in key service user service evaluations and surveys such as those emanating from the Mental Health Foundation (2000; Rose 2002). This report is unequivocal on this matter, stating as it does,

> The overwhelmingly predominant theme running through peoples' 'most helpful' supports was the role and value of relationships with other people, in all their different forms. For some people it was individuals, family or friends, ... for still others, the important people in their lives were mental health professionals: counsellors, CPNs, support workers or social workers.
>
> (Mental Health Foundation 2000: 34)

This body of literature clearly draws attention to the dominance of the 'medical model' (with its focus on diagnosis, symptomotology and associated pharmacological response[1]) posits this as the orthodoxy of contemporary mental health care and yet this is repeatedly highlighted as a bone of contention for service users. Similar focused research undertaken by mental health academics, educationalists and clinicians produces comparable findings (see, for example, Forrest *et al.* 2000; Coffey *et al.* 2004).

The second theme refers to the over-zealous reliance on medication, the desire for 'talking therapies' in place of (or in addition to) medication and the (extensive) level of dissatisfaction with this overuse of medication (and its associated iatrogenic effects). Once more, this might serve as a focus for reflection, exploration and discussion in CS: does the client feel there is an over-emphasis on one domain of psychosocial care at the expense of others? In addition to the literature already cited, more recent and methodologically robust evidence continues to identify the same issues. The Service User Research Enterprise (2007) document identifies five priority areas for research (in mental health care): social and welfare issues, involvement in services, medication, alternative treatments and ethnicity. This document declares that many service users feel there is an over-reliance on medication; experience of and concerns with side-effects are commonplace. Service users would like to see research to investigate the effectiveness and appropriateness of medication. Moreover, many service users are concerned about this over-reliance on medication and feel they have limited access to psychological therapies.

Similarly, the latest findings from the Healthcare Commission (2007) regarding the views of mental health service users reinforce these perceptions. According to the report the survey produced 15,900 completed questions (with a healthy response rate of 38 per cent). The interpersonal aspects of the care received were well regarded by most service users with 81 per cent saying that their community psychiatric nurse (CPN) definitely listened to them and 86 per cent saying their (CPN) definitely treated them with respect and dignity. Moreover, just over half (52 per cent) who had received counselling (though it is not made clear what constituted this counselling) said they had definitely found it useful. As with previous studies, the report indicates that there is continuing evidence of a substantial unmet need for talking therapies, with over a third (35 per cent) of service users who had not received counselling reporting that they would have liked to. Furthermore, medications continue to be identified as an issue with one-third of service users who were prescribed new medications not being told about possible side effects.

As a result, there is a sizeable (and growing) body of robust literature which clearly highlights the emphases that service users wish to see in their mental health care service, yet this is difficult to reconcile with the contemporary mental health policy (see Boardman 2005) and the contemporary emphases in P/MH nursing curricula (see Delaney *et al.* 1999; Perraud *et al.* 2006). Given the well-documented concerns of service users, one could be forgiven for expecting that this would be explored in CS sessions on a regular basis.

Unresolved debates/issues

1. An agreed definition of clinical supervision and the creation of an accepted nomenclature

Examination of the extant literature, both contemporary and of a recognised vintage, indicates that confusion still clearly abounds as to the nature and purpose of CS; and for that matter, that despite several attempts to produce one, there is currently no universally accepted definition. This, at least in part, accounts for the well-documented confusion, miscomprehension and lack of understanding as to the nature and purpose of CS. This may look like a semantic argument yet science is dependent upon a shared, agreed nomenclature (McGraw-Hill's *Encyclopedia of Science and Technology Online*, recovered 2009). Indeed, science's need for understandable, stable and internationally-accepted systems for naming and categorising phenomena has given rise to the existence of many such systems (Michon, recovered 2010). A shared nomenclature refers to a list of agreed names, definitions, principles, rules and recommendations that govern the formation, use and application of a particular domain of science. For example, biology as a meaningful science is prefaced by the five codes of biological nomenclature (i.e. the Latinised scientific naming and classification of organisms, Winston 1999). Chemistry has the International Union of Pure and Applied Chemistry nomenclature captured in a number of key publications (IAUPC 1979, 1993, 2007; Connelly and McCleverty 2001). Physics, astronomy and medicine all have shared nomenclatures that transcend international boundaries. Even relatively esoteric areas of science such as suicidology have made significant advances towards achieving a shared nomenclature (see Silverman *et al.* 2007).

Evidence presented in this book and elsewhere shows that we are stymied in our efforts to advance the evidence base of CS in many aspects because of the lack of this shared nomenclature. Without this, we are unable to assert, with a degree of empirical confidence, that we are referring to the same phenomena; that we are measuring the same thing(s), or that we are even educating/training our colleagues in the same practice. *Movement towards a shared, agreed, international nomenclature for CS can then be considered to be the most pressing 'scientific' challenge facing all those in the academe who wish to advance the science of CS.*

2. Cross-disciplinary (inter-professional) CS or CS only within one's own discipline?

Chapters in this book and existing literature in the substantive area indicate that there are (broadly speaking) two apparently polarised positions on this issue. The first suggests that one's supervisor should share the same discipline as the supervisee. Such views are commonly encountered when practitioners are first introduced to CS (see Chapter 19, for example). Furthermore, such a position is entirely understandable and appears to be linked to the notion that only practitioners who share the same discipline can really understand what it is like to be in that discipline and thus are better placed to be supervisors. Similar related findings can be located in surveys of whom practitioners want to be their line managers and the associated rationales for those choices (see, for example, Thompson 2008). There may also be a relationship here between the supervisee's knowledge and awareness of the actual purposes of CS. For example, when supervisees hold the (inappropriate?) view that supervisors should be experts in the disciplinary area of the supervisee and exist to impart their expertise to them, the desire to have a supervisor who shares the same discipline as the supervisee should not come as a surprise. Additional evidence in this book (see for example Chapters 12 and 28) appears to underscore this relationship; the relative state of the science in different parts of the world and especially a lack of a shared nomenclature (definition of the purposes of CS) appear to be linked to views of who can and should be one's supervisor.

However, there appears to be an increasing evidence base, bound up (to a greater or lesser extent) with related changes in contemporary health care delivery, that cross-disciplinary or inter-professional models of CS are more befitting of and in keeping with twenty-first century health care challenges. As Arthur and Russell-Mayhew point out in Chapter 31, the complexity of patient care issues often means that a variety of health care professionals are inevitably involved in the care-giving scenario; solutions to problems and seamless (interfaced) health care service delivery inevitably require a multi-disciplinary approach, and human problems as expressed as health care issues rarely (if ever) fall within the man-made (artificial?) boundaries of one health care profession or another. One merely has to look at one of the reports produced as a result of an enquiry into so-called health care 'failures' to see that those reports' recommendations invariably exhort greater (and more efficient) communication within the multi-disciplinary team, fewer artificial barriers between different disciplines and a more effective 'team'-based approach to delivering health care (see, for example, Coid 1994). Evidence reported in Chapter 24 in this book indicates that following engagement in a formal CS educational experience, the various disciplinary groups in the study held the view that the supervisor and supervisee sharing the same theoretical background was regarded as low importance and this is an encouraging sign. It appears that exposure to high quality CS training/education can open the minds of practitioners to the benefits of cross-disciplinary (inter-professional) CS. As a result, this might be one area where additional research could be undertaken in the next decade.

The editors of this book have previously stated (see Chapter 1) that seeking to homogenise all CS experiences and posit the existence of only one appropriate way to operationalise CS is an ill-advised policy. Nevertheless, there is evidence to suggest that some approaches appear to have more utility than others and it is difficult to ignore the wider health care delivery context of the twenty-first century. Given the arguments above, the editors argue that cross-disciplinary (inter-professional) approaches to CS appear to have more utility than uni-disciplinary approaches. Such approaches are more congruent with the reality of twenty-first century, Western health care systems and they are more in keeping with approaches to CS that emphasise the growth and development of the supervisee (rather than the expert supervisor providing answers to the supervisee's problems).

3. What records, if any, should be maintained regarding CS and who should be responsible for these?

A further issue that the authors would argue needs attention during the next decade is that of record keeping in CS. The limited literature that exists in this area indicates three principal positions regarding recording in CS namely:

1   That the supervisor records minimum data to meet the needs of audit;
2   That the supervisee makes extensive notes for their learning journal, reflective diary;
3   The supervisor records headings or key words to be used as an aide memoire (Cutcliffe 2000).

There are those who argue that minimal records need to be maintained (e.g. Clark *et al.* 1998; Bond and Holland 1998; Gilmore 1999; Powers 1999) for a variety of reasons, though many questions still remain regarding this minimal recording including: what is to be recorded (and what is not); how often do records need to be made; who decides what is recorded/not recorded; and who has access to these records? More support is evident in the extant literature for the supervisee to make notes (some advocate for extensive notes) that are used in conjunction with his/her reflective diary/learning journal (see, for example, Rolfe *et al.* 2001). In other words, the linkage between reflective practice and the educational (developmental – formative: see Chapter 3) domain of CS is reinforced but in addition, enacting such linkage requires notes to be taken by the supervisee. Importantly, despite the positioning of some (e.g. Johns 1996) most contributors to this debate firmly locate the responsibility for determining what is included in a reflective journal with the supervisee (and this is certainly the view of the editors). The third discrete position is that of minimal record keeping on the part of the supervisor. The case for this position seems even more logical when one starts to factor in scenarios where the supervisor has many supervisees.

The editors suggest that arriving at some form of resolution to this issue, as with many CS related matters, is prefaced by first arriving at an understanding of the nature and purpose of CS. While bedeviled by various re-interpretations, CS was designed (originally) as a democratic, emancipatory process concerned with the growth and development of the supervisee (see Chapter 24). As has been pointed out in several other places in this book, CS was never originally intended to be (another) a form of managerial oversight. It was never intended to be a supervisor-driven or supervisor-led process. It was not created with the interests and/or agenda of the supervisor and/or organisation as the primary concern (though there are obvious and well-documented positive outcomes for both the supervisor and the organisation). The history of CS in the United States, in the United Kingdom, in Scandinavian countries and in Australia/New Zealand all show that CS was designed to occur in a wholesome atmosphere of partnership, permissiveness and support; it was principally concerned with supporting the nurse–patient relationship. The editors are of the view that many of the unresolved debates in CS would be very well served (and informed) by returning to the original idea(s) that drove the introduction of CS. Accordingly, the issue of what to record in CS and whom should do the recording then is prefaced by the statement: given that CS is designed to occur in an atmosphere of permissiveness and support, and is a supervisee-led process designed to ultimately improve patient care.... In the view of the editors it then becomes abundantly clear that the supervisee can/should decide what he/she records. There would appear to be a place for (and we would argue merit in) supervisor-initiated discussion around what the supervisee has chosen to record and not to record (as this can, in and of itself, be a very useful educational and awareness-raising tool).

4. The creation (or otherwise) of a minimum set of core competencies for supervisors

It is reasonable to suggest that one current trend in higher education is an emphasis on competency acquisition, and furthermore examination of the extant literature indicates that this is an international phenomenon (see, for example, Dearing 1997; Faris 1995; US Department of Education 2001). Programmes, courses, modules (whatever vernacular term is used) increasingly refer to specific competencies that successful graduates can expect to obtain as a result of completing the education. Voorhees (2001) captures this shift succinctly when he states that pathways to learning, "lead most directly to learning opportunities in which competencies are defined explicitly" and that "this new paradigm will ultimately redefine the roles of faculty, institutions and accreditors". Several chapters within this book have drawn attention to the wide variation that exists in curricula (such as they are) for courses designed to train/prepare practitioners to become supervisors. Similarly, the length of such courses varies considerably and these differences can be located within the same country. That is to say that course length and curricula content do not appear to be determined primarily by their country of origin.

More disturbingly, several of the chapters in this book illustrate how there is no apparent consensus in the literature as to what is required to prepare practitioners (adequately) to become supervisors. There are a number of implications arising out of this lack of similarity (let alone consistency) including: are practitioners being prepared in (or for) the same phenomenon? Does this lack of consistency and similarity preclude researchers from engaging in any methodologically meaningful comparisons? While there are some commonalities with other interpersonal-focused activities and disciplines/professions, there appears to be a growing consensus that there is a specific skill set for CS; though there is currently no consensus on what these skills are. It can be argued that the issue of the lack of common, shared views of core competencies for CS is another matter that is bedevilled by the misunderstanding of the nature and purpose of CS. Chapters in this book indicate that frequently encountered misunderstandings include:

- The expectation that providing supervision requires one to be more knowledge-able and technically proficient than the people one is supervising (see for example Chapter 18). Such a conceptualisation would then require a certain skill set (and curriculum to be offered) and the editors would argue that this approach has more to do with instructing/informing the practice of a more junior colleague rather than CS per se.
- The expectation that supervision will be driven by monitoring adherence to pro-fessional codes of conduct, individual organisational policies and procedures. Such a conceptualisation would then require the supervisor to be more familiar and conversant with professional codes of conduct, ethical guidelines and codes, and organisational policies and procedures.
- That CS is more akin to a form of personalised psychotherapy wherein the supervisor acts as a psychotherapist for the supervisee; as a result any and all kinds of intra- or interpersonal angst and issues can be brought to the CS session by the supervisee and the supervisor then needs to help to address these. Such a conceptualisation would then require the supervisor to be famil-iar with one (or more) theoretical approaches to psychotherapy (e.g. person-centred, cognitive behavioural), and in terms of core competencies, the supervisor would need to have the skill set associated with the particular theo-retical approach used.

In closing

> The most exciting phrase to hear in science, the one that heralds the most dis-coveries, is not 'Eureka!' (I found it!) but 'That's funny…'
>
> (Isaac Asimov)

> Everything that can be counted does not necessarily count; everything that counts cannot necessarily be counted.
>
> (Albert Einstein)

> To raise new questions, new possibilities, to regard old problems from a new angle, requires creative imagination and marks real advance in science.
>
> (Albert Einstein)

With apologies to these two scientific masters (and thanks to brainyquote.com) the editors would like to draw on these quotations and use them as the basis for our closing comments; believing as we do that these quotations hold as much wisdom and applicability for the substantive area of CS science as they did when they were first uttered.

Future research endeavours into CS, while seeking answers and a degree of cer-tainty, are more than likely to create new, hitherto unasked questions. The editors welcome this situation and uphold the view that the statement 'I don't know' is the foundation of wisdom and knowledge development.

The editors will not belabour the argument that we have included previously in this book (in more than one place); but we find comfort in Einstein's words. If the need to accept methodological pluralism and the different, though potentially com-plimentary, forms of knowledge has the support of Einstein, who are we to differ?

Lastly, we uphold the view and regard it as sacrosanct, that good science and advances in our knowledge (and practice) of CS require imagination, creativity, and a willingness to view issues from multiple perspectives. We look forward to engaging in such activities ourselves over the next decade and beyond and accessing/reading the work of others in the scientific academe of CS scholars. We hope that in some small way, this book has advanced our knowledge base, maybe adopted a number of different views and perspectives to enhance our understanding and stimulated the imagination and creativity of CS around the globe.

Note

1 Some might even say reflex.

References

Akerjordet, K. and Severinsson, E. (2004), Emotional intelligence in mental health nurses talking about practice, *International Journal of Mental Health Nursing*, 13(3): 164–170.

Alleyne, J. and Jumaa, M.O. (2007), Building the capacity for evidence-based clinical nursing leadership: the role of executive co-coaching and group clinical supervision for quality patient services, *Journal of Nursing Management*, 15(2): 230–243.

Appleby, J., Walshe, K. and Ham, C. (1995), *Acting on the Evidence*, research paper, Birmingham: National Association for Health Authorities and Trusts.

Avis, M., Bond, M. and Arthur, A. (1994), *Patient satisfaction and the management of outpatient consultation*, unpublished report, University of Nottingham, Nottingham.

Barker, P. (1994), Points of view, *Nursing Times*, 90(8): 66–68.

Barriball, L., While, A. and Much, U. (2004), An audit of clinical supervision in primary care, *British Journal of Community Nursing*, 9(9): 390–396.

Beech, P. and Norman, I.J. (1995), Patients' perceptions of the quality of psychiatric nursing care: findings from a small-scale descriptive study, *Journal of Clinical Nursing*, 4(2): 117–123.

Bloom, B.S. (ed.) (1956), *Taxonomy of Educational Objectives, the classification of educational goals – Handbook I: Cognitive Domain*, New York: McKay.

Boardman, J. (2005), New services for old: an overview of mental health policy, in A. Bell and P. Lindley (eds), *Beyond the Water Towers: The Unfinished Revolution in Mental Health Services 1985–2005*, London: The Sainsbury Centre for Mental Health.

Bond, M. and Holland, S. (1998), *The Skills of Clinical Supervision*, Oxford: Open University Press.

Butterworth, T., Carson, J., White, E., Jeacock, J., Clements, A. and Bishop, V. (1997), *It is Good to Talk: An Evaluation of Clinical Supervision and Mentorship in England and Scotland*, Manchester: The School of Nursing Studies, The University of Manchester.

Clark, A., Dooher, J., Fowler, J., Phillips, A.M. and Wells, A. (1998), Individual sessions of clinical supervision, in J. Fowler (ed.), *The Handbook of Supervision*, London: Quay Books, pp. 85–107.

Coffey, M., Higgon, J. and Kinnear, J. (2004), 'Therapy as well as tablets': an exploratory study of service users' views of community mental health nurses' (CMHNs) responses to hearing voices, *Journal of Psychiatric and Mental Health Nursing*, 11(4): 435–444.

Coid, J.W. (1994), The Christopher Clunis enquiry, *Psychiatric Bulletin*, 18: 449–452.

Connelly, N.G. and McCleverty, J.A. (2001), *Nomenclature of Inorganic Chemistry II: Recommendations 2000*, Cambridge: Royal Society of Chemistry.

Cutcliffe, J.R. (1997), Evaluating the success of clinical supervision, *British Journal of Nursing*, 6(13): 725.

Cutcliffe, J.R. (2000), To record or not to record: documentation in clinical supervision, *British Journal of Nursing*, 9(6): 350–355.

Cutcliffe, J.R. (2003), Clinical supervision and reflective practice: symbient and integral aspects of the role of community psychiatric nurses, in B. Hannigan, M. Coffey and P. Burnard (eds), *A Handbook of Community Mental Health Nursing*, London: Routledge, pp. 132–144.

Cutcliffe, J.R. and Epling, M. (1997), An exploration of the use of John Heron's confronting interventions in clinical supervision: case studies from practice, *Psychiatric Care*, 4(4): 174–180.

Cutcliffe, J.R. and McFeely, S. (2001), Practice nurses' 'lived experiences' of clinical supervision: a hermeneutic study, *British Journal of Nursing*, 10(5): 312–323.

Cutcliffe, J.R. and Proctor, B. (1998a), An alternative training approach in clinical supervision: part one, *British Journal of Nursing*, 7(5): 280–285.

Cutcliffe, J.R. and Proctor, B. (1998b) An alternative training approach in clinical supervision: part two, *British Journal of Nursing*, 7(6): 344–350.

Cutcliffe, J.R., Dukintis, J., Carberry, J., Tilley, C., Turner, S., Anderson-Moll, D. and Cooper, W. (1997), User's views of their continuing care community psychiatric services, *The International Journal of Psychiatric Nursing Research*, 3(3): 382–394.

Dearing, R. (1997), *Higher education in the learning society: report of the national committee*, London: HMSO.

Deery, R. (1999), Professional issues: improving relationships through clinical supervision 2, *British Journal of Midwifery*, 7(4): 251–254.

Delaney, K.R., Chisholm, M., Clement, J. and Merwin, E.I. (1999), Trends in psychiatric mental health nursing education, *Archives of Psychiatric Nursing*, 13(2): 67–73.

Department of Health (1994) *Independent Inquiry Relating to Deaths and Injuries on the Children's Ward at Grantham and Kesteven General Hospital during the period February to April 1991* (Clothier Report), London: HMSO.

Elbeck, M. and Fecteau, G. (1990), Improving the validity of measures of patient satisfaction with psychiatric care and treatment, *Hospital and Community Psychiatry*, 41(9): 998–1001.

Evans, D. (2003), Hierarchy of evidence: a framework for ranking evidence evaluating healthcare interventions, *Journal of Clinical Nursing*, 12(1): 77–84.

Faris, R. (1995), *Reforms in Training Systems in Three Countries*, Victoria, Canada: Ministry of Skills, Training and Labour.

Finnish Ministry of Health and Social Services (1983), Työnohjaustyötyhmän muistio [Memorandum of Supervision Committee] Sosiaali ja terveysministeriö [Ministry of Social Affairs and Health],*Työryhmämuistio [Report of the working group of clinical supervision]*, Helsinki, Finland.

Florence, Z., Schulz, T. and Pearson, A. (2005), Inter-reviewer agreement: an analysis of the degree to which agreement occurs when using tools for the appraisal, extraction and meta-synthesis of qualitative research findings, *The Cochrane Collaboration*, online, available at: www2.cochrane.org/colloquia/abstracts/ melbourne/O-69.htm [accessed 2009].

Forrest, S., Risk, I., Masters, H. and Brown, N. (2000), Mental health service user involvement in nurse education: exploring the issues, *Journal of Psychiatric and Mental Health Nursing*, 7(1): 51–57.

Gilmore, A. (1999), *Review of the United Kingdom Evaluative Literature on Clinical Supervision in Nursing and Health Visiting*, London: United Kingdom Central Council.

Glasziou, P., Vandenbrouche, J. and Chalmers, I. (2004), Assessing the quality of research, *British Medical Journal*, 328(7430): 39–41.

Gordon, D., Alexander, D.A. and Dieztan, J. (1979), The psychiatric patient: a voice to be heard, *British Journal of Psychiatry*, 135: 115–121.

Greene, J. (2007), *Mixed Methods approaches in social inquiry*, San Francisco, CA: Wiley & Sons.

Healthcare Commission (2007), *Community Mental Health Services – Views of Mental Health Service Users: Key Findings from the 2007 Survey*, London: Healthcare Commission.

Holm, A.K., Lantz, I. and Severinsson, E. (1998), Nursing students' experiences of continual process-oriented group supervision, *Journal of Nursing Management*, 6(2): 105–113.

Holm, A.K., Lantz, I. and Severinsson, E. (2003), A theoretical perspective of the core concepts of nursing supervision, *Norsk tidskrift for sykepleieforskning*, 2: 71–82.

Hyrkäs K., Appleqvist-Schmidlechner K. and Kivimäki K. (2005), First-line managers' views of the long-term effects of clinical supervision: how does clinical supervision support and develop leadership in health care? *Journal of Nursing Management*, 13(3): 209–220.

Hyrkäs K., Appelqvist-Schmidlechner K. and Metsänoja R. (2006), Efficacy of clinical supervision: influence on job satisfaction, burnout and quality of care, *Journal of Advanced Nursing*, 55(4): 521–535.

IUAPC (International Union of Pure and Applied Chemistry) (1979), *Nomenclature of Organic Chemistry, Sections A, B, C, D, E, F, and H*, Oxford: Pergamon Press.

IUAPC (1993), *A Guide to IUPAC Nomenclature of Organic Compounds (Recommendations 1993)*, Oxford: Blackwell.

IUAPC (2007), *Quantities, Units and Symbols in Physical Chemistry*, 3rd edn, Oxford: Blackwell.

Johns, C. (1996), Visualising and realising caring in practice through guided reflection, *Journal of Advanced Nursing*, 24(6): 1135–1143.

Jones, A. (2003), Clinical supervision in promoting a balanced delivery of palliative nursing care, *Journal of Hospice and Palliative Nursing*, 5(3): 168–175.

Jones, A. (2009), Fevered love, in L. de Raeve, M. Rafferty and M. Paget (eds), *Nurses and Their Patients: Informing Practice through Psychodynamic Insights*, London: M&K Publishing.

Kelly, B., Long. A. and McKenna, H.P. (2001), A survey of community mental health nurses' perceptions of clinical supervision in Northern Ireland, *Journal of Psychiatric and Mental Health Nursing*, 8(1): 33–44.

Lynch, L. and Happell, B, (2008), Implementing clinical supervision: Part 1: Laying the ground work, *International Journal of Mental Health Nursing*, 17(1): 57–64.

McGraw-Hill's Encyclopedia of Science and Technology (2009), online, available at: www.access science.com [recovered 2009].

McKenna, H.P., Cutcliffe, J.R. and McKenna, P. (2000), Evidence-based practice: demolishing some myths, *Nursing Standard*, 14(16): 39–42.

McKibbon, K.A. and Walker, C.J. (1994), Beyond ACP Journal Club: how to harness Medline for therapy problems, *Annals of Internal Medicine*, 121(1): 125–127.

Malin, N.A. (2000), Evaluating clinical supervision in community homes and teams serving adults with learning disabilities, *Journal of Clinical Nursing*, 31(3): 548–557.

Mental Health Foundation (2000), *Strategies for Living: A Summary Report of User-led Research into Peoples' Strategies for Living with Mental Distress*, London: The Mental Health Foundation.

Michon, G.P. (2010), *Planet Trek: Mapping New Worlds – what is nomenclature?* online, available at: http://btc.montana.edu/ceres/Worlds/Landform/ nomenclature. htm.

Muir Gray, J.A. (1997), *Evidence-Based Health Care*, Edinburgh: Churchill Livingstone.

Murray, L. (1997), How can clients and carers become allies? *Nursing Times*, 93(27): 40–42.

Peat, J. (with Mellis, C., Williams, K. and Xuan, W.) (2001), *Health Science Research: A Handbook of Quantitative Methods*, London: Sage.

Perraud, S., Delaney, K.R., Carlson-Sabelli, L., Johnson, M.E., Shephard, R. and Paun, O. (2006), Advanced practice psychiatric mental health nursing, finding our core: the therapeutic relationship in the 21st century, *Perspectives in Psychiatric Care*, 42(4): 215–226.

Petticrew, M. and Roberts, H. (2003), Evidence, hierarchies, and typologies: horses for courses, *Journal of Edipediomol Community Health*, 57(7): 527–529.

Powers, S. (1999), *Nursing Supervision: A Guide for Clinical Practice*, London: Sage.

Pluye, P., Grad, R., Dunikowski, L. and Stephenson, R. (2004), *A Challenging Mixed Literature Review Experience*, 12th Cochrane Colloquium, The International Cochrane Collaboration, Ottawa, formerly online and available at: www. cochrane.org/colloquia/abstracts/

ottawa/0–088.htm [accessed 2009], abstract online, available at: www.imbi.uni-freiburg.de/OJS/cca/index.php/cca/article/ view/2610.

Roen, K., Rodgers, R., Arai, L., Petticrew, M., Popay, J., Roberts, H. and Sowden, H. (2004), *Narrative Synthesis of Qualitative and Quantitative Evidence: An Analysis of Tools and Techniques*, 12th Cochrane Colloquium, The International Cochrane Collaboration, Ottawa, formerly online and available at: www.cochrane.org/ colloquia/abstracts/ottawa/0–058.htm [accessed 2009], abstract online, available at: www.imbi.uni-freiburg.de/OJS/cca/index.php/cca/article/view/2580.

Rolfe, G., Freshwater, D. and Jasper, M. (2001), *Critical Reflection for Nursing and the Helping Professions: A User's Guide*, London: Palgrave Macmillan.

Rose, D. (2002), *Users' Voices: The Perspectives of Mental Health Service Users on Community and Hospital Care*, London: The Sainsbury Centre for Mental Health.

Sackett, D.L., Rosenberg, W., Gray, J.A. Haynes, R.B. and Richardson, W.S. (1996), Evidence-based medicine: what it is and what it isn't, *British Medical Journal* 312(7023): 71–72.

Sackett, D.L., Richardson, W.S., Rosenberg, W.M. and Haynes, R.B. (1997), *Evidenced-Based Medicine: How to Practice and Teach EBM*, London: Churchill Livingstone.

Service User Research Enterprise (2007), S*ervice User Priorities for Research*, London: Institute of Psychiatry/Kings College.

Severinsson, E. (2001), Confirmation, meaning and self-awareness as core concepts of the nursing supervision model, *Nursing Ethics*, 8(1): 36–44.

Shepherd, G., Murray, A. and Muijen, M. (1995), Perspectives on schizophrenia: a survey of user family carer and professional views regarding effective health care, *Journal of Psychiatric and Mental Health Nursing*, 4(4): 403–422.

Silverman, M., Berman, A., Sandal, N., O'Carroll, P.W. and Joiner, T. (2007), Rebuilding the Tower of Babel: a revised nomenclature for the study of suicide and suicidal behaviors Part I: background, rationale, *Suicide and Life-Threatening Behaviors*, 37(3): 245–247.

Smith, J.P. (1995), Clinical supervision: conference by the NHSE, *Journal of Advanced Nursing*, 21(5): 1029–1031.

Smith, P. (2001), Clinical supervision: my path towards clinical excellence, in J.R. Cutcliffe, T. Butterworth, and B. Proctor (eds), *Fundamental Themes in Clinical Supervision*, London: Routledge, pp. 159–169.

Teasdale, K., Brocklehurst, N. and Thom, N. (2001), Clinical supervision and support for nurses: an evaluation, *Journal of Advanced Nursing*, 33(2): 216–224.

Thompson, J. (2008), What perioperative and emerging workforce nurses want in a manager, *Annual Review of Nursing Education*, 78(2): 246–261.

United Kingdom Central Council (2006), *Position Statement on Clinical Supervision for Nursing and Health Visiting*, London: UKCC.

US Department of Education, National Center for Educational Statistics (2001), *Defining and Assessing Learning: Exploring Competency-based Initiatives*, Washington, DC: US Department of Education, National Center for Educational Statistics.

US Department of Health and Human Services (2010), *US Preventative Services Taskforce*, online, available at: www.ahrq.gov/CLINIC/uspstfix.htm [accessed 2010].

Voorhees, R.A. (2001) Competency-based learning models: a necessary future, *New Directions for Institutional Research*, 110(Summer): 5–13, also online, available at: www.cpass.umontreal.ca/documents/pdf/mesure/reference/11.Competency-Based_Learning_Models.pdf [accessed 2010].

Walker, J. (2009), Examining the benefits of professional clinical supervision, *Kai Tiaki Nursing New Zealand*, 15(5): 12–14.

Wallcraft, J. (2003), *The Mental Health Service User Movement in England*, London: The Sainsbury Centre for Mental Health.

Weinstein, R.M. (1979), Patient attitudes towards mental hospitalization: a review of quantitative research, *Journal of Health and Social Behavior*, 20(September): 237–258.

White E. (1996), Clinical supervision and Project 2000: the identification of some substantive issues, *NTResearch*, 1(2): 102–111.

White, E. and Winstanley, J. (2009), Implementation of clinical supervision: educational preparation and subsequent diary accounts of the practicalities involved, from an Australian mental heath nursing innovation, *Journal of Psychiatric and Mental Health Nursing*, 16(10): 895–903 with erratum in 17(1): 96.

Winston, J.E. (1999), *Describing Species: Practical Taxonomic Procedure for Biologists*, New York: Columbia University Press.

Wolsey, P. and Leach, L. (1997), Clinical supervision: a hornet's nest? *Nursing Times*, 93(44): 24–27.

Yegdich, T. (1999), Clinical supervision and managerial supervision: some historical and conceptual considerations, *Journal of Advanced Nursing*, 30(5): 1195–1204.

Index